Clinical Procedures in Veterinary Nursing

Edited by

Victoria Aspinall BVSc MRCVS
Principal, Abbeydale Veterinary Training, Gloucester, UK

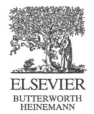

ELSEVIER
BUTTERWORTH
HEINEMANN

Edinburgh London New York Oxford Philadelphia St Louis Sydney Toronto 2003

BUTTERWORTH-HEINEMANN
An imprint of Elsevier Limited

First published 2003
  Reprinted 2004, 2005, 2006, 2007

ISBN-13: 978–0–7506–5416–6
ISBN-10: 0–7506–5416–3

British Library Cataloguing in Publication Data
A catalogue record for this book is available from the British Library

Library of Congress Cataloging in Publication Data
A catalog record for this book is available from the Library of Congress

Notice
Medical knowledge is constantly changing. Standard safety
precautions must be followed, but as new research and clinical
experience broaden our knowledge, changes in treatment and drug
therapy may become necessary or appropriate. Readers are advised to
check the most current product information provided by the
manufacturer of each drug to be administered to verify the
recommended dose, the method and duration of administration, and
contraindications. It is the responsibility of the practitioner, relying on
experience and knowledge of the patient, to determine dosages and
the best treatment for each individual patient. Neither the publisher
nor the editors assume any liability for any injury and/or damage to
persons or property arising from this publication.

The Publisher

 ELSEVIER your source for books,
journals and multimedia
in the health sciences

www.elsevierhealth.com

Working together to grow
libraries in developing countries

www.elsevier.com | www.bookaid.org | www.sabre.org

ELSEVIER   BOOK AID International   Sabre Foundation

The publisher has made every effort to obtain permission to reproduce
all borrowed material

The
publisher's
policy is to use
paper manufactured
from sustainable forests

Printed and bound in China

Clinical Procedures in Veterinary Nursing

For Butterworth-Heinemann:

Senior Commissioning Editor: Mary Seager
Development Editor: Catharine Steers
Project Manager: Morven Dean
Design: George Ajayi
Illustrations Manager: Bruce Hogarth

Contents

Contributors

Victoria Aspinall BVSc MRCVS
Principal, Abbeydale Veterinary Training,
20 Glevum Way, Abbeydale, Gloucester, UK

Richard Aspinall BVSc Cert.VR MRCVS
Aspinall Auld and Clarkson, The Animal
Hospital, 20 Glevum Way, Abbeydale,
Gloucester, UK

Carole Bowden Dip AVN (Surg) VN
Head Nurse, Clifton Villa Veterinary Surgery,
Richmond Hill, Truro, Cornwall, UK

Jennifer Davis MRIPH
Laboratory Manager and Senior Technician,
Wood Veterinary Group, Gloucester
Laboratories, St Oswalds Road,
Gloucester, UK

Suzanne Easton MSc BSc
Senior Radiographer, Division of Companion
Animals, University of Bristol, UK

Jo Masters Cert Ed. VN
Veterinary Nursing Manager, Vetlink School of
Veterinary Nursing, Glastonbury, Yeovil, UK

Pip Millard VN
Lecturer in Veterinary Nursing and Practice
Manager, Woodland Veterinary Surgery,
Katherine Court, Salisbury Road, Cheltenham,
Glos., UK

Rachel Mowbray BVSc MRCVS
Vale Vets, The Animal Hospital,
Stinchcombe, Dursley, Glos., UK

Trish Samuel VN
Lecturer in Veterinary Nursing and Practice
Manager, The Crescent Veterinary Surgery,
31 Church Street, Tewkesbury, Glos., UK

Foreword

The role of the veterinary nurse is constantly changing as veterinary practice becomes more and more sophisticated. New theories, techniques, skills and tools are being used in practice to meet the current needs of a society that is highly technological, complex and dynamic. Specialisation has led to the development of new techniques. The competence-based approach of the veterinary nurse National Vocational Qualification framework and the establishment of new graduate programmes aim to give veterinary nurses the knowledge, skills and responsibilities consistent with their role.

This book describes many of the clinical procedures performed by veterinary nurses in practice.

Although it is nearly impossible for any one publication to capture all of the procedures carried out in veterinary practice, this book goes a long way to address many of the procedures that are now routinely carried out by veterinary nurses.

Clinical Procedures in Veterinary Nursing will help students develop the skills needed as part of their training and will be useful later as a quick reference guide for up-to-date information on clinical procedures. The book will also be an invaluable aid for those returning to veterinary practice after a brief career break.

Barbara Cooper
College of Animal Welfare

Preface

This book aims to provide instruction in all the practical tasks likely to be encountered in a modern small animal practice. It is designed to be of use to both qualified and student veterinary nurses and to veterinary nurses returning to practice after a prolonged interval; it may also help student veterinary surgeons who require information about ordinary everyday nursing tasks. It is also hoped that the text will act as a useful reference for student veterinary nurses preparing for their practical exams.

All the procedures have been written in a 'step-by-step' format and, where relevant, many are preceded by a list of equipment. This enables the nurse to have everything to hand before starting the task and to know exactly what is to be done before hand. Good preparation is of prime importance to the welfare of the patient and to the efficiency of the task. Each procedure is divided into a column describing the action in minute detail and a column explaining the rationale—why the particular action is performed in this situation.

The contributors to this text all have extensive experience of working in their particular field. While they all agree that the methods they have described may not be the only way of performing a procedure, these are the ones that, in their opinion, are the simplest and most reliable way of achieving the optimal result. The range of subjects included in the book reflects the breadth of work done in most practices. I have included a chapter on exotic species, as the appearance of these animals in the surgery is now becoming almost commonplace. Descriptions of handling and restraining these exotic species and dogs and cats have been included because, although not technically clinical procedures, no technique can be performed safely and to the benefit of the patient without correct restraint.

This book is not designed to be a core text, as the format does not allow coverage of all the theoretical knowledge underpinning every aspect of a nurse's work, but it is hoped that it will become a valuable source of information for all the practical aspects of work in a veterinary practice. Additional information can be found by referring to the list of suggested further reading at the end of each chapter.

I hope that *Clinical Procedures in Veterinary Nursing* will be useful to everyone who reads it and that it will become, rather like a favourite recipe book, the standard reference for all practical tasks within the surgery!

Victoria Aspinall
May 2002

Acknowledgements

This book would not have been possible if it were not for the help and support of my husband and children who put up with my bad temper and lack of attention whenever I became obsessed with writing. I would also like to thank all the contributors who put such dedication into producing their chapters on time, Catharine Steers for her work in preparing the book for publication and finally to Mary Seager without whose support this project would never have started.

Figures 1.1, 3.5, 10.1, 11.1 and 12.5 are reproduced by permission of Butterworth-Heinemann from Masters & Bowden 2001 *Pre-Veterinary Nursing Textbook*; Figures 1.4, 1.5, 1.6, 1.7, 1.8 and 1.13 are reproduced by permission of Butterworth-Heinemann from Anderson & Edney 1991 *Practical Animal Handling*; Figures 3.3, 4.1, 5.1, 5.4, 5.5, 6.10, 6.11, 6.12, 6.13, 6.14, 7.3, 7.4, 7.5, 7.6, 7.7, 7.9, 7.10 and 8.9 are reproduced by permission of BSAVA from Lane & Cooper 1999 *Veterinary Nursing*; Figures 6.5, 6.6, 6.7 and 6.8 are reproduced by permission of Mosby from McKelvey & Hollingshead 2000 *Small Animal Anesthesia & Analgesia*; Figure 7.13 is reproduced by permission of Butterworth-Heinemann from Bowden & Masters 2001 *Quick Reference Guide to Veterinary Surgical Kits*; Figure 12.10 is reproduced by permission of Butterworth-Heinemann from Lewington 2000 *Ferret Husbandry, Medicine & Surgery*; Figure 12.17 is reproduced by permission of BSAVA from Hotston Moore 1999 *BSAVA Manual of Advanced Veterinary Nursing*.

Dogs

- Tying a tape muzzle
- Lifting dogs weighing up to 15 kg
- Lifting dogs weighing over 20 kg
- Lifting small dogs with spinal damage
- Lifting large dogs with spinal damage
- To examine the cranial end of the body
- To examine the caudal end of the body or take the rectal temperature
- To examine the dog on its side or to provide firmer control
- To examine or restrain the dog on its back
- Administering a tablet
- Administering a liquid feed or medication
- Applying ear medication
- Applying eye medication
- Restraint for a subcutaneous injection
- Restraint for an intramuscular injection
- Restraint for an intravenous injection using the cephalic vein
- Restraint for an intravenous injection using the lateral saphenous vein
- Restraint for an intravenous injection using the jugular vein

Cats

- Lifting a friendly cat used to being handled (method 1)
- Lifting a friendly cat used to being handled (method 2)
- Lifting a frightened or aggressive cat
- Carrying a cat
- To examine a friendly cat
- To examine a fractious cat
- Administering a tablet
- Administering a liquid feed or medication
- Applying ear medication
- Applying eye medication
- Restraint for a subcutaneous injection
- Restraint for an intramuscular injection
- Restraint for an intravenous injection using the cephalic vein
- Restraint for an intravenous injection using the lateral saphenous vein
- Restraint for an intravenous injection using the jugular vein (method 1)
- Restraint for an intravenous injection using the jugular vein (method 2)

Handling and restraint

V. Aspinall

Introduction

No matter what procedure is to be performed, correct restraint of the patient is essential for the safety and welfare of both the animal and the handler. An animal that is securely and comfortably restrained will suffer less stress and will be less inclined to struggle and escape.

Most animals brought into a veterinary practice are used to being handled, but you may encounter stray dogs and feral cats which are wary of human contact. Their reaction to restraint may be unpredictable and even dangerous and you must protect your own safety.

It is important when handling any species of animal that you approach quietly and confidently and perform the technique correctly at the first attempt, not at the third or fourth attempt: nothing upsets an animal more than clumsy inept handling. You must know how to carry out the procedure, have all the equipment ready to hand and organise assistance if you think you are going to need it. It is also important to feel confidence in yourself. Animals are very sensitive to your mood and may detect your fear and bite you.

(For the purposes of description, the veterinary nurse restrains the patient, while the veterinary surgeon performs the task. In many cases two nurses or a nurse and the animal's owner can perform the task.)

DOGS

PROCEDURE: TYING A TAPE MUZZLE (FIG. 1.1)

This prevents the dog from biting the handler and diverts its attention away from the procedure being carried out.

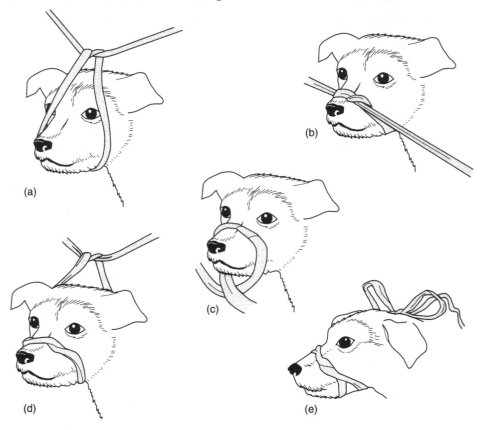

(a)

(b)

(c)

(d)

(e)

Figure 1.1 Tying a tape muzzle. Reproduced, with permission, from *Pre-Veterinary Nursing Textbook*, p. 152, by Masters and Bowden (2001). Butterworth Heinemann, UK.

ACTION

1. Place the dog in a sitting position on the floor.

2. Ask an assistant to stand astride the dog and grasp the scruff on either side of the head just behind the ears.

RATIONALE

1. In this position the dog is less likely to wriggle or bite. If the dog is small, it may be easier to place it on a table; avoid being bitten while you lift it on to the table.

2. If the dog moves its head around, the muzzle cannot be tied quickly. Be careful when scruffing a brachycephalic breed as there is a risk of prolapsing the eyes.

3. Using a length of cotton tape or bandage, tie a loop in it.

4. Approach the dog slowly and deliberately, crouching down to its level.

5. Place the looped tape over the nose and tighten quickly and firmly with the knot over the nose.
6. Bring the long ends of the tape down and cross over under the chin.

7. Take the two ends of the tape backwards and tie them in a bow behind the ears.
8. Ask the assistant holding the dog to keep the head pressed downwards.
9. If the dog is a brachycephalic or short-nosed breed, insert another piece of tape under the loop over the nose and under the piece at the back of the head.
10. Bring the two ends of this piece together and tie into a bow on the bridge of the nose.

11. Never leave a muzzled animal unattended.

3. Any long strip of material can be used, e.g. a tie or even a stocking, but it must be strong enough to hold the jaws together.
4. Crouching low helps to prevent fear aggression; standing over the dog may provoke it to jump up and bite.
5. Any delay in tightening the loop may allow the dog to shake its head free.

6. Further throws around the nose before finally crossing over will strengthen the muzzle.
7. A bow allows a quick release if the dog becomes distressed.
8. This position prevents the dog from lifting its forefeet to pull off the muzzle.
9. This prevents the muzzle from slipping off over the short nose.

10. The dog must be carefully observed as pressure over the nose may lead to respiratory distress.
11. There is a risk of asphyxiation by vomit or saliva.

PROCEDURE: LIFTING DOGS WEIGHING UP TO 15 KG

For example, cocker spaniels, beagles, etc.

ACTION

1. Keep your back straight and, with your legs slightly apart, bend your knees.
2. Place one arm around the front of the dog's chest and the other around its back end, over the tail.
3. Hold the dog close to your chest.

4. Straighten your legs, so raising the dog off the ground.
5. Place it firmly on the table.
6. Do not leave the animal unattended while it is on the table.

RATIONALE

1. This ensures that the weight of the dog is born by your spine and your pelvic girdle.

3. This will prevent the dog from struggling as it is lifted.

6. The dog may attempt to jump off the table, injuring itself, and it may then escape.

PROCEDURE: LIFTING DOGS WEIGHING OVER 20 KG (FIG. 1.2)

For example, labradors, springer spaniels, etc.

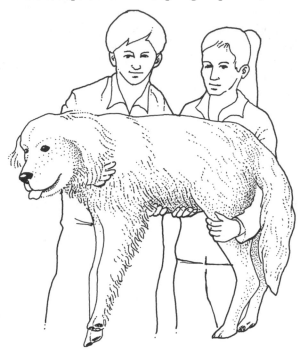

Figure 1.2 Lifting a large dog. Adapted, with permission, from *Veterinary Nursing*, 2nd edn, by Lane and Cooper (1994). Butterworth Heinemann, UK.

ACTION

1. Arrange for another person to assist you.

2. Both people stand on the same side of the dog.
3. Keep your back straight and, with your legs slightly apart, bend your knees.
4. You take the head end by placing one hand under the chest and the other under the neck.

5. Hold the head close to your chest. cannot turn its head around to bite.
6. Instruct your assistant to adopt the safe lifting position.
7. Instruct your assistant to place one hand under the abdomen and the other around the back end under the tail.
8. Both people straighten their legs simultaneously and lift the dog on to the table.

RATIONALE

1. Never attempt to lift a heavy dog by yourself. You may do permanent damage to your back!

3. This ensures that the weight of the dog is born by your spine and your pelvic girdle.
4. If possible, the person lifting the head should be familiar to the dog, e.g. the owner. This reduces the risk of anyone being bitten.
5. If the head is held close to you the dog

PROCEDURE: LIFTING SMALL DOGS WITH SPINAL DAMAGE (FIG. 1.3)

This can also be used for cats.

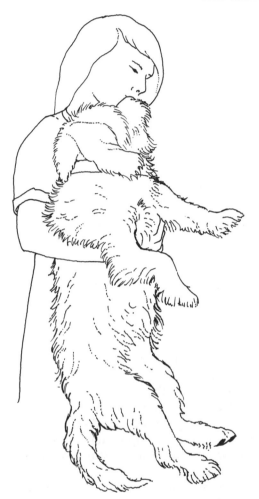
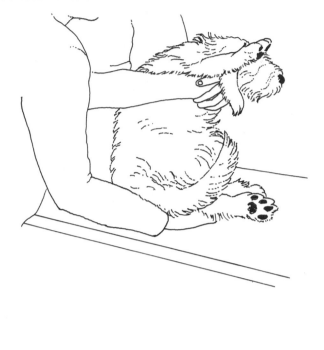

Figure 1.3 Lifting a small dog with spinal damage.

ACTION

1. Approach the animal quietly and with care.

2. If appropriate, apply a tape muzzle.

3. With a straight back and bent knees, place your arms around the animal's chest.
4. Straighten your knees and lift the animal, allowing the legs to hang downwards.

5. Gently place the animal on its side on a suitable non-slip surface ready for examination.

RATIONALE

1. It may be frightened and in extreme pain, leading to unpredictable behaviour.
2. This will prevent the dog biting you as you lift it.

4. This position prevents compression of the spine, which would cause acute pain and further damage.
5. Care must be taken to avoid causing further pain.

PROCEDURE: LIFTING LARGE DOGS WITH SPINAL DAMAGE (FIG. 1.4)

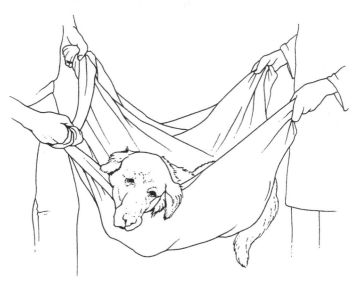

Figure 1.4 Lifting a large dog with spinal damage.

ACTION

1. Arrange for another person to assist you.

2. Find something that can be used as a 'stretcher', such as a blanket or sheet, an ironing board or a solid plank of wood.

3. Approach the animal quietly and with care.

4. If appropriate, apply a tape muzzle.

5. With the help of your assistant and adopting the correct lifting position, lift the dog on to the blanket or plank.
6. If using a plank, tie the dog on to it using tapes or bandages.

7. Gently carry the dog to the table and place it on the table, still on the blanket or plank.

RATIONALE

1. Do not attempt to lift a large injured dog by yourself. You may damage your back, get bitten or cause the condition of the patient to deteriorate.
2. The dog must be supported on something which prevents compression of the spine. This would cause acute pain and further damage.
3. It may be frightened and in extreme pain, leading to unpredictable behaviour.
4. This will prevent the dog biting you as you lift it.

6. This will prevent the dog from falling or jumping off the 'stretcher' as you lift it, with the risk of further injury.
7. The 'stretcher' can be removed from under the dog later on.

Restraint for general examination

PROCEDURE: TO EXAMINE THE CRANIAL END OF THE BODY

ACTION

1. Using the correct procedure, lift the dog on to a stable examination table covered in a non-slip mat.
2. Stand to one side of the dog.
3. Place one arm under the dog's neck and pull the head close to your chest with your hand.
4. Place the other arm over the dog's back with your elbow pointing towards the far side.
5. Apply pressure with your elbow and forearm along the spine, making the dog sit down.

RATIONALE

1. If the table does not shake and the dog's paws do not slip, the dog will feel secure and be less inclined to try and jump off the table.

3. If the head is held firmly against your chest, the dog cannot move to bite you.

5. In a sitting position the dog will feel secure.

PROCEDURE: TO EXAMINE THE CAUDAL END OF THE BODY OR TAKE THE RECTAL TEMPERATURE

(Continuing from the previous procedure.)

ACTION

1. Keep one arm under the neck pulling the head close to your chest.
2. Move the other arm and place it under the abdomen, gently lifting the dog into a standing position.
3. Pull the body close to your chest by bringing your forearm up under the abdomen.

4. If you are required to restrain the dog for a long period of time, move your hand to lie over the spine, but be careful that the dog does not sit down again.
5. If the dog starts to move or object to the examination, quickly return to the previous position.

RATIONALE

1. If the head is held firmly against your chest the dog cannot move to bite you.

3. This position holds the dog securely against you, reducing the risk of you being bitten and preventing it from moving during the examination.
4. This position may be more comfortable for you, while you still maintain control over the dog.
5. You must be aware of the dog's 'mood' and respond quickly to prevent anyone being bitten.

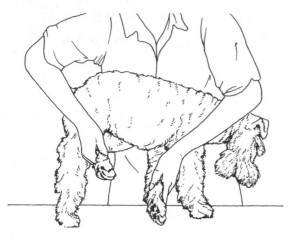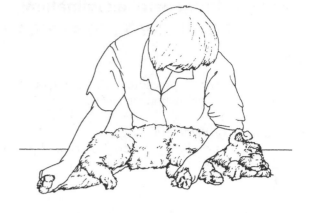

Figure 1.5 Restraining a dog on its side.

PROCEDURE: TO EXAMINE THE DOG ON ITS SIDE OR TO PROVIDE FIRMER CONTROL (FIG. 1.5)

ACTION

1. Apply a tape muzzle if appropriate.

2. Using the correct lifting procedure lift the dog and place it on a stable table covered in a non-slip mat.

3. With the dog in a standing position, stand to one side of the dog.

4. Reach over the dog and grasp the foreleg and hindleg furthest away from you at the level of the radius and tibia.

5. As quickly and as firmly as possible, pull the legs away from you, supporting the dog's spine against your chest.

6. Gently lower the body down to the table.

7. Place your arm across the chest and neck and apply firm pressure to keep the dog's head on the table.

RATIONALE

1. This method is used to restrain more difficult dogs and you should be prepared for an aggressive response.

2. If the table does not shake and the dog's paws do not slip, the dog will feel secure and be less inclined to struggle and escape.

4. It may be difficult to reach over the back of larger dogs, especially if you are short or the table is high.

5. This move must be done quickly before the dog begins to struggle and change position.

6. Avoid letting the body drop to the table as it may injure or frighten the animal.

7. Most dogs will become submissive in this position, but some will try to stand up again and you must be prepared. With large dogs, you may have to lean quite heavily but you must always observe the condition of the animal.

PROCEDURE: TO EXAMINE OR RESTRAIN THE DOG ON ITS BACK

ACTION

1. Place the dog on its side as previously described.
2. Ask an assistant to hold both the back legs and you hold both the forelegs.
3. Roll the dog over until it is lying on its back.
4. Extend the fore- and hindlegs, presenting the ventral abdomen for examination.
5. The sides of the neck can be grasped between the forelegs to give greater restraint if necessary.

RATIONALE

2. If the dog is small, this may be performed by one person.

5. Most dogs will feel quite comfortable in this position and will only struggle if they feel insecure or in pain.

Restraint for the administration of drugs
PROCEDURE: ADMINISTERING A TABLET

ACTION

1. Place the dog in a sitting position or in sternal recumbency on a suitable non-slip surface.

2. If necessary ask an assistant to hold the tail end of the dog.
3. Place one hand over the top of the muzzle and, using your fingers and thumb, gently raise the head and open the mouth.
4. Hold the tablet in the fingers of your other hand and with your forefinger pull down the lower jaw.
5. Place the tablet on the back of the tongue.

6. Close the mouth and hold it closed with one hand.
7. Stroke the neck until you feel the dog swallow the tablet.

RATIONALE

1. If the dog feels secure it will be less inclined to attempt to escape. Select a surface of a suitable height for you. Bending over for long periods may injure your back: place small dogs on a table, but larger dogs can be dosed on the floor.
2. This will prevent the dog from standing up or moving backwards.
3. Raising the head makes the lower jaw relax, making it easier to open.

5. If the tablet is placed as far back on the tongue as possible the swallowing reflex is initiated and the dog cannot spit it out.
6. This also prevents the dog from spitting the tablet out.
7. The dog may hold the tablet in the side of its mouth and spit it out as soon as you relax your grip. If swallowing has occurred, the tablet should be passing down the oesophagus!

PROCEDURE: ADMINISTERING A LIQUID FEED OR MEDICATION

ACTION	RATIONALE
1. Place the dog in a sitting position or in sternal recumbency on a suitable non-slip surface.	1. If the dog feels secure it will be less inclined to attempt to escape. Select a surface of a suitable height for you. Bending over for long periods may injure your back: place small dogs on a table, but larger dogs can be dosed on the floor.
2. If necessary ask an assistant to hold the tail end of the dog.	2. This will prevent the dog from standing up or moving backwards.
3. Place one hand over the top of the muzzle and, using your fingers and thumb, gently tilt the head upwards and to one side.	3. This position restrains the head while encouraging the jaw to relax and open.
4. Open the mouth slightly, creating a pocket at the angle of the jaw.	4. The pocket holds the liquid as it runs into the main part of the oral cavity.
5. Using a syringe filled with the liquid, insert it into the side of the mouth.	5. Try to avoid scraping the syringe over the gums as you may damage the mucous membranes.
6. Slowly depress the plunger so that the liquid trickles into the back of the mouth.	6. If you depress the plunger too quickly the liquid will squirt out over you and the dog.
7. Continue until the syringe is empty and repeat as necessary.	
8. When the procedure is complete, wipe the mouth clean and wipe up any spillage on the dog's coat.	8. Never leave the dog covered in liquid as it will become wet and cold, and in summer dried food may attract flies.

PROCEDURE: APPLYING EAR MEDICATION

ACTION	RATIONALE
1. Place the dog in a sitting position or in sternal recumbency on a suitable non-slip surface.	1. If the dog feels secure it will be less inclined to attempt to escape. Select a surface of a suitable height for you. Bending over for long periods may injure your back: place small dogs on a table, but larger dogs can be dosed on the floor.
2. If necessary apply a tape muzzle.	2. Some dogs may object to the application of ear medication.
3. Stand to one side of the dog.	
4. Place one arm under the dog's neck and over the muzzle. Pull the head towards your chest.	4. This prevents the head from moving suddenly when the medication is applied. Avoid holding the head in the area of the ear as this will interfere with the treatment.
5. Place the other arm over the dog's back with your elbow pointing towards the far side.	5. If the dog starts to struggle you can apply extra pressure by pressing your elbow closer to your side.

6. The veterinary surgeon will stand on the other side of the dog and apply the medication to the nearest ear.
7. The ear is gently massaged to disperse the drops or ointment.
8. To treat the other ear, exchange places.

Note. Many dogs do not object to the application of ear medication and can be treated single-handedly.

6. The applicator is introduced down the vertical part of the ear canal and squeezed.

PROCEDURE: APPLYING EYE MEDICATION

ACTION

1. Place the dog in a sitting position or in sternal recumbency on a suitable non-slip surface.

2. If necessary apply a tape muzzle.

3. Stand to one side of the dog.
4. Place one arm under the dog's neck and over the muzzle. Pull the head towards your chest.

5. Place the other arm over the dog's spine with your elbow pointing towards the far side.
6. The veterinary surgeon should stand in front of the dog and cup the head in both hands. Using the thumb of one hand the lower eyelid can be pulled down and the medication can be applied around the edge of the conjunctiva.
7. Release the tension on the eyelid and close the eyelids over the medication.
8. As you relax your hold on the dog, make sure that it does not rub at its eye with its paws or rub its head on the ground.

Note. Eye medication may be applied single-handedly, but if the dog moves suddenly there is a risk of damaging the eye.

RATIONALE

1. If the dog feels secure it will be less inclined to attempt to escape. Select a surface of a suitable height for you. Bending over for long periods may injure your back: place small dogs on a table, but larger dogs can be dosed on the floor.
2. Some dogs may object to the application of eye medication.

4. This prevents the head from moving suddenly when the medication is applied. Avoid holding the head in the area of the eye as this will interfere with the treatment.
5. If the dog starts to struggle you can apply extra pressure by pressing your elbow closer to your side.
6. You must ensure that the head is held firmly as sudden movement may result in damage to the eye.

7. This allows the medication to spread over the tissues of the eye and eyelid.
8. After about a minute most medication will have dispersed and will no longer cause any discomfort.

PROCEDURE: RESTRAINT FOR A SUBCUTANEOUS INJECTION

ACTION	RATIONALE
1. Place the dog in a sitting position or in sternal recumbency on an examination table with a non-slip surface.	1. If the dog feels secure and comfortable it will be less inclined to move or try to escape.
2. Apply a tape muzzle if necessary.	2. This is usually a quick and painless procedure, but some dogs may object and should be muzzled to prevent you being bitten.
3. Grasp the scruff firmly with one hand.	3. This restrains the head and tents the skin ready for injection.
4. Using the other hand insert the point of the needle with the bevel uppermost into the raised skin of the scruff.	4. Be careful to avoid pushing the point of the needle through the skin on the opposite side of the raised scruff.
5. Inject the contents of the syringe into the subcuticular space and withdraw the needle.	5. If you wish, you may draw back on the syringe, before injecting, to check that you have not penetrated a small blood capillary, but the blood supply to this area is relatively poor and the risk is low.
6. Gently massage the site of injection to disperse the drug.	6. Absorption from this site takes about 30–45 minutes.

Note. If the dog is likely to object to this procedure, it may be safer to arrange for an assistant to restrain the animal.

PROCEDURE: RESTRAINT FOR AN INTRAMUSCULAR INJECTION

ACTION	RATIONALE
1. The dog should be placed in a standing position on the floor or on a suitable table with a non-slip surface.	1. If the dog feels secure it will be less inclined to attempt to escape. Select a surface of a suitable height for you. Bending over for long periods may injure your back: place small dogs on a table, but larger dogs can be injected on the floor.
2. Apply a tape muzzle if necessary.	2. This injection may be slightly painful and some dogs may object.
3. Stand to one side of the dog.	
4. Place one arm under the neck and pull the head close to your chest.	4. If the head is firmly restrained, the dog cannot move suddenly or turn to bite.
5. Place your other arm over the dog's chest.	5. Be prepared to restrain the dog firmly in this position as sudden movement may cause damage and pain at the site of injection.
6. The veterinary surgeon will stand to one side of the dog and towards the hind end of the body.	

7. The quadriceps group of muscles lies on the cranial aspect of the femur and the veterinary surgeon will fix them between the fingers and thumb of the hand lying closest to the caudal end of the dog.

8. Using the other hand, the veterinary surgeon should introduce the needle through the skin and the muscle mass in a direction running towards the femur and almost at right angles to the lateral aspect of the thigh.

9. The veterinary surgeon should draw back slightly on the plunger to ensure that a blood vessel has not been penetrated.

10. If there is no blood present in the needle, inject the contents slowly.

11. Withdraw the needle and massage the site gently.

7. The quadriceps group are the most common site for intramuscular injections but the lumbodorsal muscles and the triceps of the forelimb can also be used.

8. At this angle the needle is unlikely to penetrate any major blood vessels or nerves.

9. Muscle tissue has a good blood supply and there is a risk of vascular penetration.

10. Muscle tissue is very dense and rapid injections of any volume of fluid may be very painful. Avoid giving any more than 2 ml at a time.

11. Gentle massage will help to disperse the drug into the bloodstream. The effect usually takes place in about 20–30 minutes.

PROCEDURE: RESTRAINT FOR AN INTRAVENOUS INJECTION USING THE CEPHALIC VEIN (FIG. 1.6)

(Assume that the skin has been clipped and sterilised ready for venepuncture.)
The cephalic vein runs over the dorsal aspect of the lower foreleg.

ACTION

1. Place the dog in sternal recumbency on a stable examination table with a non-slip surface.

2. Apply a tape muzzle if necessary.

3. Stand to one side of the dog.
4. Place one arm under the dog's chin and around the head, holding the head close to your chest.
5. Using your other hand, extend the foreleg on the opposite side towards the veterinary surgeon.
6. Cup the elbow in the palm of your hand, bringing the thumb across the crook of the elbow.

RATIONALE

1. If the dog feels secure it will be less inclined to attempt to escape. Select a surface of a suitable height for you: bending over for long periods may injure your back.
2. Some dogs will object to this procedure and a tape muzzle will protect you and the veterinary surgeon from being bitten. It also diverts the dog's attention from the injection.

4. If the head is held firmly and as close to you as possible, the dog is less likely to be able to bite you or the veterinary surgeon.
5. Your hand can rest on the table, ensuring that the foreleg is supported and held firmly.

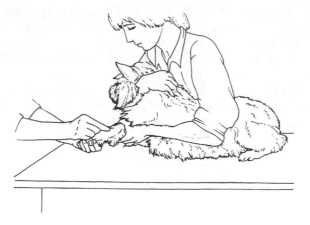

Figure 1.6 Holding a dog for intravenous injection using the cephalic vein.

7. Apply gentle pressure with your thumb and rotate your hand slightly outwards.

8. Maintain this pressure while the veterinary surgeon inserts the needle through the skin and into the underlying cephalic vein.

9. The veterinary surgeon should draw back on the syringe to check that the vein has been penetrated.

10. If blood appears at the hub of the needle, raise your thumb a little and the veterinary surgeon will slowly inject the contents of the syringe into the vein.

11. When the procedure is complete, and the needle has been slowly withdrawn, you should apply gentle pressure to the injection site for about 30 seconds.

   Note. If a blood sample is to be collected, maintain pressure on the vein until there is enough blood in the syringe.

7. This pressure acts as a tourniquet, trapping blood passing up the foreleg and resulting in dilation of the vein—referred to as 'raising the vein'.

8. The cephalic vein should be clearly visible lying just under the skin.

9. Perivascular injection may lead to tissue damage and a check must be made that the vein has been penetrated before attempting the injection.

10. Releasing the pressure allows the drug to flow into the vein.

11. This prevents haemorrhage into the area around the vein.

PROCEDURE: RESTRAINT FOR AN INTRAVENOUS INJECTION USING THE LATERAL SAPHENOUS VEIN

(Assume that the skin has been clipped and sterilised ready for venepuncture.)
The lateral saphenous vein runs over the lateral aspect of the hock.

ACTION

1. Apply a tape muzzle if necessary.

2. Place the dog in lateral recumbency on a stable examination table with a non-slip surface.
3. Stand on the dorsal side of the dog, so that the legs are directed away from you.
4. Using the arm closest to the head, place your forearm across the dog's neck and use this hand to hold both forepaws.
5. Place the other hand around the uppermost hindleg at the level of the mid-tibia/fibula.

6. Stretch out the leg and apply gentle pressure.
7. Maintain this pressure while the veterinary surgeon inserts the needle through the skin and into the underlying saphenous vein.
8. The veterinary surgeon should draw back on the syringe to check that the vein has been penetrated.

9. If blood appears at the hub of the needle, raise your thumb a little and the veterinary surgeon will slowly inject the contents of the syringe into the vein.
10. When the procedure is complete, and the needle has been slowly withdrawn, you should apply gentle pressure to the injection site for about 30 seconds.

Note. If a blood sample is to be collected, maintain pressure on the vein until enough blood is in the syringe.

RATIONALE

1. Some dogs may object to this procedure and should be muzzled. This must be done before putting the dog into lateral recumbency.
2. If the dog feels secure and comfortable it will be less inclined to struggle and attempt to escape.

4. In this position you can use the weight of your body to hold the cranial end of the dog on the table.
5. The lateral saphenous vein collects blood from the hindpaw and runs superficially on the caudal aspect of the hock and distal tibia. Pressure applied around the distal tibia acts as a tourniquet, trapping venous blood and causing the vein to dilate—known as 'raising the vein'.

7. The saphenous vein should be clearly visible lying just under the skin.

8. Perivascular injection may lead to tissue damage and a check must be made that the vein has been penetrated before attempting the injection.
9. Releasing the pressure allows the drug to flow into the vein.

10. This prevents haemorrhage into the area around the vein.

PROCEDURE: RESTRAINT FOR AN INTRAVENOUS INJECTION USING THE JUGULAR VEIN

(Assume that the skin has been clipped and sterilised ready for venepuncture.)
The jugular vein runs in the jugular furrow on either side of the trachea.

ACTION	RATIONALE
1. Place the dog in a sitting position on a stable examination table with a non-slip surface.	1. If the dog feels secure and comfortable it will be less inclined to struggle and attempt to escape.
2. Apply a tape muzzle if necessary.	2. Some dogs may object to this procedure.
3. Stand to one side of the dog and place one hand under the dog's chin, raising the head and bringing it close to your chest.	3. Firm restraint is essential for this procedure to prevent the dog moving suddenly and causing injury to itself or to you.
4. Place your other arm over the dog's back and round to the front of its chest, holding it close to your body.	
5. The veterinary surgeon will stand in front of the dog and apply pressure at the base of the jugular furrow with the fingers of one hand.	5. The jugular vein on each side of the trachea runs in a groove known as the jugular furrow. It collects venous blood from the head and carries it towards the heart. Pressure applied at the base of the vein will prevent the flow of blood towards the heart, causing the vein to dilate—known as 'raising the vein'.
6. Using the other hand the veterinary surgeon should insert the needle through the skin into the underlying vein.	6. The jugular vein should be clearly visible lying just under the skin.
7. The veterinary surgeon should draw back on the syringe to check that the vein has been penetrated.	7. Perivascular injection may lead to tissue damage and a check must be made that the vein has been penetrated before attempting the injection.
8. If blood appears at the hub of the needle, raise your thumb a little and the veterinary surgeon will slowly inject the contents of the syringe into the vein.	8. Releasing the pressure allows the drug to flow into the vein.
9. When the procedure is complete, and the needle has been slowly withdrawn, you should apply gentle pressure to the injection site for about 30 seconds.	9. This prevents haemorrhage into the area around the vein.

Note. If a blood sample is to be collected, maintain pressure on the vein until enough blood is in the syringe. This vein is rarely used in the dog as the other veins are more convenient and usually provide a sufficient volume of blood.

CATS

Most cats are used to being handled and will respond to being stroked
and spoken to quietly. These cats do not pose much of a problem
but many, particularly feral cats, can be extremely difficult to handle
and you must be prepared to exercise varying degrees of restraint,
depending on the individual. It is important to remember that cats have
five weapons of assault—four sets of claws and a set of sharp teeth!

PROCEDURE: LIFTING A FRIENDLY CAT USED TO BEING HANDLED (METHOD 1)

ACTION

1. Approach the cat calmly and confidently, talking to it quietly.
2. Assess whether the cat is safe to stroke.

3. If safe, gently stroke the top of the cat's head and run your hand along its back.

4. Gently but firmly grasp the scruff of the neck with one hand and lift the cat.

5. Place the other hand under the sternum and support the cat.
6. Place the cat on a stable non-slip surface.

RATIONALE

1. Most cats are used to human noise and will be reassured by a low quiet tone of voice.
2. A frightened or aggressive cat will warn you by hissing or growling as you approach, while a friendly cat may rub itself against your hand and even purr!
3. This will reassure the cat, and may elicit a purr. If the cat hisses, use another method of lifting and restraint.
4. Picking a cat up by the scruff mimics the way in which the queen carries her kittens. It initiates an innate relaxation response, which in the 'wild' would enable the queen to move the kittens safely from place to place without the risk of them struggling and escaping.
5. Kittens and smaller cats may be lifted by the scruff, but heavier cats need added support.
6. If the cat feels insecure, it may try to scratch, bite or escape.

PROCEDURE: LIFTING A FRIENDLY CAT USED TO BEING HANDLED (METHOD 2)

ACTION

1. Approach the cat calmly and confidently, talking to it quietly.
2. Assess whether the cat is safe to stroke.

3. If safe, stroke the cat and gently run one hand over the chest and under the sternum.
4. Place the other hand under the abdomen to support it from the other side.
5. Lift the cat on to a stable examination table with a non-slip surface.

RATIONALE

1. Most cats are used to human noise and will be reassured by a low quiet tone of voice.
2. A frightened or aggressive cat will warn you by hissing or growling as you approach.

4. In this position the cat feels supported and secure and is unlikely to struggle.

PROCEDURE: LIFTING A FRIGHTENED OR AGGRESSIVE CAT

ACTION

1. Grasp the scruff of the cat quickly and firmly.

2. Lift the cat by the scruff, letting the hind end of the body hang down.

3. Place the cat on a table and restrain in an appropriate way.

RATIONALE

1. If you do not take enough scruff or make any mistake in handling you are likely to get bitten or scratched.
2. Do not leave the cat 'hanging' for more than a few seconds as this is unpleasant for the cat, particularly if large.
3. Aggressive cats may have to be restrained using such equipment as a crusher cage or a restraining bag.

PROCEDURE: CARRYING A CAT

ACTION

1. Place the body of the cat under one elbow and forearm holding it close to your side. Let the hindlegs gently dangle.

2. Hold the forepaws together between the thumb and fingers of the hand on that side.
3. Hold the scruff of the cat firmly with your free hand.

RATIONALE

1. The body is supported by the angle of your arm, but the hindlegs are unable to push the cat's body up in order to escape. Watch out for the hindlegs getting caught in side pockets.
2. This prevents the forelegs from scratching you.
3. In this position, the cat feels secure and comfortable. If it tries to escape, you have control of the head via the scruff and you can apply stronger pressure to the body with your elbow.

Note. Avoid carrying aggressive or frightened cats around in your arms as their movements are often unpredictable. They should be carried in a wire cat basket which allows them to see out while providing you with clear visibility of their condition.

Restraint for general examination

Cats that are used to being handled respond to minimal restraint, but you should be prepared to use firmer methods on more difficult cats, particularly if you are single-handed.

PROCEDURE: TO EXAMINE A FRIENDLY CAT

ACTION

1. Place the cat on a stable examination table in a sitting position.
2. Stand to one side of the cat.
3. Run the hand closest to the cat over its back and under the cat's jaw, gently raising the head up a little.
4. Place the other hand over the forelegs.

5. If the cat begins to struggle or object to examination, move the hand from under the chin and grasp the scruff.
6. Use the elbow on this side to press the cat's body firmly against your side.

7. Use the other hand to hold the forelegs firmly down on to the table.

Note. This position uses minimal restraint, allowing examination of the whole body and

RATIONALE

1. The cat will feel secure and comfortable and will be less inclined to try and escape.

3. If the cat is relaxed this hand can be placed on the chest, but you should be ready to move to restrain the head if necessary.
4. This prevents the cat from raising its forepaws to scratch.
5. This controls the head, allowing examination of the body.

6. In this position, the cat is unable to move or gain enough grip to make an escape. It may be more comfortable to lift the cat supporting it against your body rather than leaning over the examination table.
7. This controls the forepaws and prevents scratching.

enabling the rectal temperature to be taken safely.

PROCEDURE: TO EXAMINE A FRACTIOUS CAT

ACTION

1. Firmly grasp the scruff of the cat with one hand.

2. Pick up the cat and with the other hand, grasp its hindlegs.
3. Place the cat on the table in lateral recumbency, extending its head and hindlegs.

4. As the cat struggles, make sure that you keep your arms wide apart to maintain the position.

This position allows examination of most of the body but it is inadvisable to use it to take the rectal temperature, as the cat may struggle and damage itself. For the welfare of the cat, another method of restraint should be adopted as soon as possible.

Restraint equipment available for use with more aggressive cats includes crusher cages, cat

RATIONALE

1. Some fractious cats seem to have the ability to 'use up' their scruffs by hunching their shoulders and letting their heads sink down, making the scruff very difficult to grasp. Adult toms also have thickened scruffs which are difficult to hold for any length of time.

3. The cat is unable to move against the strength of the handler's arms, but a really angry cat will continue to attempt to escape and a great deal of growling and miaowing will be heard!
4. As the forelegs are not restrained you must be careful to avoid being scratched.

grabbers and cat bags out of which the head or legs can be extended while the rest of the body is retained inside. Wrapping an aggressive cat in a towel and extending the head or a leg is also a useful means of restraint. Chemical restraint is widely used, but some form of contact with the cat will still be necessary to administer the drug.

Restraint for the administration of drugs

PROCEDURE: ADMINISTERING A TABLET (FIG. 1.7)

ACTION

1. Place the cat in a sitting position on a suitable non-slip surface.
2. Grasp the cat's head by placing one hand over the head and your thumb and forefinger at the angle of the jaw.
3. Apply gentle pressure at the angle of the jaw.
4. Gently but firmly, tilt the head backwards.

5. Hold the tablet between the thumb and forefinger of your other hand.
6. Use your second and third fingers to apply gentle downwards pressure to the cat's lower jaw.

7. As the jaw opens, place or drop the tablet on to the back of the tongue.

8. Keeping the head tilted vertically, close the mouth and hold it closed with your hand.
9. Gently stroke the throat until the cat is seen to swallow.

RATIONALE

1. The cat will feel secure and less inclined to escape.
2. Be aware that the cat may raise its forepaws at this point.

4. As the head is tilted the jaw will naturally relax and the mouth should be easier to open.

6. At the first attempt the jaws should open easily. At later attempts, the cat may clench its jaws tightly closed, making the procedure more difficult—an experience often reported by owners!
7. If the tablet is placed as far back as possible on the tongue, the swallowing reflex will be induced.
8. It is important to hold the mouth closed as this prevents the cat from spitting the tablet out.
9. Some cats may learn to hold the tablet in the side of their cheeks until the head is released when they then spit the tablet out!

Note. If you have an assistant, the cat can be further restrained by holding the forelegs while you administer the tablet as described (Fig. 1.7).

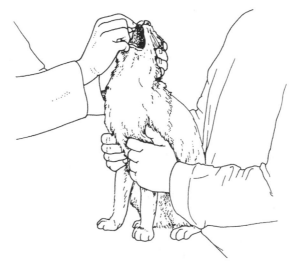

Figure 1.7 Administering a tablet.

PROCEDURE: ADMINISTERING A LIQUID FEED OR MEDICATION (FIG. 1.8)

ACTION

1. Sit on a chair with a towel or other absorbent material covering your knees.
2. Take the cat on to your knee with its head pointing away from you.
3. Grasp the cat's head with one hand, with your thumb and forefinger at the angle of the jaw, and slightly tilt the head to one side.
4. Open the mouth slightly, creating a pocket at the angle of the jaw.
5. Using a small syringe filled with the liquid, gently insert the end of the barrel into the mouth at the angle of the jaw.
6. Slowly depress the plunger so that the liquid trickles into the mouth.
7. Continue until the syringe is empty and repeat as necessary.
8. When the procedure is complete, clean the cat's mouth, paws and any other parts which are wet or covered in liquid.

RATIONALE

1. This procedure can be messy and the towel will absorb any spilt liquids.
2. In this position, the cat will be comfortable and easy to restrain.
3. If the cat raises its forepaws, ask an assistant to hold them down or wrap them in the towel.
4. This pocket holds the liquid as it runs into the main part of the oral cavity.
5. Be as gentle as possible: rough handling can easily damage the mouth.

6. If you depress the plunger too quickly, the liquid may squirt out over you and the cat.

8. Never leave the cat covered in liquid as it will become wet and cold. Drying food may attract flies.

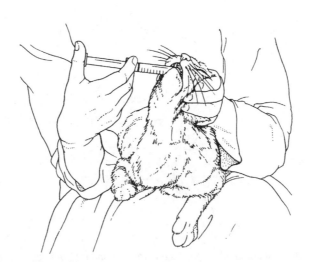

Figure 1.8 Administering a liquid feed or medication.

PROCEDURE: APPLYING EAR MEDICATION (FIG. 1.9)

ACTION

1. Place the cat in a sitting position on a stable examination table with a non-slip surface.
2. Standing to one side, place your hands on either side of the cat bringing them forward to restrain the forelegs on the table.

3. The veterinary surgeon will stand in front of the cat and take hold of the pinna of the ear to be treated, with the finger and thumb of one hand.
4. The veterinary surgeon will gently twist the head so that it faces upwards.

5. Using the other hand, the veterinary surgeon can apply the medication to the ear.

RATIONALE

1. The cat will feel secure and less inclined to escape.
2. Cats used to being handled prefer minimal restraint. This procedure does not usually cause too much discomfort and the cat is unlikely to struggle; however, if struggling does occur be prepared to grasp the scruff with one hand and restrain the forelegs with the other.
3. In this position, the veterinary surgeon can gain maximum access to the affected ear.

4. This brings the ear uppermost so that any medication runs down the ear canal by gravity. It also helps to restrain the head.

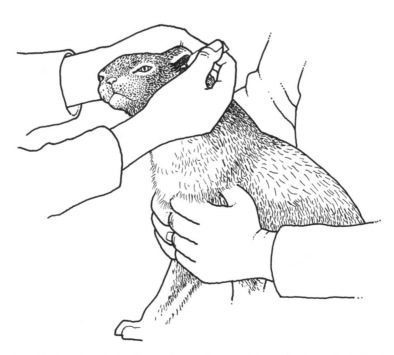

Figure 1.9 Applying ear medication. Adapted, with permission, from *Veterinary Nursing*, 2nd edn, by Lane and Cooper (1994). Butterworth Heinemann, UK.

PROCEDURE: APPLYING EYE MEDICATION

ACTION

1. Place the cat in a sitting position on a stable examination table with a non-slip surface.
2. Place one hand on either side of the cat's rump.
3. The veterinary surgeon should stand in front of the cat and take the cat's head in one hand, placing the thumb over the cranium and the fingers under the chin. The affected eye should be on the far side of the head away from the palm of the hand.
4. The skin around the affected eye is gently stretched with the forefinger and thumb of this hand.
5. Using the other hand, the medication is applied around the edges of the conjunctiva.
6. Relax the stretching around the eyes and eyelids.
7. Gently close the eyelids over the medication.

8. You must maintain control of the forepaws the a short while to prevent the cat from clawing at the eye or rubbing its head on the table.

RATIONALE

1. The cat will feel secure and less inclined to escape.
2. This prevents the cat from trying to go backwards and escape.
3. In this position, the head is held still, reducing the risk of damage to the eye. If the cat struggles, the nozzle of the tube may scratch or penetrate the eye.

4. This will open the eyelids, allowing examination of the eye and conjunctiva.
5. If you are too rough you may cause damage to the delicate conjunctiva.
6. This enables the eyelids to close.

7. This allows the drops or ointment to spread around the tissues of the eye and eyelids.
8. After a minute or so, the ointment will have dissipated and the cat should not feel any discomfort.

PROCEDURE: RESTRAINT FOR A SUBCUTANEOUS INJECTION (FIG. 1.10)

ACTION

1. Place the cat in sternal recumbency on an examination table with a non-slip surface. The cat should face away from you.
2. Grasp the scruff firmly with one hand.

3. Using the other hand, introduce the point of the needle with the bevel uppermost, into the raised skin of the scruff.
4. Inject the contents into the subcuticular space and withdraw the needle.

5. Gently massage the site of injection to disperse the drug.

Note. Most cats will not object to this procedure and it can usually be performed single-handedly provided that you give the injection

RATIONALE

1. In this position, the cat feels secure and cannot slip.

2. This gives control of the head, as the cat is unable to turn and bite. It also tents the skin ready for injection.
3. Be careful to avoid pushing the point of the needle through the skin on the opposite side of the raised scruff.
4. If you wish, you may draw back on the syringe, before injecting, to check that you have not penetrated a small blood capillary, but the blood supply to this area is relatively poor and the risk is low.
5. Absorption from this site takes about 30–45 minutes.

quickly; however, some cats will need to be restrained by an assistant to prevent struggling.

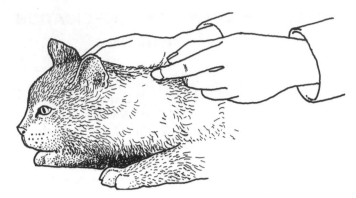

Figure 1.10 Restraint for a subcutaneous injection. Adapted, with permission, from *Veterinary Nursing*, 2nd edn, by Lane and Cooper (1994). Butterworth Heinemann, UK.

PROCEDURE: RESTRAINT FOR AN INTRAMUSCULAR INJECTION (FIG. 1.11)

ACTION

1. Place the cat in a standing position on an examination table with a non-slip surface.

2. Standing to one side of the cat, restrain the head firmly by grasping the scruff.

3. The veterinary surgeon should take the nearest hindleg and locate the quadriceps group of muscles lying on the cranial aspect of the femur. The muscles should be fixed between the thumb and fingers of the hand closest to the caudal end of the cat.

4. Using the other hand, the veterinary surgeon should introduce the needle through the skin and the muscle mass in a direction running towards the femur and almost at right angles to the lateral aspect of the thigh.

5. The veterinary surgeon should draw back slightly on the plunger to ensure that a blood vessel has not been penetrated.

6. If there is no blood present in the needle, inject the contents slowly.

7. Withdraw the needle and massage the site gently.

RATIONALE

1. In this position, the cat is held firmly but is quite comfortable. It is essential to restrain the cat adequately, as sudden movement may result in damage to the muscle tissues.

2. The head must be held tightly, as this potentially painful procedure could cause the cat to bite.

3. The quadriceps group is a large muscle mass which provides easy access for injection. The hamstring group and the gluteals should not be used as there is a risk of bone and sciatic nerve damage.

4. At this angle the needle is unlikely to penetrate any major blood vessels or nerves.

5. Muscle tissue has a good blood supply and there is a risk of vascular penetration.

6. Muscle tissue is very dense and rapid injections of any volume of fluid may be very painful. Avoid giving more than 2 ml at a time.

7. Gentle massage will help to disperse the drug into the bloodstream. The effect usually takes place in about 20–30 minutes.

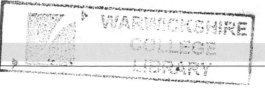

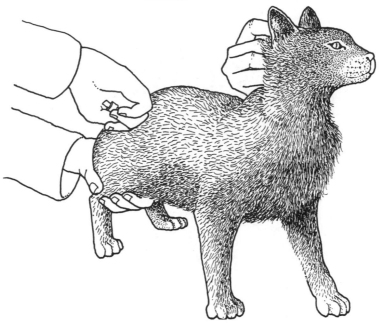

Figure 1.11 Restraint for an intramuscular injection. Adapted, with permission, from *Veterinary Nursing*, 2nd edn, by Lane and Cooper (1994). Butterworth Heinemann, UK.

PROCEDURE: RESTRAINT FOR AN INTRAVENOUS INJECTION USING THE CEPHALIC VEIN (FIG. 1.12)

(Assume that the skin has been clipped and sterilised ready for venepuncture.)
The cephalic vein runs over the dorsal aspect of the lower foreleg.

ACTION

1. Place the cat on a stable examination table with a non-slip surface, in sternal recumbency or in a sitting position.
2. With one hand take a firm grasp of the scruff, facing the cat towards the veterinary surgeon.
3. Use your forearm and elbow to hold the remainder of the body close to you.
4. Using the other hand, extend a foreleg towards the veterinary surgeon.
5. Support the cat's elbow in the palm of your upturned hand and place your thumb across the crook of the elbow.
6. Apply gentle pressure with your thumb and rotate your hand slightly outwards.

7. Maintain this pressure while the veterinary surgeon inserts the needle through the skin

RATIONALE

1. In this position the cat will feel secure and comfortable and will be less likely to move or try to escape.
2. It is vital that the cat is held firmly as sudden movement may cause injury to the patient, to yourself or to the vet.
3. Extra control can be achieved by changing the pressure exerted by your elbow.

5. Your hand can rest on the table, ensuring that the foreleg is supported and held firmly.
6. This pressure acts as a tourniquet, trapping blood passing up the foreleg and resulting in dilation of the vein—referred to as 'raising the vein'.
7. The cephalic vein should be clearly visible lying just under the skin.

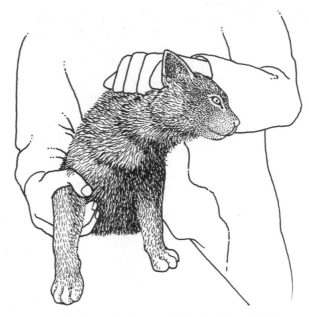

Figure 1.12 Restraint for an intravenous injection using the cephalic vein. Adapted, with permission, from *Veterinary Nursing*, 2nd edn, by Lane and Cooper (1994). Butterworth Heinemann, UK.

and into the underlying cephalic vein.

8. The veterinary surgeon should draw back on the syringe to check that the vein has been penetrated.

8. Perivascular injection may lead to tissue damage and a check must be made that the vein has been penetrated before attempting the injection.

9. If blood appears at the hub of the needle, raise your thumb a little and the veterinary surgeon will slowly inject the contents of the syringe into the vein.

9. Releasing the pressure allows the drug to flow into the vein.

10. When the procedure is complete, and the needle has been slowly withdrawn, you should apply gentle pressure to the injection site for about 30 seconds.

10. This prevents haemorrhage into the area around the vein.

Note. If a blood sample is to be collected, maintain pressure on the vein until enough blood is in the syringe.

PROCEDURE: RESTRAINT FOR AN INTRAVENOUS INJECTION USING THE LATERAL SAPHENOUS VEIN

(Assume that the skin has been clipped and sterilised ready for venepuncture.)
The lateral saphenous vein runs over the lateral aspect of the hock.

ACTION

1. Place the cat in lateral recumbency on a stable examination table with a non-slip surface.
2. With one hand grasp the scruff firmly.

3. With the other hand, extend the uppermost hindleg, at the same time stretching out the body.

4. Position your hand around the lower leg at the level of mid-tibia/fibula and apply gentle pressure.

5. Maintain this pressure while the veterinary surgeon inserts the needle through the skin and into the underlying saphenous vein.
6. The veterinary surgeon should draw back on the syringe to check that the vein has been penetrated.

7. If blood appears at the hub of the needle, release the pressure a little and the veterinary surgeon will slowly inject the contents of the syringe into the vein.
8. When the procedure is complete, and the needle has been slowly withdrawn, you should apply gentle pressure to the injection site for about 30 seconds.

RATIONALE

1. The cat will feel secure and comfortable and will be less likely to move or try to escape.
2. The head must be restrained firmly to prevent the cat wriggling or biting.
3. If the cat struggles or is aggressive, it may be necessary to exert extra control by wrapping the cat in a towel with the head out. The hindleg can be extended from the towel.
4. The lateral saphenous vein collects blood from the hindpaw and runs superficially on the caudal aspect of the hock and distal tibia. Pressure applied around the distal tibia acts as a tourniquet, trapping venous blood and causing the vein to dilate—known as 'raising the vein'.
5. The saphenous vein should be clearly visible lying just under the skin.

6. Perivascular injection may lead to tissue damage and a check must be made that the vein has been penetrated before attempting the injection.
7. Releasing the pressure allows the drug to flow into the vein.

8. This prevents haemorrhage into the area around the vein.

PROCEDURE: RESTRAINT FOR AN INTRAVENOUS INJECTION USING THE JUGULAR VEIN (METHOD 1) (FIG. 1.13)

(Assume that the skin has been clipped and sterilised ready for venepuncture.)
The jugular vein runs in the jugular furrow on either side of the trachea.

ACTION	RATIONALE
1. Sit on a chair and place the cat on your lap.	1. This ensures that you are comfortable and able to support and restrain the cat more easily.
2. Turn the cat over into dorsal recumbency.	2. In this position there is easy access to the ventral part of the neck. If the cat feels secure in your lap it will be more likely to relax.
3. Take all four legs in one hand.	3. Control of the legs prevents the veterinary surgeon from being scratched.
4. The veterinary surgeon should gently extend the head with one hand, placing the thumb under the chin and cupping the cranium in the palm of the hand.	4. Extending the head and neck stretches out the jugular vein as it runs beside the trachea and tenses the overlying skin, making it easier to penetrate the vein with the needle.
5. You can now place the thumb of your other hand at the base of the jugular furrow at the point where the trachea enters the thoracic cavity.	5. The jugular vein on each side of the trachea runs in a groove known as the jugular furrow. It collects venous blood from the head and carries it towards the heart.
6. Apply gentle pressure.	6. Pressure applied at the base of the vein will prevent the flow of blood towards the heart, causing the vein to dilate—known as 'raising the vein'.

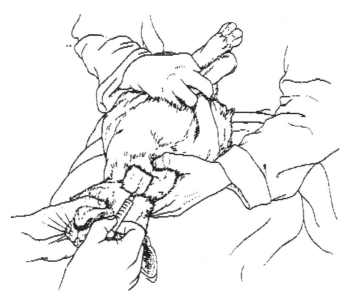

Figure 1.13 Restraint for an intravenous injection using the jugular vein. Reproduced, with permission, from *Practical Animal Handling*, p. 128, by Anderson and Edney (1991). Butterworth Heiremann, UK.

7. Maintain this pressure while the veterinary surgeon inserts the needle through the skin and into the underlying jugular vein.

8. The veterinary surgeon should draw back on the syringe to check that the vein has been penetrated.

9. If blood appears at the hub of the needle, raise your thumb a little and the veterinary surgeon will slowly inject the contents of the syringe into the vein.

10. When the procedure is complete, and the needle has been slowly withdrawn, you should apply gentle pressure to the injection site for about 30 seconds.

7. The jugular vein should be clearly visible lying just under the skin.

8. Perivascular injection may lead to tissue damage and a check must be made that the vein has been penetrated before attempting the injection.

9. Releasing the pressure allows the drug to flow into the vein.

10. This prevents haemorrhage into the area around the vein.

Note. The jugular vein is more often used for blood sampling. During this procedure, pressure is maintained until enough blood has collected in the syringe.

PROCEDURE: RESTRAINT FOR AN INTRAVENOUS INJECTION USING THE JUGULAR VEIN (METHOD 2)

(Assume that the skin has been clipped and sterilised ready for venepuncture.)

ACTION

1. Place the cat in a sitting position on a stable examination table with a non-slip surface.
2. It may be necessary to ask an assistant to place a hand on either side of the cat's rump to maintain it in this position.

3. You should bring one hand over the cat's back and restrain the forelegs and paws on the table.

4. Place your the other hand under the chin and raise the cat's head so that the neck and chin are in a straight line.

5. The veterinary surgeon should apply pressure at the base of the jugular furrow with the fingers of one hand.

6. Using the other hand the veterinary surgeon should insert the needle through the skin into the underlying vein.

RATIONALE

1. The cat will feel secure and comfortable and will be less likely to move or try to escape.
2. This should prevent the cat from struggling during the procedure. If the cat struggles, the assistant should be prepared to use extra force.
3. If the cat struggles you may have to use the scruff to restrain and extend the head. However, this leaves the forelegs free and the cat may scratch the veterinary surgeon.
4. In this position the jugular vein and overlying skin are tensed, making it easier to penetrate the vein with the needle.
5. The jugular vein on each side of the trachea runs in a groove known as the jugular furrow. It collects venous blood from the head and carries it towards the heart.
6. The jugular vein should be clearly visible lying just under the skin.

7. The veterinary surgeon should draw back on the syringe to check that the vein has been penetrated.

8. If blood appears at the hub of the needle, the veterinary surgeon will release the pressure on the vein and slowly inject the contents of the syringe into the vein.

9. When the procedure is complete, and the needle has been slowly withdrawn, you should apply gentle pressure to the injection site for about 30 seconds.

Note. The jugular vein is more often used for blood sampling. During this procedure, pressure

7. Perivascular injection may lead to tissue damage and a check must be made that the vein has been penetrated before attempting the injection.

8. Releasing the pressure allows the drug to flow into the vein.

9. This prevents haemorrhage into the area around the vein.

is maintained until enough blood has collected in the syringe.

FURTHER READING

Anderson RS, Edney ATB (eds) 1991 Practical Animal Handling. Pergamon, Oxford
Cooper B, Lane DR (eds) 1999 Veterinary Nursing, 2nd edn. Butterworth-Heinemann, Oxford

Dallas S (ed.) 1999 Manual of Veterinary Care. BSAVA, Gloucester

- To measure the body temperature
- To measure the pulse rate by palpation of the femoral artery
- To measure the pulse rate using a stethoscope
- To measure the pulse rate by palpation of the chest
- To measure the pulse rate using an oesophageal stethoscope
- To measure the respiratory rate by direct observation
- To measure the respiratory rate using a stethoscope
- To measure the respiratory rate using an oesophageal stethoscope
- To assess capillary refill time
- To measure the electrical activity of the heart using an electrocardiogram
- To measure the percentage of oxygen (oxygen saturation) in the blood using a pulse oximeter
- To measure central venous pressure
- To measure arterial blood pressure using a non-invasive technique
- To measure carbon dioxide levels using a mainstream capnograph
- To measure carbon dioxide levels using a sidestream capnograph
- To measure urine production
- To measure tear production
- To measure intraocular pressure

2

Measuring clinical parameters

R. Aspinall

Introduction

Diagnosis of a patient's condition is based on a thorough clinical examination followed by a range of diagnostic tests. Part of the clinical examination includes the measurement of certain basic indicators of the body's function, known as the clinical parameters (Table 2.1). Among the easiest to measure and therefore the most commonly performed are body temperature, pulse or heart rate and respiratory rate. Once these are known, they are compared with normal values for that species and the significance of the result is evaluated in the context of the symptoms. Later, once treatment has started, the parameters can be monitored and used as indicators of the progress of the disease.

Clinical parameters such as the percentage of blood gases or blood pressure require the use of complicated equipment but are essential measurements during anaesthesia and for monitoring the progress of the critically ill and hospitalised patient.

Measurement of clinical parameters and the monitoring of changes in their levels are an essential part of patient care. The veterinary surgeon must be able to rely on the veterinary nurse being able to perform the procedure correctly and accurately and to know that the nurse understands that, when the results are abnormal, some action must be taken to return them to normal.

This chapter describes the methods of measuring these parameters in detail so that the veterinary nurse can approach the process with a degree of understanding and use the more complicated apparatus without fear.

Table 2.1 Normal clinical parameters in the dog and cat

Clinical parameter	Dog	Cat
Body temperature (°C)	38.3–38.7	38.0–38.5
Pulse rate (beats/min)	60–180	110–180
Respiratory rate (breaths/min)	10–30	20–30
Capillary refill time (s)	1–2	1–2
Oxygen saturation	Close to 99%	Close to 99%
Arterial blood pressure:	Puppy—108/60	Kitten—123/63
systolic/diastolic (mmHg)	Adult—141/81	Adult—129/70
Central venous pressure (mm H_2O)	3–7.5	3–7.5
Carbon dioxide concentration (mmHg)	End tidal: 35–54	End tidal: 32–35
	Inspired: less than 8	Inspired: less than 8
Volume of urine produced (ml/kg/h)	1–2	1–2
Volume of tears produced (ml)	15–25	15–25
Intraocular pressure (mmHg)	25	25

PROCEDURE: TO MEASURE THE BODY TEMPERATURE (TABLE 2.1)

Equipment. Mercury or digital thermometer.

ACTION

1. Place the animal in a comfortable standing position on a table.
2. Ask an assistant to restrain a dog gently by placing one arm around the neck and the other around the chest. Ensure that the dog is relaxed and quiet. Cats should be held lightly with both hands around the shoulders or place one hand under the chin and the other around its chest, pulling it close to your body.
3. Select either a mercury or digital thermometer.
4. Lubricate the end with KY jelly or a similar lubricant.
5. Shake the mercury down to the bulb or check that the digital thermometer is switched on and displaying a reading.
6. Gently but firmly, insert the instrument into the rectum through the anus. A slight rotating action may help entrance through the rectal sphincters. Cats, particularly, may require patient gentle pressure before the sphincters relax.
7. Leave the thermometer in position for at least 30 seconds.
8. Clean the end of the thermometer by wiping with a paper cloth or cotton wool.

RATIONALE

1. If the patient feels uncomfortable or insecure it will try to escape.
2. In this position, the animal will feel comfortable and unrestricted; however, the assistant will be able to react quickly if it tries to jump off the table.

3. Choice of instrument depends on availability.
4. Lubrication reduces the discomfort of insertion into the rectum.
5. If the mercury is not shaken down the new reading will be inaccurate.

6. In animals, the oral route is not practical but the rectal route is easy and well tolerated.

7. The mercury has to have time to warm up and expand.
8. This prevents transmission of disease to the next animal for which the thermometer is used.

9. Read the mercury thermometer by looking for the line of mercury against the scale. Read off the figures on the digital thermometer.
10. Record the reading on the hospital record or clinical record.
11. Shake down the mercury or reset the digital reading.
12. Place the bulb of the instrument in the disinfectant container.

9. The glass of the thermometer magnifies the mercury line and makes it easier to read.
10. To monitor rises or falls in the body temperature.
11. To prepare the thermometer for use in the future.
12. This prevents transmission of disease to the next animal for which the thermometer is used.

PROCEDURE: TO MEASURE THE PULSE RATE BY PALPATION OF THE FEMORAL ARTERY (TABLE 2.1)

ACTION

1. Place the animal in a comfortable standing position on a table.
2. Ask an assistant to restrain the dog gently by placing one arm around the neck and the other around the chest. Ensure that the dog is relaxed and quiet. Cats should be held lightly with both hands around the shoulders or place one hand under the chin and the other around its chest, pulling it close to your body.
3. Standing on one side of the animal, place the fingers of one hand on the medial aspect of the thigh. Locate the femoral artery as it runs down the medial aspect of the femur.
4. Press gently against the artery with the second and third fingers and feel the pulse.

5. Count the beats of the pulse for 60 seconds.

6. Record the pulse rate.

RATIONALE

1. If the patient feels uncomfortable or insecure it will try to escape.
2. In this position, the animal will feel comfortable and unrestricted; however, the assistant will be able to react quickly if it tries to jump off the table.

3. The pulse can be palpated at any point where an artery runs over a bone and close to the body surface. The femoral pulse is the easiest to detect.
4. The tips of the fingers are sensitive to touch. The thumb and the forefinger have a pulse of their own which may be mistaken for the dog's pulse.
5. This is enough time in which to detect any abnormalities.
6. If there any irregularities in rate and rhythm, inform the veterinary surgeon.

PROCEDURE: TO MEASURE THE PULSE RATE USING A STETHOSCOPE (TABLE 2.1)

ACTION

1. Place the animal in a comfortable standing position on a table.
2. Ask an assistant to restrain the dog gently by placing one arm around the neck and the other around the chest. Ensure that the dog is relaxed and quiet. Cats should be held lightly with both hands around the shoulders or place one hand under the chin and the other around its chest, pulling it close to your body.
3. Place the earpieces of the stethoscope in your ears and place the stethoscope head on the lower left chest caudal to and just dorsal to the elbow—between the third and sixth ribs.
4. Listen to the rhythm of the heart and count the heart beats for 60 seconds.
5. Record the pulse rate.

RATIONALE

1. If the animal is quiet and comfortable the heart can be heard more easily.
2. In this position, the animal will feel comfortable and unrestricted; however, the assistant will be able to react quickly if it tries to jump off the table.

3. This is close to the left ventricle where the heart beat can be best heard.

4. This is enough time in which to detect any abnormalities.
5. If there any irregularities in rate and rhythm, inform the veterinary surgeon.

PROCEDURE: TO MEASURE THE PULSE RATE BY PALPATION OF THE CHEST (TABLE 2.1)

ACTION

1. This method is best used for narrow-chested breeds of dog, such as whippets, greyhounds or lurchers, or most cats.
2. Place the animal in a comfortable standing position on a table.
3. Ask an assistant to restrain the dog gently by placing one arm around the neck and the other around the chest. Ensure that the dog is relaxed and quiet. Cats should be held lightly with both hands around the shoulders or place one hand under the chin and the other around its chest, pulling it close to your body.
4. Either put the flat of the hand on the lower left chest caudal to and just dorsal to the elbow or stretch the hand across to the other side over the sternum and feel the heart beating.
5. Count the beats over 60 seconds.

6. Record the pulse rate.

RATIONALE

1. The hand will reach across the sternum more easily in such animals.

2. If the animal is quiet and comfortable the heart can be heard more easily.
3. In this position, the animal will feel comfortable and unrestricted; however, the assistant will be able to react quickly if it tries to jump off the table.

4. To feel the heart beating within the chest.

5. This is enough time in which to count the rate.
6. If there any irregularities in rate, inform the veterinary surgeon.

PROCEDURE: TO MEASURE THE PULSE RATE USING AN OESOPHAGEAL STETHOSCOPE (TABLE 2.1)

ACTION

1. The patient is anaesthetised with a cuffed endotracheal tube in place.

2. Select the correct diameter of oesophageal stethoscope.
3. Lay the stethoscope tube on the outside of the dog or cat and measure the approximate length from the mouth to the heart. Mark the tube with a pen or adhesive bandage at the mouth end.
4. Lubricate the end of the stethoscope with KY jelly and introduce it through the patient's mouth and into the oesophagus using gentle pressure. Push it in up to the premarked part of the tube.
5. Insert the earpieces of the stethoscope into your ears and listen to the rhythm of the heart.
6. Count the heart beats for 60 seconds

7. Record the pulse rate on the patient's anaesthetic chart.

RATIONALE

1. A conscious animal will not tolerate the placing of the tube through the mouth and into the oesophagus.
2. Small dogs require a smaller bore of tube than larger dogs.
3. This ensures that the tube is best placed to hear the heart when inside the oesophagus.

4. Gentle pressure enables the tube to enter the oesophagus. Pushing the tube up as far as the mark ensures that the end of the tube lies close to the heart.

5. If there any irregularities in rate and rhythm, inform the veterinary surgeon.
6. This is enough time in which to count the rate and detect any abnormalities.
7. The use of the oesophageal stethoscope helps to monitor any cardiac changes during the anaesthetic.

PROCEDURE: TO MEASURE THE RESPIRATORY RATE BY DIRECT OBSERVATION (TABLE 2.1)

ACTION

1. Place the animal in a comfortable standing position on a table.
2. Observe the movement of the rib cage.

3. Count the number of breaths taken over 60 seconds.
4. Record the respiration rate on the patient's hospital chart or clinical case record.

RATIONALE

1. If the patient feels uncomfortable or insecure it will try to escape.
2. The chest expands and contracts once with each breath.
3. This is enough time to obtain an accurate measurement of the rate.
4. To produce a permanent record of any changes, which may indicate a need for treatment.

PROCEDURE: TO MEASURE THE RESPIRATORY RATE USING A STETHOSCOPE (TABLE 2.1)

ACTION

1. Place the animal in a comfortable standing position on a table.
2. Place the earpieces of the stethoscope in your ears and place the diaphragm of the stethoscope on the upper half of the chest just caudal to the scapula.
3. Count the breaths taken over 60 seconds.

4. Record the respiration rate on the patient's hospital chart or clinical case record.

RATIONALE

1. If the patient feels uncomfortable or insecure it will try to escape.
2. This position ensures that the diaphragm of the stethoscope lies over the trachea and bronchi. This is the best place to hear air movement into and out of the lungs.
3. This is enough time to obtain an accurate measurement of the rate.
4. To produce a permanent record of any changes, which may indicate a need for treatment.

PROCEDURE: TO MEASURE THE RESPIRATORY RATE USING AN OESOPHAGEAL STETHOSCOPE (TABLE 2.1)

ACTION

1. The patient is anaesthetised with a cuffed endotracheal tube in place.

2. Select the correct diameter of oesophageal stethoscope.
3. Lay the stethoscope tube on the outside of the animal and measure the approximate length from the mouth to the heart. Mark the tube with a pen or adhesive bandage at the mouth end.

4. Lubricate the end of the stethoscope with KY jelly and introduce it through the patient's mouth and into the oesophagus using gentle pressure. Push it in up to the premarked part of the tube.
5. Insert the earpieces of the stethoscope into your ears and listen to the rhythm of the heart.
6. Record the respiration rate on the anaesthetic chart of the patient.

RATIONALE

1. A conscious animal will not tolerate the placing of the tube through the mouth and into the oesophagus.
2. Small dogs require a smaller bore of tube than larger dogs.
3. This ensures that the tube is best placed to hear the heart when inside the oesophagus.

4. Gentle pressure enables the tube to enter the oesophagus. Pushing the tube up as far as the mark ensures that the end of the tube lies close to the heart.

5. If there any irregularities in rate and rhythm, inform the veterinary surgeon.
6. The use of an oesophageal stethoscope helps to monitor depth of anaesthetic.

PROCEDURE: TO ASSESS CAPILLARY REFILL TIME (CRT) (TABLE 2.1)

ACTION

1. Ask an assistant to hold, and gently restrain, the animal on the table.
2. Keeping the animal's mouth closed, raise the lip and look at the gum over the upper dental arch.
3. Gently press on the gum with the ball of your thumb.
4. Lift your thumb and observe the time it takes to become pink again.
5. The gum should take approximately 1–2 seconds to return to normal.
6. Report any abnormalities to the veterinary surgeon.

RATIONALE

1. If the animal is held securely it will not try to jump off the table or become stressed.
2. To assess the colour and general appearance of the gum.

3. Pressure will push all the blood out of the squeezed area.
4. Releasing the pressure allows the blood to flow back into the gum capillaries.

6. So that prompt action can be taken, e.g. a dehydrated dog may have an increased CRT so needs to be given intravenous fluids.

CRT is a quick and useful way of assessing the circulation. Generally, a dehydrated animal will have a prolonged CRT because of the reduction in circulating blood volume. The technique also allows assessment of the colour of the mucous membranes: paler gums might indicate anaemia; a blue tinge or cyanosis might indicate respiratory problems; and yellow coloration or jaundice might indicate liver problems or haemolytic anaemia.

PROCEDURE: TO MEASURE THE ELECTRICAL ACTIVITY OF THE HEART USING AN ELECTROCARDIOGRAM (ECG)

An ECG trace (Fig. 2.1) measures the electrical activity of the heart muscle and is produced by attaching electrical contacts to two set points on the outside of the body. One of the leads is the earth wire, which is clipped on to the right hind-leg. In animals, the other contacts are on each of the other three limbs and provide three different measurements of the electrical waves produced as the heart muscle contracts.

Equipment. ECG machine and leads, surgical spirit.

ACTION

1. Place the animal in right lateral recumbency. Some cats may resent this position and it may be better to have them in a normal upright sitting position. Do not sedate the animal.
2. Ask an assistant to hold the animal's front and back legs so that it lies comfortably on the table.
3. Attach the four leads to the four limbs as follows:
   red to the right foreleg
   yellow to the left foreleg
   black to the right hindleg
   green to the left hindleg.

RATIONALE

1. This is the standard position for performing ECG recordings. The use of sedatives may affect the ECG trace.

2. If the patient is comfortable it will not struggle and affect the resulting trace.

3. The clips should be attached just below the elbows and below the hocks and should be allowed to hang down to minimise movement.

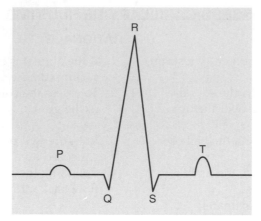

Figure 2.1 A normal lead II ECG trace.

4. Soak the crocodile clips with surgical spirit.
5. Make sure that the room is quiet and stress-free. Set the ECG machine to manual control and switch it on.
6. Using the markings on the machine, select lead I and do a test trace. Set the electrical filters if required.

7. Record a 1 mV deflection on the test trace.

8. Set the paper speed to 2.5 mm/s and record traces from leads I, II, III, AVR, AVL and AVF. Record each lead for 30 seconds.

9. Increase the paper speed to 5 mm/s and record lead II for a further 30 seconds.

10. Read the trace and look for abnormalities of rhythm and abnormalities in the PQRST waves.
11. The veterinary surgeon may require longer traces if an abnormality does not appear in the allocated time.

12. Label the trace by writing on the client's name, date, age and sex of the animal and the case number.

4. To ensure good electrical contact.
5. Any noise or movement will affect the ECG trace.

6. The filters reduce excessive electrical interference from other electrical circuits in the room, e.g. electric lights or plugged-in appliances, which would affect the trace.
7. This helps to calibrate the measurements of the actual trace.
8. This routine forms a standard initial survey for the detection of any obvious irregularities; 30 seconds provides enough time for frequent abnormalities to be identified.
9. The most useful and diagnostic measurement is taken across the heart on lead II, from the left foreleg to right hindleg. Faster paper speed will show abnormalities of rhythm or waveform more clearly by stretching the recording over a longer piece of paper.
10. Arrythmias, chamber size irregularities and blocks of the cardiac conduction pathways can be diagnosed by the use of an ECG.
11. Some arrythmias may be intermittent, e.g. in an animal showing signs of fainting. In some cases special small portable ECG units may have to be worn by the animal when exercised. These record digitally and can be used to recall traces from when the dog showed symptoms (e.g. fainting).
12. This enables the trace to be identified. If traces are taken at a later date it enables them to be related to the earlier readings.

PROCEDURE: TO MEASURE THE PERCENTAGE OF OXYGEN (OXYGEN SATURATION) IN THE BLOOD USING A PULSE OXIMETER (TABLE 2.1)

The pulse oximeter works by transmitting a pulsed infrared light across a thin flap of tissue to a sensor on the other side of a clip. Small pulsing arterioles within this tissue alter the passage of the light and allow the machine to record a pulse rate. Oxygen tension is calculated by using the difference in light absorption by deoxygenated blood compared with that of oxygenated blood. The machine expresses this difference as a percentage.

Equipment. Portable pulse oximeter and sensor lead (Fig. 2.2).

ACTION	RATIONALE
1. Set up the pulse oximeter near to the patient and either plug it in to the mains or, if battery operated, ensure that the battery is charged.	1. The pulse oximeter must be clearly visible to the anaesthetist.
2. Set the pulse oximeter to sound its alarm if the pulse rate and oxygen tension go above or below the normal range.	2. To ensure that action can be taken if the oxygen level falls or the heart rate is too slow or too fast.
3. Select the correct sensor for the size of patient.	3. Smaller animals require smaller clips.

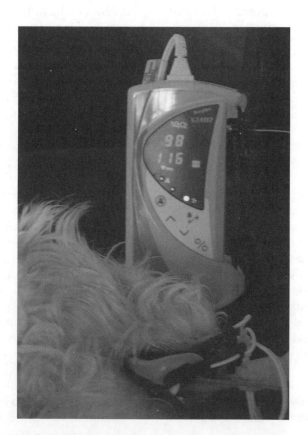

Figure 2.2   A pulse oximeter.

4. Select the correct site on which to attach the sensor.
5. Select a site that does not interfere with the surgical procedure.
6. Switch the machine on and monitor the oxygen tension and pulse rate.

7. Record the readings on the patient's anaesthetic chart.

4. Sites include the tongue, interdigital web, lip, vulva or prepuce.
5. For instance, using the tongue would interfere with a dental extraction.
6. In order to identify and correct any reduction in blood oxygen levels or changes in the pulse rate.
7. Pulse oximetry is used to monitor any changes in anaesthetic level. The heart rate may rise if the depth of anaesthesia is lightening or start to slow if depth is increasing. Oxygen tension may fall if there is a problem with the anaesthetic machine or if the blood in pulmonary circulation is unable to take up the gas, e.g. in cases of pulmonary oedema.

PROCEDURE: TO MEASURE CENTRAL VENOUS PRESSURE (CVP)

Equipment. 1 litre bag of saline, an infusion set, intravenous catheter (14F or smaller), no. 15 scalpel blade, may also need a specially designed 'through the needle' jugular catheter, chlorhexi-dine solution, swabs, spirit and bandaging materials, three-way tap, 2×0.5 m of sterile drip tubing to connect to the catheter and to the three-way tap, a metric ruler and a stand to hold it vertically.

ACTION

1. Assemble the apparatus required (Fig. 2.3)

2. Ask an assistant to restrain the animal for a jugular puncture.
3. Clip, swab and wipe with spirit an area of the jugular furrow near to the thoracic inlet on the selected side of the neck.
4. Put on disposable gloves.
5. Ask your assistant to raise the jugular vein by applying digital pressure to the base of the jugular furrow at the thoracic inlet.
6. When the vein is raised, gently push the needle and catheter into the vein with the point towards the head. Check that blood is flowing out of the needle hub and remove the needle while holding the catheter firmly in place.
7. An alternative method is to make a small stab incision through the skin over the vein. If you go too deep you may cut into the vein

RATIONALE

1. CVP can be measured by using simple apparatus usually found in a veterinary practice. Manometers are available but are not a necessity.
2. A calm gentle approach will prevent the animal struggling.
3. To ensure maximum sterility. The site is at a similar level to the right atrium of the heart, which is where the CVP is measured.
4. To ensure maximum sterility.
5. This will cause the vein to engorge by blocking blood return to the heart—known as 'raising the vein'.
6. This will leave the flexible plastic catheter inside the vein. A rigid needle would be likely to dislodge and lacerate the vein if the animal was to move.

7. Cutting the skin allows the thin 'through the needle' catheter to be placed in the vein with minimal resistance. If the skin is not cut first,

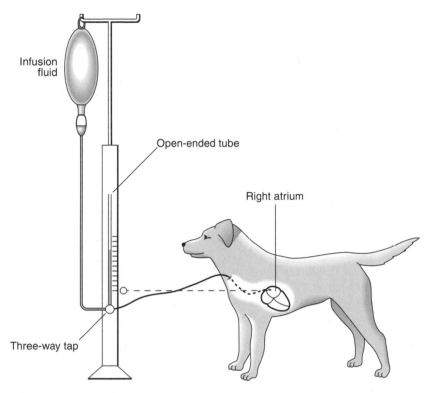

Figure 2.3 Method of measuring central venous pressure.

itself. It can be helpful to mark the spot over the vein and then ask the assistant to release pressure. Move the skin (and spot mark) away from the vein and make the incision.

8. Set the three-way tap to allow saline to flow out of the free end of the infusion set, allowing air bubbles in the saline to disperse. Connect the tubing to the end of the catheter once all air bubbles have dispersed.

9. Fix the catheter in place using a bandage or adhesive tape strips.

10. Turn the three-way tap to exclude the patient and allow saline to flow up the vertical tubing until halfway up its length (25 cm)

11. Check that there are no air bubbles in the pressure tube.

12. Set the three-way tap to exclude the drip bag so that the catheter is now connected, via the tubing and the tap, to the vertical open tubing stretched over the ruler.

the catheter may fray or roll back over the needle and may damage the vein.

8. Air bubbles might cause an air embolism or a block in the circulation and threaten the patient's life. Check that the tube has no blockages or kinks.

9. Under local anaesthetic a butterfly bandage could be placed around the catheter hub or tubing and sutured to the animal's skin.

10. This primes and checks the patency of the tubing and removes any possibility of air entering the patient.

11. This prevents air inadvertently entering the patient's bloodstream. Bubbles will reduce the accuracy of the measurement.

12. Allows the patient's blood pressure to be measured.

13. The level in the vertical tube will fall rapidly and settle at a certain mark. Here it will oscillate up and down in time with the patient's breathing.
14. Make sure that the zero line on the ruler is level with the right atrium of the heart in the chest.
15. Read the CVP in centimetres of water against the ruler.
16. Reconnect the drip to the animal by turning the three-way tap to exclude the pressure arm of the tubing.
17. Repeat the readings hourly, using the procedure as described from point 10.

13. This is the central venous pressure. The pressure of the column of water will equal the pressure in the patient's right atrium.
14. This is only a rough guide. A spirit level can be used for greater accuracy.
15. Ask the veterinary surgeon for an interpretation.

17. This is used to monitor the CVP during the day, usually in an animal on prolonged intravenous therapy.

Central venous pressure is the pressure of the blood entering the right atrium. The jugular catheter must be level with the right atrium of the heart at the time of the measurement. CVP measurement can be useful to determine whether too much fluid is being given to an animal being kept on a drip for a long time:

- A raised CVP may indicate overperfusion and a raised blood volume.

- A lowered CVP might reflect a failing heart or loss of blood pressure from shock or blood loss. A faster drip rate is required to increase blood volume.

Monitoring such a case might show an increase in CVP as shock improves or blood volume increases. The absolute measurement is less important than the trend shown by the CVP results.

PROCEDURE: TO MEASURE ARTERIAL BLOOD PRESSURE USING A NON-INVASIVE TECHNIQUE (TABLE 2.1)

Invasive (direct) techniques of blood pressure measurement, where arteries are catheterised and linked to a pressure transducer, are more accurate and may be a more common method of blood pressure measurement in university and referral practices. In general veterinary practice non-invasive (indirect) techniques of measurement are more likely to be used.

ACTION

1. Place the animal in a comfortable standing position on a table.

2. Set up the instrument.
3. Choose a cuff of an appropriate size for the animal.

RATIONALE

1. If the animal feels uncomfortable or insecure it will try to escape. A distressed animal may have an artificially raised blood pressure. This is particularly important in conscious cats.

3. If the cuff is the wrong size the measurement will be inaccurate. Too large a cuff will produce a lower blood pressure reading than is actually shown by the animal; too small a cuff will produce a higher blood pressure reading than the actual pressure.

4. Choose a suitable site on a distal limb or the tail (see below).

5. Shave the transducer site or wet thoroughly with spirit. Lubricate with gel and place transducer over artery while listening for the pulse on the instrument's loudspeaker or earphones. Inflate the cuff until the pulse stops, then, while looking at the pressure dial slowly deflate the cuff until the pulse restarts.

6. Take a number of readings over several minutes.

7. Record the measurement on the patient's anaesthetic chart or clinical case record.

4. The cuff is placed over a peripheral artery where a pulse can be palpated. The chosen site must be almost cylindrical for the cuff to sit comfortably and maximise the accuracy of the measurements.

5. Shaving and use of a gel reduce air interference between transducer and skin and improve the signal. The cuff pressure at which the pulse restarts in the systolic pressure.

6. This allows for variations caused by anxiety or movement, which can produce an artificially raised result.

7. Blood pressure measurement is used to monitor an anaesthetic or as part of a health check.

Cuff-positioning sites. These include:

- Tail base (coccygeal artery)—best in conscious dogs and cats
- Forelimb proximal to carpus (median artery)
- Forelimb distal to carpus (common palmar digital artery)
- Hindlimb proximal to hock (saphenous artery)—best in anaesthetised dogs
- Hindlimb distal to hock (medial plantar artery).

In the dog, blood pressure measurement is usually part of anaesthetic monitoring.

Anaesthetic drugs can cause a lowered pressure (hypotension) and fluctuations in the pressure can reflect change in the depth of anaesthesia or blood volume. Monitoring allows necessary treatment to be taken to correct the altered blood pressure. In the cat, raised blood pressure (hypertension) is reasonably common in older animals and is often a consequence of diseases such as renal failure. Routine monitoring of older cats may detect hypertension and allow corrective treatment. Conditions such as retinal haemorrhage and blindness can be directly caused by a raised blood pressure.

PROCEDURE: TO MEASURE CARBON DIOXIDE LEVELS USING A MAINSTREAM CAPNOGRAPH (TABLE 2.1)

A mainstream instrument measures end-tidal CO_2 levels (i.e. it samples the last bit of expired air from each breath). The technique is used during anaesthesia to monitor the inspired and expired CO_2.

ACTION

1. Set up the capnograph.
2. After turning off the anaesthetic gas supply, disconnect the endotracheal tube from the gas delivery tube.

3. Connect the CO_2 sensor between the endotracheal tube and the gas delivery tube.
4. Restart the anaesthetic gases and set the vaporiser to the correct concentration, as required by the veterinary surgeon.
5. Read the CO_2 levels from the digital display.
6. Record the levels on the patient's anaesthetic record or print a graph directly from the machine.
7. Take readings every minute throughout the anaesthetic procedure.

RATIONALE

2. In order to insert mainstream sensor into the gas flow to and from the animal. Turning off the gas first will help prevent spillage of anaesthetic gases into the environment.
3. Inspired and expired gases pass through the sensor.
4. To maintain the level of anaesthesia.

6. To allow monitoring of anaesthesia and early corrective action should the levels start to rise.
7. To identify any trends and to allow early corrective treatment.

PROCEDURE: TO MEASURE CARBON DIOXIDE LEVELS USING A SIDESTREAM CAPNOGRAPH (FIG. 2.4)

A sidestream instrument measures end-tidal CO_2 and inspired CO_2 concentrations.

ACTION

1. Set up the capnograph.
2. Without disconnecting the endotracheal tube, attach the small tube leading to the instrument to the special port on the end of the gas delivery tube.
3. Read the levels of inspired and expired CO_2 from the digital display. They are displayed as a scrolling graph showing the changes of CO_2 concentration with each breath.
4. Record the levels on the patient's anaesthetic record or print a graph directly from the machine.
5. Take readings every minute throughout the anaesthetic procedure.

RATIONALE

2. This machine sucks a small sample of gas out of the gas flow rather than being positioned in the midst of the flow.

3. Both inspired and end-tidal CO_2 levels are measured.

4. To allow monitoring of anaesthesia and early corrective action should the levels start to rise.
5. To identify any trends and to allow early corrective treatment.

The sidestream instrument is more accurate and is useful in monitoring both the patient's anaesthetic progress and the efficiency of the anaesthetic equipment. The mainstream type of capnograph has disadvantages compared with the sidestream type:

- It is more vulnerable to accidental damage as the sensor lies close to the animal during use. The sidestream capnograph can be placed a safe distance away and is less likely to be disturbed.
- It only measures expired end-tidal CO_2 and is useful for identifying a pulmonary problem and a consequent rise in CO_2. However, if the level of CO_2 is high in the inspired gases (e.g. exhausted soda lime in a circuit), the mainstream machine cannot specify whether the cause of the problem is the patient or the apparatus. In a dangerous, life-threatening situation, time may be lost trying to decide the cause of the problem.

Capnographs that measure both the CO_2 levels and the respiratory rate are available and may be combined with a pulse oximeter.

Hypercapnia (raised CO_2 levels). This may be caused by:

- Faulty anaesthetic equipment, e.g. blocked endotracheal tube, excessive dead space, faulty valves, exhausted soda lime.
- Patient problems, e.g. hypoventilation (reduced respiratory rate, breath-holding), any lung condition that prevents the normal exchange of oxygen and carbon dioxide.

Hypocapnia (lowered CO_2 levels). This may be caused by:

- Patient problems, e.g. hyperventilation caused by panting, or excessive respiratory rate.

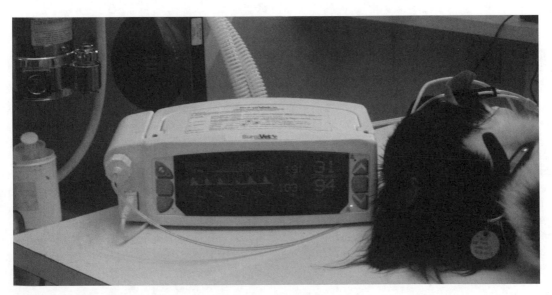

Figure 2.4   A sidestream capnograph with a pulse oximeter.

PROCEDURE: TO MEASURE URINE PRODUCTION (TABLE 2.1)

Equipment. Sterile urinary catheter, empty used drip bag, infusion set.

ACTION	RATIONALE
1. Catheterise the patient as described in Chapter 3.	
2. Drain the bladder with a 50 ml syringe until it is empty.	2. To get an accurate measure of future urine production.
3. Connect the needle end of the infusion set to the urinary catheter.	
4. Make sure that the empty drip bag is level with, or preferably below the level of, the animal's bladder.	4. This uses gravity to fill the bag and to prevent inadvertent reflux of stale urine back into the bladder.
5. Once an hour either weigh the bag on accurate scales or empty it with a 50 ml syringe and note the volume.	5. 1 ml of urine weighs approximately 1 g. Thus the volume can be calculated by the urine weight in grams. This gives the volume of urine produced per hour.

Hourly urinary output is a useful indicator of renal function. Normal kidneys will produce 1–2 ml/kg bodyweight/hour. If urine production is less than 0.5 ml/kg/hour then the animal may be severely dehydrated or in renal shutdown.

This procedure is most likely to be performed in hospitalised and recumbent patients. The catheter may be left in place for more than 24 hours and it is very important that a sterile approach is taken to prevent the patient developing cystitis. Bladder infection in a patient that is already ill may cause its condition to deteriorate.

PROCEDURE: TO MEASURE TEAR PRODUCTION (TABLE 2.1)

Equipment. Schirmer tear measurement strips.

ACTION	RATIONALE
1. Ask an assistant to restrain the animal on the table.	1. The animal needs to be comfortable to allow the measurement to be made.
2. Remove two Schirmer test strips from their sterile plastic envelope.	2. These are packaged to keep the strips dry and sterile.
3. Fold the end of one strip at the notch near the end. Try not to touch the paper with your fingers.	3. Touching the strip may cause moisture to be absorbed from your fingers and this may affect the accuracy of the result.
4. Gently roll out the lower eyelid and hook the short end of the strip so that it rests against the junction of the cornea and the conjunctiva.	4. This ensures that the strip makes good contact with the area of tear production.
5. Gently close the eyelids.	5. To hold the strip in place.
6. Hold in place for 1 minute.	6. This is the standard time of the test.
7. Remove the strip and measure the length of the blue-stained area of wet paper.	7. The longer the length of the stain, the greater the volume of tears produced.

8. Repeat the measurement in the other eye using the second strip.

    This simple test is a useful method of assessing tear production. Keratoconjunctivitis sicca (KCS) or 'dry-eye' is a distressing problem in certain

8. To compare the two eyes.

breeds and the Schirmer test can be used to diagnose and monitor the effectiveness of treatment.

PROCEDURE: TO MEASURE INTRAOCULAR PRESSURE (IOP) (TABLE 2.1)

Equipment. Either a mechanical IOP instrument (Schiotz) or a digital instrument (Tonopen).

ACTION

1. Ask an assistant to restrain the animal on the table.

2. Put local anaesthetic drops in both eyes. (Proxymetacaine 5% disposable drops are suitable.)
3. Select the appropriate piece of equipment.

USING A SCHIOTZ TONOMETER

1. Calibrate the machine by pressing it gently on to the metal test block. Different weights can be added to the plunger.
2. Ask the assistant to hold the animal's head up so that the cornea is horizontal.

3. Gently rest the instrument on the cornea and take a reading from the needle.

4. Take at least two readings from both eyes.

5. Record the readings on the clinical case record or hospitalisation chart.

USING A TONOPEN

1. Put a new latex sheath over the end of the Tonopen using the cardboard applicator supplied by the maufacturers.

RATIONALE

1. The animal needs to be comfortable and firmly restrained to allow the measurement to be taken.
2. This desensitises the cornea so that it can be touched without the animal blinking or reacting.

1. This sets the zero pressure level.

2. Readings depend on gravity, so the instrument must be held as vertically as possible.
3. A soft eyeball will only deflect the probe a little, thus producing a reading closer to the zero baseline. Conversely, a harder eyeball will deflect the probe more, thus producing a higher reading.
4. This allows comparison of the pressure in both eyes and, by repetition, checks the accuracy of the instrument. Each reading should be the same as the previous measurement.
5. To allow the comparison with later measurements and to monitor the efficacy of treatment.

1. This protects the sensitive end of the instrument and prevents cross-infection.

2. Calibrate the machine by pushing the button near the tip with the head of the Tonopen held downwards. When it 'beeps', point the head vertically upwards. The machine should read 'good' on the display bar and readings can now be taken. If the display says 'bad', the process has to be repeated until the correct response is obtained.

2. To calibrate and ensure the accuracy of the actual readings.

3. Gently touch the latex-covered tip on to the anaesthetised cornea. This should be done several times until a 'beep' is heard.

3. The machine works by gentle corneal contact, not by deforming the surface by pressure.

4. Repeat the readings more than once and take them from both eyes.

4. This allows comparison of the pressure in both eyes and, by repetition, checks the accuracy. Each reading should be the same as the previous measurement.

5. Discard the latex sleeve.

5. To prevent cross-infection.

6. Record the readings in the clinical case record or on the hospitalisation chart.

6. To allow comparison with later measurements and to monitor the efficacy of treatment.

Intraocular pressure rises if the eye begins to suffer from glaucoma. This increase in pressure can be very destructive to the internal structures of the eye and can cause severe pain, blindness and eventual collapse of the eye. Tonometry readings are a useful method of assessing any rise and allowing time for drugs to be used to reduce the pressure. Serial readings can indicate how effective treatment has been.

The mechanical tonometer is less accurate and is used only as a guide. The Tonopen is much more accurate and reliable.

FURTHER READING

Chandler EA, Thompson DJ, Sutton JB, Price CJ 1995 Canine Medicine and Therapeutics. Blackwell Science, Oxford

Hall LW, Clarke KW 1996 Veterinary Anaesthesia, 9th edn. WB Saunders, London

Hotson-Moore A (ed.) 1999 Manual of Advanced Veterinary Nursing. BSAVA, Gloucester

Moore M (ed.) 1999 Manual of Veterinary Nursing. BSAVA, Gloucester

Peiffer RL, Petersen-Jones SM 1997 Small Animal Ophthalmology. WB Saunders, London

3

Medical nursing procedures

J. Masters

Introduction

Much of the work of the veterinary nurse is concerned with nursing medical patients. These are the patients that are not hospitalised for any type of surgical procedure. Medical conditions can be divided into those that are caused by microorganisms and are infectious, e.g. cat flu or canine parvovirus, and those that develop as a result of an upset in the normal processes of the body, e.g. renal failure, diabetes mellitus or exocrine pancreatic insufficiency. Many patients may not require hospitalisation and may be treated during a consultation or at home, but some will require further diagnostic tests and, if critically ill, will require observation and skilled nursing care. Those patients that have an infectious disease must be isolated to prevent the spread of infection and barrier nursing procedures must be instigated either at home or within the practice.

The aim of nursing the medical patient is to help the animal to return to a state of normal health as soon as possible. While in the hospital it must be kept warm and comfortable, free from pain and, remembering that this is an animal removed from its normal surroundings, free from fear and apprehension. The veterinary nurse plays an extremely important part in the recovery process and the care that she or he gives must be based on an understanding of the disease process and the aims of the treatment regimen.

This chapter describes the general techniques used in medical nursing and relates them to some of the more common conditions seen in practice. It is important to understand that most of the techniques can be used in a range of conditions: some examples of their use are given.

PROCEDURE: GENERAL EXAMINATION OF THE DOG OR CAT

ACTION

1. Observe the patient in its kennel and record any abnormalities.
2. Remove the patient and place in a comfortable position suited to a full examination.

3. Ask an assistant to reassure and restrain the patient.

4. Examine the patient, starting at the cranial end and identifying any abnormalities, including discharges, wounds, lumps, painful areas.

5. Temperature, pulse and respiration (TPR) parameters should be taken at this time.

6. Record all findings on the patient's hospital card.

RATIONALE

1. Handling the patient will involve some stress, which may influence clinical signs.
2. If the patient feels comfortable it is less likely to try to escape. A cat or small dog should be examined on a table, whereas a larger dog may be more suited to an examination on the floor.
3. Reassuring the patient will help it to relax. An assistant should be ready to restrain the patient if it tries to escape or becomes aggressive during the examination.
4. Examining a patient from head to tail as a routine will limit the likelihood of any area being excluded. Any abnormalities should be noted, however minor or unrelated to the treatment the patient is receiving.
5. TPR should be noted whenever the patient is examined as a measure of the patient's progress.
6. All findings must be recorded on the hospital card to help identify any abnormalities and communicate the patient's progress to all staff. Report any abnormalities to the veterinary surgeon.

PROCEDURE: BARRIER NURSING: AVOIDANCE OF CROSS-INFECTION

ACTION

1. Staff should be allocated solely to the isolation facility and not allowed to nurse patients in the general ward.

2. Personal protective clothing, such as disposable gloves, aprons and foot covers, should be worn. This should be placed in the clinical waste after use.
3. Patients who are most likely to spread disease should be cleaned out and treated after all other patients in the isolation facility.

RATIONALE

1. Staff could transmit infection from the patient they are nursing to others of the same species or those susceptible to infection, such as paediatric cases.
2. Protection from zoonotic disease is a high priority. The wearing of protective clothing will prevent disease being spread via staff clothing.
3. This will prevent disease being spread from the most infectious patient by the nursing staff.

4. Each patient in the isolation facility should be allocated its own equipment, i.e. food bowl, water bowl, litter tray, etc. This should be washed and disinfected or sterilised separately from others. Bedding should all be disposable and should be placed in the clinical waste.

5. All findings must be recorded on the patient's hospital sheet. Report all abnormalities to the veterinary surgeon. Barrier nursing notices should be displayed.

4. Infection can be spread from fomites such as kennel equipment. Allocation of equipment to specific kennels will limit this, as will cleaning the items separately. Keep track of equipment by numbering kennels and their applicable equipment. Most bedding cannot be sterilised satisfactorily and may pass infection on during the cleaning process.

5. The veterinary surgeon should be made aware of the patient's progress. Barrier nursing notices can prevent inadvertent cross-contamination; personnel entering the isolation area should be kept to a minimum.

PROCEDURE: APPLICATION OF AN ENEMA (DOGS)

- Examples of use include: emptying the rectum; as a diagnostic aid; administering drugs.
- Examples of solutions used: water (rectal lavage); soapy water (soap flakes); oily substances (such as liquid paraffin/mineral oil); phosphate enemas (proprietary brands). For cats a proprietary mini enema is usually the product of choice.

ACTION

1. Prepare all equipment, including enema solutions at body temperature (and associated tubing, catheters, Higginson's syringe as required), disposable gloves, aprons and absorbent tissue. Lubricant will also be required.
2. Restrain the patient in a suitable environment, near to an outside door. Two members of staff will be required for this procedure. Place the patient in a standing position.

3. The end of the tubing to be inserted into the rectum should be lubricated before insertion. The assistant should raise the patient's tail and the anal area should be cleaned with some warm water to remove any faecal material or debris.
4. Place the end of the tubing in the patient's anus and gently twist until it is in the rectum. The enema solution should be introduced slowly either by gravity or by pump, depending on the method used.

RATIONALE

1. As with all procedures, the preparation of the equipment before beginning the procedure is both an efficient and practical method of working. The solution should be warmed to prevent shock and promote tolerance.
2. Giving an enema is a messy procedure and faeces can pass on infection both to the staff and other patients. The dog will need to evacuate its bowel soon after the application of the enema and will require an area that can be cleaned and disinfected effectively.
3. Lubricating the tube end will allow easy access and prevent damage to the rectal mucosa. The anal area should be cleaned to prevent infection being introduced from the external area.

4. Gently twisting the tube end will encourage the anal sphincter to relax and allow passage of the tube into the rectum. This is more difficult in cats.

5. Once the solution has been delivered, the dog should be allowed free access to a run area to evacuate its bowels.
6. When bowel evacuation is complete, the patient should be cleaned appropriately and a note made of the amount and type of excreta passed.

5. If the solution has worked as required, bowel evacuation should commence shortly; if not, you may need to repeat the treatment.
6. The patient should be thoroughly clean, dry and comfortable before being put back into its kennel. The type of excreta passed may indicate the reason for a constipation problem, e.g. bones.

PROCEDURE: CATHETERISATION OF THE DOG

- Two people are required.
- Examples of procedures include short-term catheterisation to obtain a sterile urine sample, or indwelling catheterisation useful in recumbent patients.

- Examples of catheter types include: conventional plastic or Foley silicone dog catheters (Fig. 3.1).

ACTION

1. Prepare all the equipment, including sterile catheter and any application equipment, e.g. stylets to assist with introduction, lubricant, disposable gloves, apron, sterile sample container or collecting vessel, such as a kidney dish, syringe, three-way tap or bung. If measurement of urine output and input is required, a urine collection bag will need to be prepared. Absorbent material such as swabs/tissue will be useful and suture material may be required for indwelling catheters.
2. The assistant should restrain the patient on the examination table. Gloves and aprons should be put on. The preputial area should be cleaned and the penis extruded.

3. Remove the catheter from its outer packaging and cut the end from the inner packaging, which is used as a feeder sleeve.
4. The catheter tip should be lubricated, introduced into the urethra and then advanced using gentle pressure. Urine will flow back down the catheter when the bladder is reached and may require collection. The bladder may need flushing, depending on the procedure that is to be performed. Suturing or sticking the catheter to the prepuce will be required if the catheter is to be indwelling.

RATIONALE

1. As with any procedure, the preparation of the equipment before beginning the procedure is both an efficient and practical method of working. Ensure that you understand why the catheter is being introduced and any procedures that will be carried out after its introduction. This will enable all necessary equipment to be prepared. The catheter and collection bag should be sterile to prevent infection being introduced into the urinary tract.

2. The patient may be standing or in lateral recumbency depending on personal preference. Protective clothing should be worn to prevent the spread of zoonoses and introduction of infection to the patient.
3. The use of a feeder sleeve allows the catheter to be fed into the urethra without having to touch the sterile tubing.
4. Gentle pressure should enable the catheter to pass the narrowing of the urethra at the ischial arch or around an enlarged prostate gland. If resistance is met, the catheter size may need to be reassessed. The application of zinc oxide tape to the catheter enables it to be sutured to the preputial area.

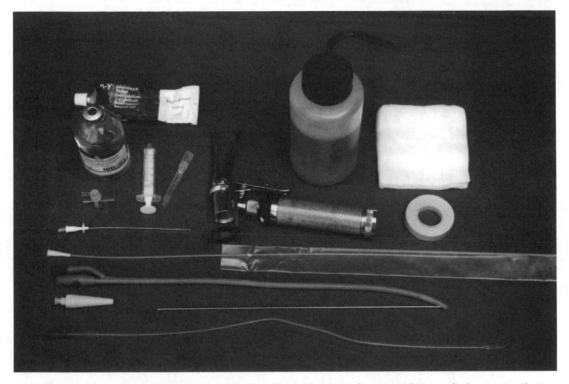

Figure 3.1 Equipment required for general catheterisation. Types of catheter from top to bottom: Jackson cat catheter, conventional dog catheter, latex Foley catheter with stylet correctly placed, Tiemans catheter.

5. Remove the catheter slowly and dispose of it correctly. Clean and dry the patient before returning it to its kennel.

5. Removing the catheter slowly will help prevent tissue damage and urine splashes, which could be a zoonotic risk. All catheters and associated equipment should be disposed of in the clinical waste. Keeping the patient clean will prevent urine scalds.

PROCEDURE: CATHETERISATION OF THE BITCH

- Two people are required.
- Examples of use include: short-term catheterisation to obtain a sterile urine sample; or indwelling catheterisation, useful in recumbent patients.
- Examples of catheter types include: Foley indwelling bitch catheters and Tiemans

catheters for the bitch. A vaginal speculum (sterile) will be required unless the insertion is to be carried out using the sterile digital method (Fig. 3.1).

ACTION

1. Prepare all the equipment, including sterile catheter and any application equipment (such as vaginal speculum and stylets to assist with introduction if required), lubricant, dispos-

RATIONALE

1. As with all procedures, the preparation of the equipment before beginning the procedure is both an efficient and practical method of working. Ensure that you have

gloves, apron, sterile sample container/ collecting vessel (such as a kidney dish), three-way tap or bung. If measurement of urine output and input is required, a urine collection bag will need to be prepared.

2. Put on gloves and an apron. Ask the assistant to restrain the patient, either in lateral or dorsal recumbency, or in a standing position, depending on the insertion method used. If the catheter is to be inserted using the digital method, sterile gloves should be worn by the person carrying out the procedure.
3. The vulval area should be cleaned and free from debris.
4. The catheter should be removed from its outer wrapping, exposing the tip from the inner sleeve, and lubricated. Do not use petroleum-based lubricants on latex catheters. If using a Foley catheter the stylet should be placed and the balloon checked for easy inflation (Fig. 3.1).

5. Place the speculum blades between the vulval lips. If working with the patient in dorsal recumbency the blades should be inserted as caudally as possible, then the speculum should be inserted vertically into the vestibule, turning the handles cranially. If working with the patient standing, the speculum should be inserted at a slight angle towards the spine, then horizontally.
6. Once the speculum is in place, open the blades and identify the urethral orifice.

7. If using the sterile digital method the first finger of one hand (usually the non-writing hand) should be lubricated and placed into the vestibule, feeling along the ventral surface for a raised area.
8. The tip of the catheter should be inserted into the urethral orifice and gradually advanced until it reaches the bladder.

disposable understand why the catheter is being introduced and any procedures that will be carried out after its introduction. This will enable all necessary equipment to be prepared. The catheter and collection bag should be sterile to prevent infection being introduced to the urinary tract. Foley catheters must not be reused as the balloon weakens after each use.

2. Protective clothing should be worn to prevent the spread of zoonoses and introduction of infection to the patient. For insertion in dorsal recumbency the patient should be in a straight position with the hindlegs flexed and drawn cranially. For all methods the tail must be firmly restrained.
3. Cleaning the area will prevent introduction of infection to the urogenital tract.
4. Aseptic technique is necessary to prevent introduction of infection. Stylets aid the introduction and placement of the catheter and should be sterile. Most stylets are placed through the tubing but stylets used with Foley catheters should be laid alongside the tubing with the stylet placed in a drainage hole at the catheter tip.
5. In dorsal recumbency the blades should be inserted to avoid the clitoral fossa.

6. The urethral orifice should be visible halfway between the vulva and the cervix. If the patient is standing, it will be on the floor of the vestibule; if in dorsal recumbency, it will be on the uppermost side.
7. The urethral orifice is just cranial to this raised area and can be identified with the finger and the catheter guided in.

8. With the patient in dorsal recumbency the hindlegs should now be extended caudally to allow straightening of the urethra for easier catheter introduction.

9. If a Foley catheter is to be indwelling, the balloon should be inflated, the stylet removed and a collection bag attached. An Elizabethan collar may be used.

10. When the appropriate procedure has been completed, remove the catheter slowly, having first deflated the balloon in the Foley catheter, and dispose of it correctly. Ensure that the patient is clean and dry before being returned to its kennel.

9. The inflated balloon keeps the catheter secure in the bladder without the need for suturing.

10. Removing the catheter slowly will prevent tissue damage and reduce the risk of urine splashes, which could carry a zoonotic disease. All catheters and associated equipment should be disposed of in the clinical waste. Keeping the patient clean will prevent urine scalds.

PROCEDURE: CATHETERISATION OF THE TOMCAT (FIG. 3.2)

This procedure is normally carried out under a general anaesthetic, as it may be painful and struggling may cause penetration of the urethra.

- Two people required.
- Examples of use include: short-term catheterisation to obtain a sterile urine sample; indwelling catheterisation, useful in recumbent patients; hydropropulsion (using water pressure to dislodge blockages).

- Examples of catheter types include: conventional cat catheters; Jackson and silicon catheters for use in the cat (Fig. 3.1).

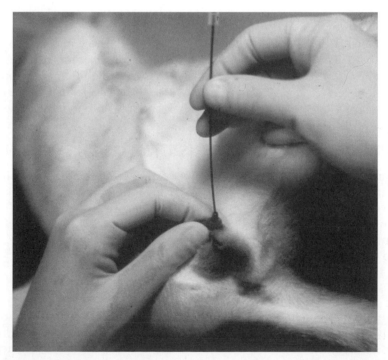

Figure 3.2 Catheterisation of a tomcat.

ACTION

1. Prepare all the equipment, including sterile catheter and any application equipment, e.g. stylets to assist with introduction if required, lubricant, disposable gloves, apron, sterile sample container or collecting vessel (such as a kidney dish), three-way tap or bung. If measurement of urine output and input is required, a urine collection bag will need to be prepared.

2. Put on gloves and apron. Position the cat in lateral or dorsal recumbency, ensuring that the tail is out of the way.

3. Remove the catheter from its outer packaging and cut the end from the inner packaging, which is used as a feeder sleeve. Lubricate the tip of the catheter.

4. Extrude the penis by applying gentle pressure on either side of the prepuce, and introduce the catheter into the urethra (Fig. 3.2). If a Jackson cat catheter is used, remove the metal stylet.

5. Continue with the procedure: collection of sample, drainage of bladder, hydropropulsion, etc.

6. Remove the catheter slowly and dispose of it correctly. Return the cat to its kennel when it is clean and dry.

RATIONALE

1. As with all procedures, the preparation of the equipment before beginning the procedure is both an efficient and practical method of working. Ensure that you understand why the catheter is being introduced and any procedures that will be carried out after its introduction. This will enable all necessary equipment to be prepared.

2. In this position the perineal area and the penis can be easily accessed.

3. The use of a feeder sleeve allows the catheter to be fed into the urethra without touching the sterile tubing. Lubrication of the tip will ensure ease of introduction and will prevent tissue damage.

4. Gentle preputial pressure should result in extrusion of the penis.

5. If an indwelling Jackson cat catheter is used, suture it to the prepuce. Attach a collection bag and use an Elizabethan collar.

6. Removing the catheter slowly will prevent tissue damage and urine splashes, which could be a zoonotic risk. All catheters and associated equipment should be disposed of in the clinical waste. Keeping the cat clean and dry will prevent urine scalds.

PROCEDURE: CATHETERISATION OF THE QUEEN

- Two people required.
- Examples of use include: short-term catheterisation to obtain a sterile urine sample; indwelling catheterisation, useful in recumbent patients; hydropropulsion (using water pressure to dislodge blockages).

- Examples of catheter types include: conventional cat catheters; Jackson and silicon catheters for use in the cat (Fig. 3.1).

ACTION

1. Prepare all the equipment including a sterile catheter and any application equipment, e.g. stylets to assist with introduction,

RATIONALE

1. As with all procedures, the preparation of the equipment before beginning the procedure is both an efficient and practical

lubricant, disposable gloves, apron, sterile sample container or collecting vessels such as a kidney dish, three-way tap or bung. If measurement of urine output and input is required, a urine collection bag will need to be prepared.

2. Put on gloves and apron. Restrain the cat and ensure that the tail is also restrained.
3. Remove the catheter from its outer packaging and cut the end from the inner packaging, which is used as a feeder sleeve. Lubricate the tip of the catheter.

4. Place the catheter between the vulval lips and introduce into the urethra by angling the catheter ventrally, using gentle pressure until the catheter enters the urethral orifice.
5. Continue with the procedure: collection of sample, drainage of bladder, hydropro-pulsion, etc.
6. Remove the catheter slowly and dispose of it correctly. Return the cat to its kennel when it is clean and dry.

method of working. Ensure that you understand why the catheter is being introduced and any procedures that will be carried out after its introduction. This will enable all necessary equipment to be prepared.

2. Restrain the cat either in a standing position or in lateral recumbency.
3. The use of a feeder sleeve allows the catheter to be fed into the urethra without touching the sterile tubing. Lubrication of the tip will ensure ease of introduction and will prevent tissue damage.
4. The use of a vaginal speculum is not necessary for this procedure. Queen catheterisation is not often performed, as blockages are rare.
5. If an indwelling Jackson cat catheter has been used, suture it in place, attach a urine collection bag and use an Elizabethan collar.
6. Slowly removing the catheter will prevent tissue damage and urine splashes, which could be a zoonotic risk. All catheters and associated equipment should be disposed of in the clinical waste. Keeping the cat clean and dry will prevent urine scalds.

PROCEDURE: MANUAL EXPRESSION OF THE BLADDER (FIG. 3.3)

- Two people required.
- Manual expression of the bladder may be required in recumbent patients or those suffering from bladder paralysis. Natural

elimination of the bladder is preferable to urinary catheterisation but it should not be attempted where there is any possibility of urethral obstruction.

ACTION

1. Put on gloves and apron and prepare urinary collection equipment (if required) and absorbent tissue.

2. An assistant should restrain the patient in a standing position in a suitable area that is clean and easy to disinfect.

RATIONALE

1. Protection of staff from zoonotic diseases transmitted by urine is essential. Urinary collection equipment, such as a kidney dish, or a sterile sample pot may be required if the urine requires analysing.
2. Restraining the patient in the standing position will ensure easy access to the bladder. The area in which the patient urinates should be easy to disinfect to prevent contamination. Dogs will often feel happier urinating outside.

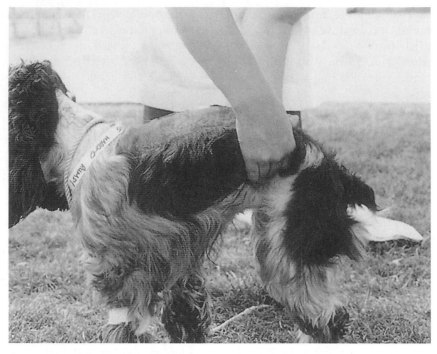

Figure 3.3 Manual expression of the bladder while supporting a recumbent patient. Adapted, with permission, from *Veterinary Nursing*, p.405, 2nd edn, by Lane and Cooper (1994). Butterworth Heinemann, UK.

3. Isolate the bladder by palpation of the caudal abdomen and place one hand either side of it on the external abdominal wall.

4. Apply gentle pressure to the abdominal wall on either side of the bladder to encourage urination. Urine should flow freely and be directed into a collection container (Fig. 3.3). Do not be tempted to squeeze the bladder: if there is any resistance and no urine flow, stop the procedure.

5. When the flow ceases, release the pressure. Measure the volume, note its colour, turbidity, smell and the time it was passed. Record your results on the patient's hospital record.

6. Ensure that the patient is clean and dry before replacing it in its kennel. All areas where urination has occurred should be cleaned and disinfected and disposable clothing placed in the clinical waste.

3. A full bladder should be easy to palpate, as it will feel like a distended sac in the caudal abdomen. If there are difficulties in isolating the bladder, ask a veterinary surgeon to examine the patient for you.

4. Gentle pressure either side of the bladder will mimic the action of the abdominal muscles and should produce a flow of urine. If there is an obstruction either in the bladder or the urethra no urine will flow. A full bladder may rupture if pressure is put on it. Squeezing a bladder with an obstructed urethra may result in rupture or bruising of the bladder wall.

5. Records should be kept of all procedures. Measuring fluid output is vital in patients on fluid therapy and a comparison of these details will enable accurate assessment of the patient's progress.

6. Ensuring that the patient is clean and dry will prevent urine scalds. Protection of staff and other patients from contamination is vital: disinfection should be a high priority.

PROCEDURE: CYSTOCENTESIS

- Two people required.
- This technique should only be performed by a veterinary surgeon and should only be carried out on a palpable bladder. It may be the only practical method of draining the bladder when obstructed.

ACTION

1. Prepare all the equipment, including disposable aprons and gloves, sterile gloves for the veterinary surgeon, a sterile syringe (5–20 ml) and needle of appropriate size (usually 23G × 2.5 cm), three-way tap and urinary collection vessel as required.

2. Put on gloves and apron and restrain the patient in lateral recumbency with the abdomen angled slightly dorsally.

3. An area of about 5 cm^2 should be clipped on the midline of the caudal abdomen. Prepare the area in an aseptic fashion using a suitable surgical preparation scrub.

4. The veterinary surgeon will put on the sterile gloves and manually locate and immobilise the bladder through the abdominal wall. Using the syringe with needle attached, the veterinary surgeon will insert the needle through the abdominal wall and into the bladder. Drawing back on the syringe, the urine will be removed.

5. Gentle pressure should be applied at the injection site when the needle is removed.

6. Collect the urine for analysis or dispose of it in the clinical waste. A note should be made of the volume, colour, smell and turbidity for the patient's records. All equipment used should be disposed of in the clinical waste.

7. The patient should be thoroughly cleaned and dried before it is placed back in its kennel.

RATIONALE

1. As with all procedures, the preparation of the equipment before beginning the procedure is both an efficient and practical method of working. For the welfare of the patient choose a syringe of suitable size and a long needle with a narrow gauge: this should ensure adequate flow. Urine collection may include the preparation of a sterile sample so a suitable pot may be required.

2. The patient should be restrained to allow easy access to the bladder.

3. This area needs to be treated as a surgical site and an aseptic technique maintained.

4. The aim is to insert the needle into the bladder causing as little trauma as possible and to prevent the introduction of infection by utilising an aseptic technique.

5. Gentle pressure around the injection site will encourage natural tissue recoil around the pierced area and prevent leakage.

6. Urine should be carefully disposed of in the clinical waste to protect staff and other patients from contamination. A record of urinary output should be noted on the patient's records to enable assessment of its progress.

7. Prevention of infection is a high priority.

PROCEDURE: PERITONEAL DIALYSIS

- Two people required.
- This technique should only be carried out by a veterinary surgeon
- Peritoneal dialysis is used to filter waste products from the blood in patients suffering from conditions such as acute renal failure. In these cases, the use of osmotic diuretics may fail to stimulate urine production.

ACTION

1. Prepare all the equipment, including disposable aprons and gloves, sterile gloves for the veterinary surgeon, a small sterile surgical pack, local anaesthetic, peritoneal catheter, trochar, giving set, and dialysis fluid warmed to body temperature. A collection vessel for the waste fluid should be available.

2. Put on gloves and apron and restrain the patient in dorsal recumbency. The hair should be clipped from the ventral abdomen and the site aseptically prepared.

3. The veterinary surgeon will inject local anaesthetic into the midline umbilical area.

4. The surgical site should be draped and a small incision made into the skin so that the catheter can be inserted into the abdomen with the aid of a trochar.

5. When the catheter is in place, the giving set and the bag containing dialysis fluid should be attached and the fluid allowed to flow into the abdominal cavity.

6. After a specified period of time (usually 30 minutes) the dialysis fluid is removed under gravity. This procedure may be repeated until the blood chemistry improves. Suture placement of the catheter may be required.

7. Ensure that the wound is clean and dry before the patient is placed back in its kennel. This patient should be closely monitored as there is a high risk of peritonitis and shock.

RATIONALE

1. As with all procedures, the preparation of the equipment before beginning the procedure is both an efficient and practical method of working. A strict aseptic technique should be used. Dialysis fluid is specific to this procedure and should be warmed to body temperature to prevent shock.

2. Restraining the patient in dorsal recumbency will result in ease of access to the ventral abdomen. The ventral area needs to be treated as a surgical site and aseptic technique maintained.

3. A general anaesthetic would be contraindicated in patients with renal failure.

4. The site should be draped to aid in asepsis. A trochar is a needle-like instrument that can be used to pierce the abdominal wall.

5. The nitrogenous waste flowing through the capillary bed of the peritoneum diffuses into the dialysis fluid.

6. The dialysis fluid carries the nitrogenous waste out with it, thus benefiting the patient by reducing urea levels. Removing the fluid by gravity can sometimes be difficult and slow but allowing the patient to move around can aid the flow. If necessary, repeat the procedure while monitoring the patient's blood urea and creatinine levels.

7. Ensure that the patient is comfortable and that there is no leakage from the wound before placing it back in its kennel. A patient in acute renal failure may be immunologically compromised and it is easy for infections such as peritonitis to develop.

PROCEDURE: PASSIVE PHYSIOTHERAPY: MASSAGE

Physiotherapy is used to maintain and improve peripheral circulation and is useful in recumbent patients. Massage is especially useful for the limbs.

ACTION

1. Restrain the patient in a comfortable position which enables access to the limbs.

2. Examine each limb in turn to check for wounds and any other abnormalities.

3. Massage each limb in turn by briskly rubbing from the feet towards the body for at least 5 minutes per limb.

4. Reassure the patient while the procedure is being carried out.

5. Regular massage should be part of the patient's daily care.

RATIONALE

1. For the procedure to be beneficial, the patient needs to feel relaxed and comfortable. It may be preferable to use the patient's kennel rather than an examination table, which it may associate with pain and discomfort.

2. Massage should not be carried out if any abnormalities are present: check with the veterinary surgeon.

3. Massaging from the feet towards the trunk of the body encourages venous return.

4. Talking to the patient will help it to relax and the massage will become not only beneficial for the circulation but a source of comfort and attention for the animal.

5. For full benefit, massage should be carried out regularly during the patient's treatment.

PROCEDURE: PASSIVE PHYSIOTHERAPY: COUPAGE

Physiotherapy is used to maintain and improve peripheral circulation and is useful in recumbent patients. Coupage promotes thoracic circulation and helps to prevent hypostatic pneumonia.

ACTION

1. Restrain the patient in sternal recumbency (or standing).

2. Examine the patient for signs of abnormality such as wounds, tumours, fractures, etc.

3. Cup your hands and slap either side of the thorax from the most caudal part of the area to the cranial part. Repeat for up to 5 minutes.

4. This procedure should be carried out up to 4–5 times daily or as recommended by the veterinary surgeon.

RATIONALE

1. The sternal position allows access to both sides of the thorax and facilitates the greatest possible lung expansion.

2. Coupage may be contraindicated with some conditions such as fractured ribs, where further damage could be caused. If in doubt, consult the veterinary surgeon.

3. This slapping promotes coughing and improves the thoracic circulation. It also assists in the removal of bronchial secretions.

4. Coupage must be carried out regularly to maintain thoracic circulation in a recumbent patient.

PROCEDURE: PASSIVE PHYSIOTHERAPY: SUPPORTED EXERCISE (DOGS)

Physiotherapy is used to maintain and improve peripheral circulation and is useful in recumbent patients. Supported exercise can be carried out using proprietary frames, but 'towel walking' is the most common method used for paraplegic patients in a practice (Fig. 3.4).

ACTION

1. Depending on the size of dog, 'towel walking' can be carried out by one or two people. A strong towel and dog lead will be required—the size is dependent on the size of the patient.

2. Restrain the dog and attach a lead. Roll the towel into a 'sausage' shape and pass under

RATIONALE

1. For large dogs one person will be needed to support the hindquarters and one to support and control the front of the patient. In giant breeds two people may be required to support the hindquarters alone. Health and safety should always be taken into consideration and the procedure should not be attempted without sufficient staff available.

2. The towel is used to support the hindquarters of the patient and mimic its

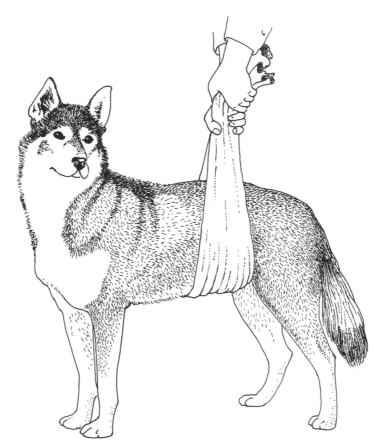

Figure 3.4 Active supported exercise using a towel.

the caudal abdomen. Hold the towel at each end, supporting the body so that the feet are on the ground (Fig. 3.4).

3. Encourage the dog to walk while supporting the hindquarters.

4. Encourage urination and defecation and improve the patient's mental attitude by carrying out this procedure in an outside environment.
5. The opportunity for a supported walk should be offered to the patient at least three times a day as part of a physiotherapy technique.

usual stance (Fig. 3.4). In a small dog, one person may be able to hold the ends of the towel with one hand and the patient's lead with the other.

3. Supported walking encourages the circulation and gives the patient confidence to try and use its limbs while they are being supported.

4. The opportunity to be outside is often invaluable in changing the patient's mental attitude and will encourage normal behaviour such as urination and defecation.
5. This procedure needs to be carried out regularly to promote improvement in the patient's condition.

PROCEDURE: PASSIVE PHYSIOTHERAPY: HYDROTHERAPY (DOGS)

Physiotherapy is used to maintain and improve peripheral circulation and is useful in recumbent patients. Hydrotherapy can be carried out for small dogs in sinks or baths available in the practice. For larger patients, referral to specialised facilities may be necessary. Hydrotherapy causes more stress than benefit in most cats!

ACTION

1. Fill a sink or bath of suitable size with warm water—ideally slightly above body temperature.

2. Gradually lower the patient into the water supporting the patient's body. Ideally the patient should start to move the limbs in a swimming action. Do not leave the patient: it will require constant support and reassurance.
3. The length of time required will vary from patient to patient but as a general rule start with approximately 5 minutes, building up the time as the patient becomes more confident.
4. The patient should be dried properly and placed in a warm kennel when each session is over.
5. As with all physiotherapy techniques, hydrotherapy sessions need to be regular to have a beneficial effect on the patient.

RATIONALE

1. The water should be deep enough to force the patient to move or swim and should be warm enough to be inviting and not chill the patient.
2. Support the patient's body at all times to prevent panic or drowning. The swimming action provides excellent physiotherapy to the limbs without weight-bearing and will help build muscle tissue and increase its strength.
3. Initially the patient will tire quickly, but as its strength builds it will tolerate a longer session in the water.

4. Do not allow the patient to become chilled as it goes back into an environment in which it cannot move.
5. Regular exercise of the limbs will build up muscle mass.

PROCEDURE: PASSIVE PHYSIOTHERAPY: PASSIVE JOINT MOVEMENT

Physiotherapy is used to maintain and improve peripheral circulation and is useful in recumbent patients. Passive joint movement will improve limb circulation and helps prevent stiffness of the joints.

ACTION

1. Ensure the patient is comfortable and relaxed: you may wish to carry out this procedure with the patient in its kennel rather than on an examination table.
2. An assistant may be required to restrain the patient's head until the patient becomes familiar with the process. It may be possible to carry out the procedure single-handed if the patient is in lateral recumbency in its kennel.
3. Slowly flex and extend the joints, one limb at a time starting with the carpal/tarsal joints and then moving upwards to the next joint.

4. The amount of time spent working on each joint should be related to the patient's condition and the degree of joint degeneration. It is usual for the timing of the sessions to increase as the patient's condition improves.
5. As with all physiotherapy techniques, joint movement sessions need to be regular to have a beneficial effect on the patient.

RATIONALE

1. A relaxed patient will benefit more from the procedure than a patient that is anxious and tense.

2. The patient may be supported in a standing position or in lateral recumbency in its kennel. This will depend on its condition. The help of an assistant may be required in some cases.
3. Slowly flexing and extending the joints will enable them to become more flexible. If a patient has been recumbent for a few days, the joints may have become very stiff. Be careful to keep within the normal range of movement to prevent joint damage. Working up the limb encourages venous return.
4. Seek advice from the veterinary surgeon.

5. Regular movement of the joints will improve circulation and prevent stiffness.

PROCEDURE: NURSING THE PATIENT WITH DIARRHOEA

A patient with diarrhoea of unknown aetiology should always be treated as a possible source of infection. Infectious diseases that may have diarrhoea as a clinical sign include canine parvovirus and feline infectious enteritis. Diseases that are also zoonotic, include campylbacteriosis and salmonellosis. If an infectious disease is suspected, barrier nursing should be maintained throughout the patient's stay.

ACTION

1. If no definite diagnosis has been made, provide isolation facilities, or choose a kennel that is easy to clean and disinfect.

RATIONALE

1. Always suspect an infectious disease if no diagnosis has been made or while diagnostic tests are being carried out. It is likely that the kennel occupied by a diarrhoeic patient will require regular cleaning and disinfection so management of this should be taken into account.

2. If an infectious disease is suspected, instigate barrier nursing techniques.

3. Provide a comfortable environment for the patient, including absorbent bedding and warmth. For cats ensure that a clean litter tray is available at all times.

4. Ensure that the medical treatment prescribed by the veterinary surgeon is carried out and recorded on the patient's record (Fig. 3.5).

5. Monitor any fluid therapy that is being given. This is likely to be administered intravenously. An example of a fluid commonly used for diarrhoeic patients is Hartmann's solution.

6. Monitor and record the usual patient parameters, i.e. temperature, pulse and respiration. An assessment of the patient's hydration status should be made and recorded.

7. Monitor and record the patient fluid intake and output, i.e. the rate and volume of fluid the patient is given as well as the amount and type of urine and faeces it produces.

8. A soiled patient should be bathed immediately with warm water and dried with disposable absorbent towel before being placed back in the clean kennel. Disposable aprons and gloves should be worn throughout the procedure and should be disposed of in the clinical waste after use.

2. Barrier nursing should be employed to protect both staff and other patients from the spread of infection.

3. These patients will be feeling uncomfortable and insecure. They may excrete diarrhoea frequently and will therefore require bedding that is absorbent and disposable. Most cats will prefer to use a clean litter tray so make sure it is cleaned every time it is used.

4. The veterinary surgeon may have prescribed drugs which must be given at the advised times to have maximum effect. The administration of any drug should be noted on the patient's records to ensure that all members of staff are aware that the treatment has been given.

5. Patients with diarrhoea lose water and electrolytes, which need to be replaced by the appropriate fluid. In cases of chronic diarrhoea a metabolic acidosis may occur and sodium bicarbonate may be required.

6. Patient parameters are required to assess progress. Clinical signs of dehydration include slightly sunken eyes, dry mucous membranes and a loss of skin elasticity.

7. Monitoring fluid intake and output gives us the information to gauge the hydration status and progress. The amount, colour and type of faeces passed should be recorded to assess the recovery process.

8. Clip away heavily soiled hair, ensuring that it is easy to clean the area if further diarrhoea occurs. The patient may be sore in places: check this with the veterinary surgeon. Thoroughly drying the patient before returning it to its kennel will prevent further soreness and the patient will not become chilled. All contaminated equipment should be regarded as a possible source of infection and be disinfected or placed in the clinical waste. Faecal material should be disposed of in the clinical waste unless required for analysis.

9. Diagnostic tests may be planned for this patient. Blood samples may be taken to measure the patient's hydration status. Faecal material may be required to aid in the diagnosis of the condition and may require collection at regular intervals. Check with the veterinary surgeon before disposing of any faecal material from the patient.

9. Packed cell volume (PCV) and blood electrolyte levels will help monitor the hydration status of the patient. Analysis of the components of the faecal material may include bacteriology.

10. The nutritional requirements of the patient will depend on the severity of the condition. Initially 'nil by mouth' is likely to be advised, with feeding starting gradually once the veterinary surgeon has approved this. A bland diet is then offered, with a gradual reintroduction of the patient's usual food.

10. Nil by mouth is instigated to rest the gastrointestinal tract. Once the inflammatory reaction has begun to subside, food may gradually be reintroduced. The use of a bland diet is less likely to inflame the gastrointestinal tract; a proprietary diet may be used in the practice. Once this diet is being tolerated without causing diarrhoea the patient's usual diet can be reintroduced.

11. If you have any concern over the condition of the patient, notify the veterinary surgeon immediately.

11. These patients can develop problems very rapidly and require constant veterinary care.

PROCEDURE: NURSING THE VOMITING PATIENT

A patient with vomiting of unknown aetiology should always be treated as a possible source of infection. Infectious diseases that have diarrhoea as a clinical sign include canine parvovirus and feline infectious enteritis. Zoonotic diseases include leptospirosis. If an infectious disease is suspected, barrier nursing should be maintained throughout the patient's stay. Vomiting can range from a minor episode, such as that resulting from scavenging, to a major attack, as occurs with some forms of poisoning. Each type will require different degrees of nursing.

ACTION

1. If no definite diagnosis has been made, provide isolation facilities, or choose a kennel that is easy to clean and disinfect.

2. If an infectious disease is suspected, use barrier nursing techniques.

3. Provide a comfortable environment for the patient, including absorbent bedding and warmth.

RATIONALE

1. Always suspect an infectious disease if no diagnosis has been made or while diagnostic tests are being carried out. It is likely that the kennel occupied by a vomiting patient will require regular cleaning and disinfection so management of this should be taken into account.

2. Barrier nursing should be employed to protect both staff and other patients from infection.

3. These patients will be feeling uncomfortable and insecure. Vomiting may occur frequently and will require efficient cleaning. The patient may be shocked and will need to be kept warm.

Kennel Chart

Animal		Owner		Case Number	
Species		Clinician		Student	
Breed		Clinical Summary			
Colour					
Sex					
Age					

Date	Day No.	Date	Day No.
Weight	Diet	Weight	Diet

	AM	PM		AM	PM
Temp			Temp		
Pulse			Pulse		
Resp			Resp		
Fed			Fed		
Ate			Ate		
Drank			Drank		

Taken Out					Taken Out				
Urine					Urine				
Faeces					Faeces				

MEDICATION		MEDICATION	
PROCEDURES		PROCEDURES	
COMMENTS		COMMENTS	

Figure 3.5 Example of a hospitalisation kennel chart. Adapted, with permission, from *Preveterinary Nursing Textbook*, p. 201, by Masters and Bowden (2001). Butterworth Heinemann, UK.

4. Ensure that the medical treatment prescribed by the veterinary surgeon is carried out and recorded on the patient's record (Fig. 3.5).

4. The veterinary surgeon may have prescribed drugs for this patient that must be given at the advised times to have maximum effect.

5. Monitor any fluid therapy that is being given. This is likely to be administered intravenously. An example of a fluid commonly used for vomiting patients is 0.9 % sodium chloride solution. Oral electrolyte replacement may be used in minor cases.

6. Monitor and record the usual patient parameters, i.e. temperature, pulse and respiration. An assessment of the patient's hydration status should be made and recorded.

7. Monitor and record the patient fluid intake and output, i.e. the rate and volume of fluid the patient is given as well as the amount and type of vomit, urine and faeces it produces.

8. Diagnostic tests may be planned for this patient. Blood samples may be taken to measure the patient's hydration status. Prepare equipment as required.

9. Nutritional requirements of the patient will depend on the severity of the condition. Initially, 'nil by mouth' is likely to be advised, with feeding starting gradually once the veterinary surgeon has approved this. A bland diet is then offered, with gradual reintroduction of the patient's usual food. Oral fluids may require monitoring initially, being given 'little and often' until the vomiting has ceased.

10. If you have any concern over the condition of the patient, notify the veterinary surgeon immediately.

The administration of any drug should be noted on the patient's records to ensure that all members of staff are aware that the treatment has been given.

5. Patients that are persistently vomiting will lose water and electrolytes, which need to be replaced by an appropriate fluid.

6. Patient parameters are required to assess progress. Clinical signs of dehydration include slightly sunken eyes, dry mucous membranes and a loss of skin elasticity.

7. Monitoring fluid intake and output gives us the information to gauge its hydration status and progress. The amount, colour and type of vomit should be recorded to make an assessment of progress.

8. Packed cell volume (PCV) and blood electrolyte levels will help monitor the hydration status of the patient.

9. 'Nil by mouth' is instigated to rest the gastrointestinal tract. Once the inflammatory reaction has begun to subside, food may gradually be reintroduced. This may begin as a bland diet, which is less likely to inflame the gastrointestinal tract; a proprietary diet may be used in the practice. Once this diet is being tolerated without causing vomiting, the patient's usual diet is gradually reintroduced.

10. These patients can develop problems very rapidly and require constant veterinary care.

PROCEDURE: NURSING THE PARAPLEGIC OR RECUMBENT PATIENT

Examples of conditions that may result in paraplegia include spinal trauma, spinal neoplasia, head injuries, pelvic fractures and medical diseases such as cardiac disease.

ACTION

1. Choose a kennel that is of a size in which the patient can lie comfortably on its side. Waterproof bedding such as a foam mattresses is ideal, with absorbent bedding material placed on top. Try to prop the patient in sternal recumbency with foam pads or sandbags. Remember that these patients may be lying in the same kennel for some time so try to place them in an area where they can see some activity to keep them stimulated.

2. Monitor and record the usual patient parameters, i.e. temperature, pulse and respiration. Urinary and faecal outputs should be recorded as well as any progress. Any abnormalities should be recorded and the veterinary surgeon notified.

3. Provide a concentrated highly digestible diet. Ensure that food and water are placed within reach of the patient. Some of these patients may refuse to eat and tempting them with their usual favourite foods may stimulate the appetite. Water must be available at all times; intake should be measured.

4. Even if the patient is incontinent, dogs should be taken outside for a change in environment on a regular basis, using 'towel walking' techniques (Fig. 3.4).

5. Turn the patient in its kennel every 4 hours to prevent hypostatic pneumonia and decubitus ulcers. Apply padding to bony prominences to prevent decubitus ulcers. Make sure that the patient is clean and dry every time it is turned to prevent urine scalding; the patient may have an indwelling catheter and this should be cared for accordingly.

RATIONALE

1. The patient needs to be able to lie comfortably but the kennel should not be so large that the patient could move around and damage itself. Sternal recumbency will help to prevent hypostatic pneumonia. Foam mattresses are comfortable for the patient and help to prevent the formation of decubitus ulcers. Absorbent bedding is required, as these patients are often incontinent.

2. Patient parameters are required to assess progress. Recumbent patients will loose heat quickly and may require covering with blankets, or use an infrared lamp or other heating device. Heat pads are not recommended for patients that are unable to move as the animal may be burnt.

3. Energy requirements are low and recumbent patients require a diet that will supply enough energy for tissue repair and the stress of being kennelled over a long period. Some of these patients may be overweight and a reducing diet may be introduced if advised by the veterinary surgeon. It is important to keep the appetite stimulated.

4. A change in the patient's environment will be stimulating. Supported exercise techniques promote good circulation and enable the patient to gain confidence.

5. Hypostatic pneumonia occurs when there is pooling of the blood in the lungs and is seen in patients left in lateral recumbency for long periods without turning. Decubitus ulcers occur on the bony prominences and are extremely slow to heal. Urine scalds are easily prevented with good nursing. The patient must be kept clean and dry at all times; barrier creams can be applied to the most susceptible areas.

6. Carry out physiotherapy techniques.

6. Simple physiotherapy such as supported exercise, passive joint movement and massage should be carried out. If equipment is available, hydrotherapy may be used.

PROCEDURE: NURSING THE EPILEPTIC PATIENT

Epilepsy is a condition of the central nervous system in which the brain sends out confused electrical messages, which result in convulsions. The convulsions consist of three phases, pre-ictal, ictal and post-ictal, with collapse occurring during the ictal phase. These convulsions or 'fits' will often take place at home and advice will initially be given to the owner (often over the telephone). Personal safety must be taken in account: an animal that is fitting may inadvertently bite.

ACTION

1. Advise the owner not to touch the animal and to ask all people to leave the room. Move all furniture away from the animal to prevent injury. Reduce noise and darken the environment. Observe the animal until the fit is over and then reassure the animal.

2. If the fit becomes continuous, or repeated fits occur one after the other, the animal must be brought to the surgery. A padded kennel should be prepared.

3. The veterinary surgeon may wish to give intravenous anticonvulsants. The patient's pulse, respiration and mucous membrane colour should be monitored frequently. An oxygen supply should be readily available in case of respiratory difficulties. Do not touch the patient until the fitting has subsided. The temperature should be taken regularly to monitor for hypothermia.

4. The progress and continuing nursing care of these patients depends on the aetiology of the fit. Some patients (i.e. those with idiopathic epilepsy) can be stabilised and may be discharged with anticonvulsive therapies. Other patients may have signs of an underlying disease of which the fit is one of the symptoms; diagnostic tests may be required to confirm this.

RATIONALE

1. A fitting animal should not be brought down to the surgery as this stimulation could prolong the fit. Transporting a fitting animal in the car could cause an accident. All stimulation should be removed from the animal, i.e. people, noise, light: a quiet environment will help the animal recover more quickly. The animal will be confused after the fit and will require comfort.

2. Prolonged fitting is known as status epilepticus: these patients will require anticonvulsant therapies and constant observation. Padding around the kennel will prevent the animal damaging itself during convulsions.

3. Anticonvulsants will depress the central nervous system and control the fit; however, they may also cause respiratory problems, so constant observation is required. These patients will essentially be sedated and lying still for long periods, which could lead to a situation in which hypothermia develops.

4. Idiopathic epilepsy can be treated with oral anticonvulsants but other disease conditions, such as renal disease or poisoning, may cause fitting and will be treated differently.

PROCEDURE: NURSING THE PATIENT WITH CARDIAC FAILURE: CONGESTIVE HEART FAILURE

Congestive heart failure occurs when the heart fails to function effectively—it compensates by changing its rate, leading to clinical signs which will indicate the side of the heart that is affected. Right-sided heart failure will result in poor venous return to the heart, congestion of organs such as the liver and spleen, and possibly the development of ascites. Left-sided heart failure will result in poor venous return from the lungs, causing pulmonary congestion and oedema, tachypnoea and coughing.

ACTION	RATIONALE
1. Choose a kennel that is of a size in which the patient can lie comfortably. Bedding should be comfortable and absorbent. The kennel needs to be in a quiet area.	1. The patient needs to be able to lie comfortably. It may be on drug therapy that results in an increase in urination, so acrylic bedding or incontinence pads may be useful in case of leakage. These patients require a stress-free environment.
2. Monitor and record the usual patient parameters, i.e. temperature, pulse and respiration. Urinary and faecal output should be recorded. Note any progress. Any abnormalities should be recorded (Fig. 3.5) and the veterinary surgeon notified.	2. Patient parameters are required to assess progress. Geriatric patients will loose heat quickly and may require covering with blankets or the use of an infrared lamp or other heating device. Heat pads are not recommended for patients that are unable to move away from the heat as they may be burnt.
3. Cardiac patients need a diet that is low in salt, contains protein of high biological value and is highly digestible; however, it is important to stimulate the patient's appetite, which may mean that salt is added to improve the taste. Cardiac patients are often overweight and a diet with reducing capabilities may be utilised at the discretion of the veterinary surgeon. Potassium supplementation may be required. Water must be available at all times; intake should be measured.	3. A diet that is low in salt will help to reduce pulmonary oedema and ascites, which occur as a result of hypertension and venous congestion; however, salt does increase the palatability of the diet and these patients must be prevented from becoming anorexic. Potassium levels may drop in patients on diuretic therapy as it is lost in the urine.
4. Ensure that the medical treatment prescribed by the veterinary surgeon is carried out and recorded on the patient's record. Cardiac drug therapy includes the use of diuretics, bronchodilators, vasodilators and glycosides.	4. The veterinary surgeon may have prescribed drugs for this patient which must be given at the advised times to have the maximum effect. The administration of any drug should be noted on the patient's records to ensure that all members of staff are aware that the treatment has been given.
5. Canine patients must be taken outside on a lead to urinate or defecate. Cats must have access to a clean litter tray at all times.	5. The patient must be rested as much as possible; it should not be exercised.

PROCEDURE: NURSING THE PATIENT WITH RENAL DISEASE

Renal diseases include acute renal failure (complete/almost complete lack of renal function), chronic renal failure (progressive loss of renal function) and nephrotic syndrome, which is associated with the development of glomerulonephritis. Leptospirosis, a zoonotic disease, can be a differential in acute renal failure and barrier nursing may be instigated until a diagnosis is made.

ACTION

1. Choose a kennel that is of a size in which the patient can lie comfortably. Bedding should be comfortable and absorbent.

2. Monitor and record the usual patient parameters, i.e. temperature, pulse and respiration. Urinary and faecal output should be recorded. Note any progress. Any abnormalities should be recorded (Fig. 3.5) and the veterinary surgeon notified.

3. Renal patients require a diet that is low in protein and phosphorus. The protein used must be of high biological value. Patients may have oral ulceration and may require much encouragement to eat. Hand-feeding or tube-feeding may be considered.

4. Ensure that the medical treatment prescribed by the veterinary surgeon is carried out and recorded on the patient's record. Drugs that may be used include anti-emetics, antibiotics, anabolic steroids and diuretics.

5. The continuing nursing care will be dependent on the disease condition. Patients with renal failure will require intravenous fluid therapy and this must be carefully monitored. Treatment for patients with acute renal failure may include peritoneal dialysis.

6. It is likely that the veterinary surgeon will require samples for diagnostic assessment of the patient's progress.

7. Canine patients must be taken outside to urinate or defecate. Cats must have access to a clean litter tray at all times.

RATIONALE

1. The patient needs to be able to lie comfortably. Acrylic bedding or incontinence pads may be useful in cases of incontinence. White bedding is useful in identifying the colour of the urine absorbed: the presence of blood will be especially noticeable.

2. Patient parameters are required to assess progress. Measure urinary output and fluid intake. This will be vital in assessing the progress of treatment.

3. Low protein levels will help to reduce levels of nitrogenous waste. The protein must be of a high biological value to enable it to be utilised for maintenance and repair. Phosphorus levels will be elevated in uraemic patients so the diet must contain low levels of phosphorus.

4. Drugs prescribed for this patient by the veterinary surgeon must be given at the advised times to have maximum effect. The administration of any drug should be noted on the patient's records to ensure that all members of staff are aware that the treatment has been given.

5. Fluid therapy will be given to correct electrolyte loss and maintain hydration.

6. Blood and urine analyses may be utilised to monitor the patient's progress.

7. Urine may require collection: check with the veterinary surgeon.

PROCEDURE: NURSING THE PATIENT WITH HEPATIC DISEASE

Hepatic disease is usually caused by a bacterial or viral infection. Examples include adenovirus, which causes infectious canine hepatitis, and *Leptospira icterohaemorrhagiae*, which causes leptospirosis. Both of these are infectious diseases and, if they are suspected, barrier nursing should be instigated until a definitive diagnosis is made. Leptospirosis is a zoonosis, so extra care should be taken to protect all personnel involved. Toxic damage caused by poisoning or prolonged drug therapy can sometimes result in hepatitis.

ACTION

1. Choose a kennel that is of a size in which the patient can lie comfortably. Bedding should be comfortable and absorbent.
2. Monitor and record the usual patient parameters, i.e. temperature, pulse and respiration. The mucous membranes may be jaundiced and ascites may develop. Urinary and faecal output should be recorded. Note any progress. Any abnormalities should be recorded (Fig. 3.5) and the veterinary surgeon notified.
3. Most hepatic patients need an energy-dense diet with moderate amounts of protein with a high biological value and increased levels of water-soluble vitamins. These patients are often anorexic and good nutritional support is essential. Hand-feeding or tube-feeding may be required.
4. Ensure that the medical treatment prescribed by the veterinary surgeon is carried out and recorded on the patient's record. Drugs that may be used are of a supportive nature.

5. The continuing nursing care will depend on the cause of the disease. Patients are likely to require intravenous fluid therapy and this must be carefully monitored.
6. It is likely that the veterinary surgeon will require samples to confirm the diagnosis and assess the patient's progress. Diagnostic imaging techniques may be used. If a liver biopsy is required, the patient will have to be prepared for surgery.
7. Canine patients must be taken outside to urinate or defecate. Cats must have access to a clean litter tray at all times.

RATIONALE

1. The patient needs to be able to lie comfortably. Acrylic bedding or incontinence pads may be useful in cases of incontinence.
2. Patient parameters are required to assess progress. Jaundice occurs where there are excessive levels of bilirubin in the blood—a result of the hepatitis affecting the biliary system. Ascites is the result of fluid accumulation (due to portal hypertension) in the abdomen; this could include blood, urine, transudates and exudates.
3. Protein is required to supply the patient's basic needs and support regeneration of damaged tissue.

4. Drugs prescribed for this patient by the veterinary surgeon must be given at the advised times to have maximum effect. The administration of any drug should be noted on the patient's records to ensure that all members of staff are aware that the treatment has been given.
5. Fluid therapy will be given to correct electrolyte loss and maintain hydration.

6. Blood biochemistry will be monitored to assess the patient's progress.

7. Supportive therapies must include good nursing techniques.

PROCEDURE: NURSING THE PATIENT WITH PANCREATIC DISEASE

Disease conditions of the exocrine part of the pancreas include pancreatitis
and exocrine pancreatic deficiency.

ACTION

1. Choose a kennel that is of a size in which the patient can lie comfortably. Bedding should be comfortable and absorbent.
2. Monitor and record the usual patient parameters, i.e. temperature, pulse and respiration. Any abnormalities should be recorded (Fig. 3.5) and the veterinary surgeon notified.
3. Patients with pancreatitis vomit persistently and quickly become dehydrated. Intravenous fluid therapy is required and should be monitored closely; use Hartmann's solution.
4. Initially patients should be kept on 'nil by mouth'. After 3–5 days, gradually introduce a low-fat diet with additional replacement enzymes.This diet may be required for a long period.
5. Pancreatitis is an extremely painful condition and peritonitis may develop as a complication. Ensure that the medical treatment prescribed by the veterinary surgeon is carried out and recorded on the patient's record. Drugs that may be used include analgesics and antibiotics.
6. Tests will be carried out to confirm the diagnosis and to assess the patient's progress. Blood and faecal samples may be required.
7. Once hospital treatment has finished, the patient will require strict dietary management and may need the provision of proprietary enzymes to aid digestion for the remainder of its life.

RATIONALE

1. The patient needs to be able to lie comfortably. Acrylic bedding or incontinence pads may be useful in cases of incontinence.
2. Patient parameters are required to assess progress.
3. The fluid and electrolytes that have been lost must be replaced with a suitable fluid such as Hartmann's.
4. Patients with pancreatic disease are unable to digest fat, so a low-fat diet is required. Added enzyme supplementation will aid the digestive process.
5. Drugs prescribed for this patient by the veterinary surgeon must be given at the advised times to have maximum effect. The monitoring of the analgesic regimen is vital as these patients will be in extreme pain if the dose of analgesic is insufficient. The administration of any drug should be noted on the patient's records to ensure that all members of staff are aware that the treatment has been given.
6. Diagnostic tests for pancreatitis include haematology (a leucocytosis may be present), biochemistry (to assess serum amylase and lipase) and abdominal radiography (to assess the degree of peritonitis). For patients with suspected exocrine pancreatic insufficiency a serum raised trypsin-like immunoreactivity (TLI) test may be carried out.
7. Once the pancreas has been damaged it is unlikely to return to normal function.

PROCEDURE: NURSING THE PATIENT WITH DIABETES MELLITUS

Diabetes mellitus is caused by degeneration of the endocrine part of the pancreas. This normally secretes the hormone insulin, which stimulates glucose uptake by the cells and storage of excess glucose in the liver as glycogen. In patients with diabetes mellitus, insufficient amounts of insulin are released, resulting in hyperglycaemia (raised blood glucose) and excretion of glucose in the urine.

ACTION

1. The patient may be admitted with keto-acidosis and will require immediate intravenous fluid therapy. Initially Hartmann's solution is used, followed by 0.9 % saline to maintain the patient once it is stable. The veterinary surgeon will also administer a short-acting soluble insulin intravenously.

2. Choose a kennel that is of a size in which the patient can lie comfortably. Bedding should be comfortable and absorbent.

3. Monitor and record the usual patient parameters, i.e. temperature, pulse and respiration. Any abnormalities should be recorded and the veterinary surgeon notified.

4. Maintenance of a patient with diabetes mellitus requires a strict routine. First thing each morning a urine sample should be collected and its glucose level tested using a simple dipstick test. A blood sample may also be collected to test for blood glucose levels.

5. Use the level of the glucose in the urine to calculate the dose of insulin to be given to the patient.

RATIONALE

1. Ketoacidosis occurs when the patient starts to break down proteins to use as a source of energy. The cells are unable to use the more normal glucose as a source of energy as this requires the presence of insulin. A metabolic acidosis occurs and ketones build up in the circulation. Hartmann's solution will correct the metabolic acidosis, while saline is used for maintenance. Soluble insulin begins working rapidly and the utilisation of glucose can begin.

2. The patient needs to be able to lie comfortably.

3. Patient parameters are required to assess progress.

4. Testing the urine glucose gives a level on which to base the dose of insulin. Urine may also be tested for ketones but these should not be present unless the condition of the patient has become unstable. Blood glucose levels can be monitored to give baseline levels but are not usually used except in a practice, as owners find it difficult to collect a blood sample.

5. Calculations are based on an initial dose of 0.5 iu (international units) per kg bodyweight. If the morning urine glucose is more than 1%, give the previous day's dose plus 2 iu. If the urine glucose is 0%, give the previous day's dose less 2 iu. If the glucose is 0.1%, give the previous day's dose. Check all dosages with the veterinary surgeon before administering the insulin.

6. Before administering the insulin, give the patient one-quarter of its daily food ration. If the patient eats this, inject the prepared dose of insulin. Insulin is usually given subcutaneously in proprietary insulin syringes. Ensure that the subcutaneous injection has been given correctly to enable the insulin to work efficiently. If the patient does not eat its food, seek advice from the veterinary surgeon.

7. All treatments must be noted on the patient's record.

8. The remainder of the patient's food ration should be given 8 hours after the insulin injection. A blood sample may be taken at this time to monitor levels of glucose.

9. Nutritional support of the diabetic patient includes a high-fibre diet. It is vital that the patient is kept to a strict regimen and that no extra food or titbits are offered.

10. Hypoglycaemia can be a complication and may occur around the time of the peak of insulin activity. Clinical signs include tremors, weakness, ataxia, collapse and coma. A conscious patient should be given oral glucose in the form of glucose powder, sugar, honey, etc. An unconscious patient will require intravenous glucose as soon as possible.

11. Diabetic patients must continue with a strict regimen in order to keep their condition stable. This includes a consistent amount of food of a consistent formula. Exercise must be monitored and should be the same amount at the same time each day. Some cases of diabetes mellitus are transient, while other patients may require insulin for the remainder of their lives.

6. The insulin will require some glucose in the blood to metabolise, so food is given before the insulin to provide this. The dose of the insulin must be calculated and administered accurately. Proprietary syringes that are calibrated in international units ensure this.

7. If the patient does not respond or there is an excessive response to the insulin injection, the record can be checked and used to adjust the dose.

8. The maximum effect of the insulin will coincide with peak blood glucose levels from the digested food.

9. High-fibre diets reduce the speed and prolong the time of glucose absorption from the small intestine. This helps the insulin control the blood glucose by preventing the glucose surges that can occur after a meal.

10. Hypoglycaemia (low blood glucose) can occur when too much insulin has been given, if the patient has failed to eat or if the peak effect of the insulin has occurred before the patient has received the major part of its daily food ration.

11. High levels of blood glucose or high levels of insulin may cause the condition of the patient to become unstable. Unusual energy demands, such as a very long walk, can also result in instability. Some patients may have diabetes as a secondary condition, e.g. a bitch may develop diabetes after her 'season'. If she is spayed she may not require insulin in the future.

PROCEDURE: NURSING THE PATIENT WITH DIABETES INSIPIDUS

Diabetes insipidus results from either a failure of the pituitary gland to produce antidiuretic hormone (ADH) or of the kidneys to respond to ADH. Either type leads to an inability to control the concentration of urine and so to conserve body fluid.

ACTION

1. The patient will present with a marked polydipsia and polyuria.
2. Choose a kennel of a size that allows the patient to lie comfortably. Bedding should be comfortable and absorbent. Water must be available and canine patients must frequently be taken outside to urinate.
3. Monitor and record the usual patient parameters, i.e. temperature, pulse and respiration. Fluid intake and output should be noted. Any abnormalities should be recorded and the veterinary surgeon notified.
4. Diagnosis of diabetes insipidus involves the use of the water deprivation test. The patient must be well hydrated and have good renal function.

5. Empty the patient's bladder and measure the specific gravity using a refractometer. Record the results.
6. The patient should be weighed and 5% of its bodyweight calculated. It should then be placed in a kennel without food and water for 1 hour.
7. After an hour the patient's bladder should be emptied, it should be weighed and the urine specific gravity measured. Repeat this process until 5% of the patient's bodyweight is lost.

8. When the testing is finished the patient should be allowed free access to water.
9. Ensure that the medical treatment prescribed by the veterinary surgeon is carried out and recorded on the patient's record.

RATIONALE

1. The patient is unable to concentrate the urine so will pass dilute urine frequently.
2. The patient needs to be able to lie comfortably. If the patient is not offered water it will dehydrate quickly as it will still exhibit polyuria.

3. Patient parameters are required to assess progress. Fluid intake and output will indicate the degree of the problem.

4. The water deprivation test assesses the ability of the patient to concentrate its urine. The patient can become dehydrated quickly and this test should only be carried out by a veterinary surgeon. Assessment of the patient's hydration status should be made throughout the test. The renal function of the patient should be taken into consideration as further complications could occur.
5. The specific gravity measurement will assess the concentration of the urine before water deprivation.
6. This provides a measurement on which to base the subsequent results.

7. When a normal patient loses 5% of its bodyweight it will concentrate its urine to a specific gravity of more than 1.020. If the patient has diabetes insipidus it will still produce dilute urine of a specific gravity of less than 1.007 and a diagnosis can be made.
8. The patient may become severely dehydrated if water is withheld for too long.
9. The veterinary surgeon may have prescribed drugs for this patient that must be given at the advised times to have

maximum effect. The administration of any drug should be noted on the patient's records to ensure that all members of staff are aware that the treatment has been given.

FURTHER READING

Agar S 2001 Small Animal Nutrition. Butterworth-Heinemann, Oxford
Blood DC and Studdert VP 2000 Comprehensive Veterinary Dictionary. WB Saunders, London

Cooper B, Lane DR (eds) 1999 Veterinary Nursing, 2nd edn. Butterworth-Heinemann, Oxford

4

Administration of fluid therapy

C. Bowden

Introduction

The healthy body contains between 60 and 70% of water, found inside and surrounding all the cells. This fluid maintains a balanced state within the body so that the normal metabolic processes can function efficiently—a process known as homeostasis. Dissolved in the body fluids are chemical materials that are essential for the body's metabolism and which play a part in controlling the movement of fluid around the body. Many medical conditions and surgical procedures cause an upset in fluid balance and if nothing is done to correct this the animal may become severely dehydrated or go into shock and die. The purpose of fluid therapy is to replace any deficit so that the circulating fluid volume is restored and renal function is improved.

There are many types of fluid used in fluid therapy and the replacement fluid must be as close as possible, in terms of the chemical constituents and volume, to that lost from the general circulation. This chapter explains the theory that underpins the selection of fluids and describes in detail the procedures involved in supplying the fluid to the patient.

PROCEDURE: APPRECIATION OF WATER CONTENT OF THE BODY (FIG. 4.1)

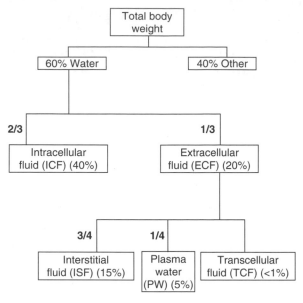

Figure 4.1 The distribution of body water into its principal compartments. Adapted, with permission, from *Veterinary Nursing*, p. 569, 2nd edn, by Lane and Cooper (1994). Butterworth Heinemann, UK.

ACTION

1. 100% total bodyweight.
2. Intracellular fluid (ICF) = 2/3 of body fluid.
3. Extracellular fluid (ECF) = 1/3 of body fluid.

4. Body fluids contain electrolytes, which yield ions.

5. Ions are small water-soluble particles carrying one or more negative or positive charges. Sodium chloride (NaCl) is an electrolyte that dissociates into sodium ions and chloride ions when dissolved in water.

6. Water balance and concentration needs to be maintained equally within the body.

RATIONALE

1. 60% water + 40% other body structures.
2. ICF is located within the cells.
3. ECF is located outside the cells: plasma—water contained within blood, interstitial fluid bathing cells, transcellular fluid within specialised areas.

4. It is important to know the electrolyte and ion composition of body fluids to ensure the correct fluid is administered.

5. It is important to know which ions are in ICF and ECF to ensure that the correct fluid therapy is administered. Cations are ions that are positively charged; the main cations in ICF are potassium and magnesium, and sodium in ECF. Anions are ions that are negatively charged; the main anions in ECF are chloride and bicarbonate.

6. Osmosis is the process by which water moves from a low concentration to a high concentration through a semipermeable membrane. Osmotic pressure is the pressure needed to prevent osmosis from happening. Osmotic pressure is maintained in the healthy animal by various homeostatic mechanisms.

PROCEDURE: APPRECIATION OF WATER BALANCE IN THE BODY

ACTION

1. Water intake: ingestion.
2. Water intake: metabolism.
3. Water loss: 50 ml/kg/24 h

4. Sensible water loss: 25 ml/kg/24 h.
5. Insensible water loss: 25 ml/kg/24 h.

6. Water replacement: 50 ml/kg/24h.
7. Electrolyte replacement:
   sodium 1 mmol/kg/24 h;
   potassium 2 mmol/kg/24 h.
8. Metabolic acidosis = loss of alkaline ions.

9. Metabolic alkalosis = loss of acidic ions.

RATIONALE

1. Ingestion of fluids and foods.
2. Metabolism of fats and carbohydrates.
3. This is the amount that needs to be replaced daily to ensure water balance.
4. Sensible loss via urine.
5. Insensible losses: respiratory, cutaneous and faeces.
6. To balance water loss.
7. To balance electrolyte loss.

8. Replace loss with fluid containing alkaline ions to correct acid–base imbalance.
9. Replace loss with fluid containing acidic ions to correct acid–base imbalance.

PROCEDURE: ASSESSING LEVEL OF DEHYDRATION OF THE PATIENT

ACTION

1. Normal physical appearance despite a history of fluid loss.
2. Mild to dry mucous membranes, slight decrease in skin turgor.
3. Decrease in skin turgor; dry mucous membranes; mild tachycardia; sunken eyes; slight increase in capillary refill time.
4. Marked decrease in skin turgor; dry mucous membranes; sunken eyes; weak pulse; increased capillary refill time; oliguria; cold extremities.
5. Very marked decrease in skin turgor; pale and dry mucous membranes; sunken eyes; tachycardia; cold extremities; muscle weakness; collapse; depression; anuria.

RATIONALE (degree of dehydration as a percentage of bodyweight)

1. Slight: > 5%.

2. Mild: 5–6%.

3. Mild: 6–8%.

4. Moderate: 10–12%.

5. Severe: 12–15%.

PROCEDURE: SELECTION OF FLUIDS IN RELATION TO THEIR ACTION IN THE BODY

ACTION	RATIONALE
1. Isotonic fluid.	1. Equal osmotic pressure to blood—no fluid movement, thereby maintaining equilibrium.
2. Hypertonic fluid.	2. Greater osmotic pressure than blood—thereby encouraging movement of fluid from cells into circulation.
3. Hypotonic fluid.	3. Lower osmotic pressure than blood—thereby encouraging movement of fluids into cells.
4. Crystalloids.	4. These fluids contain small molecules that enter and temporarily increase the blood volume before passing into the cells and equilibrating with the ICF.
5. Colloids.	5. These fluids contain large molecules that remain within the circulation, thereby increasing osmotic pressure and expanding plasma volume.
6. Blood product—plasma.	6. This helps to expand plasma volume and treat hypoproteinaemia.
7. Whole blood.	7. Used in cases where replacement of red blood cells and plasma volume expansion is required.

PROCEDURE: SELECTION OF FLUID FOR SPECIFIC NEEDS

ACTION	RATIONALE
1. 0.9% NaCl—normal saline (isotonic crystalloid).	1. Replace ECF; gastric losses or loss of acidic ions from vomiting.
2. 0.18% NaCl + 4% dextrose (isotonic crystalloid).	2. Maintenance requirements; primary water deficit replacement; neonatal ECF replacement.
3. 5% dextrose (isotonic crystalloid).	3. Primary water deficit replacement.
4. Hartmann's solution (isotonic crystalloid).	4. Replace ECF; diarrhoea and postgastric losses/alkaline ions.
5. Ringer's solution (isotonic crystalloid).	5. Replace ECF; gastric losses from vomiting.
6. Haemaccel/Gelofusine (isotonic colloids).	6. Expand plasma volume; moderate to severe fluid loss and blood loss where no blood products are available.
7. Plasma (blood product).	7. Replace plasma proteins; expand plasma volume as above; clotting defects.
8. Whole blood.	8. Replace blood loss; meet any ongoing or anticipated blood loss; anaemia; circulatory insufficiency.

PROCEDURE: ORAL FLUID THERAPY

Indications. Animal willing to drink, not vomiting, absence of intestinal obstruction.

Fluid choice. Hypotonic electrolyte solution or water.

ACTION

1. Select equipment: dosing syringe with catheter tip, towel, assistant, fluid.

2. Measure correct volume of fluid in the syringe.
3. Request assistance to hold the patient.

4. Support the patient's nose and mouth with hand in normal position.

5. Introduce the catheter tip syringe into the mouth between upper and lower premolars above the tongue surface.
6. Slowly introduce 5–10 ml of fluid into the mouth and allow the patient to swallow. Stroke the ventral aspect of the pharynx to encourage swallowing.
7. Continue until required volume has been delivered or the patient becomes agitated.

8. Dry the patient's mouth and surrounding area and replace in ready prepared clean kennel.
9. Record total fluid volume given and the frequency on the hospital record.
10. Dispose of equipment safely and appropriately.

RATIONALE

1. A dosing syringe is the most suitable method of accurate administration. It is important to select all equipment prior to procedure to ensure efficient method of administration.
2. Important to measure fluid replacement accurately to avoid excess or insufficient.
3. Ensure that the patient is kept at ease and feels safe.
4. Firm but sympathetic handling will ensure fluid is delivered safely and effectively. The head must be in the normal position to prevent aspiration pneumonia.
5. This area is the most suitable to administer fluid safely and accurately.

6. Avoid giving too much fluid at any one time as this may induce choking. Allow the patient to swallow and breathe between administrations.
7. Only continue if the patient is taking fluid well and swallowing between doses. If the patient gets distressed at any time or fails to swallow, stop the procedure immediately.
8. Always dry the area to help prevent heat loss and make the patient comfortable.

9. Ensure record keeping is accurate to prevent over- or under-administration.
10. It is essential to dispose of equipment correctly to avoid contamination and accidents.

PROCEDURE: SUBCUTANEOUS FLUID THERAPY

Indications. Mild dehydration with adequate peripheral circulation.

Fluid choice. Any crystalloid isotonic or hypotonic solution such as 0.9% NaCl; 0.18% NaCl + 4% dextrose; Hartmann's solution.

ACTION

1. Select and prepare equipment: prewarmed fluid, measured volume in sterile syringe with new sterile needle attached (maximum 10–20 ml/kg/site), clippers, surgical skin scrub, gloves, swabs (Fig. 4.2).
2. Request assistant to restrain patient in lateral recumbency.

3. Clip an area of approximately 3 cm × 3 cm on either side of the thorax over the ninth rib, midway between the ventral and dorsal borders.
4. Prepare skin aseptically with surgical scrub solution. Wear gloves.
5. Infiltrate local anaesthetic into the prepared site as instructed by the veterinary surgeon. Drape the area.

RATIONALE

1. Fluid must be prewarmed to prevent shock and discomfort and aid absorption. Isotonic or hypotonic fluid is used to promote absorption. Ensure all equipment is prepared in advance to allow for efficient procedure.
2. Firm effective handling ensures that the patient remains comfortable throughout the procedure.
3. Area must be free of hair to reduce the risk of infection. This area allows effective movement and absorption of fluid.

4. Skin must be cleaned aseptically to reduce the risk of infection.
5. Local anaesthetic will desensitise the area, preventing pain and discomfort. Draping the movement area will help to maintain asepsis.

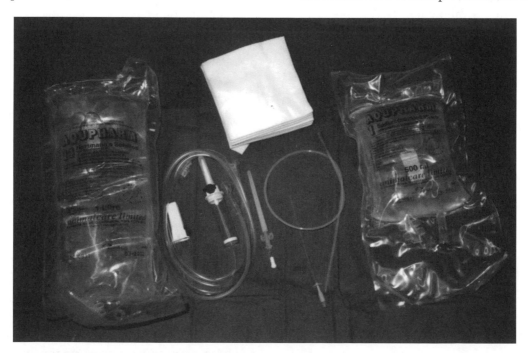

Figure 4.2 Selection of disposable equipment for fluid therapy. From left to right: Hartmann's solution, giving set, intravenous catheter, Jackson cat catheter, dog urinary catheter, normal saline (lavage).

6. Tent the skin and introduce the needle, attached to the fluid-filled syringe, subcutaneously.
7. Withdraw the plunger of the syringe.

8. Administer the volume of fluid slowly and withdraw the needle (maximum 10–20 ml/kg/site).
9. Massage the area.
10. Repeat the procedure on the other side of the thorax.
11. Remove the drapes and dry the area. Allow the patient to resume sternal recumbency and replace it in the kennel.
12. Dispose of equipment safely and appropriately.

6. Administration must be subcutaneous, avoiding any puncture of the thoracic cavity.
7. To check that a vein has not been punctured by accident.
8. Fast infusion of fluid can cause considerable discomfort.
9. To ensure even and effective distribution.
10. To ensure equal distribution in the body.
11. Ensure the patient is comfortable in the kennel.

12. It is essential to dispose of equipment correctly correctly to avoid contamination and accidents.

PROCEDURE: INTRAPERITONEAL FLUID THERAPY

Indications. Mild dehydration where fluids cannot be administered orally; where larger volumes need to be infused rapidly; neonatal and exotics.

Fluid choice. Any isotonic crystalloid fluid such as 0.9% NaCl; 0.18% NaCl+4% dextrose; Hartmann's solution.

ACTION

1. Select and prepare equipment: prewarmed fluid, measured volume in sterile syringe with sterile new needle attached, clippers, surgical skin scrub solution, swabs, gloves.
2. Assistant to restrain the patient in dorsal recumbency and reassure the patient throughout procedure.

3. Clip area surrounding umbilicus.

4. Prepare skin aseptically and drape the area.
5. Infiltrate local anaesthetic into the prepared site—region of umbilicus, as instructed by the veterinary surgeon.
6. Introduce the sterile needle attached to the fluid syringe through the skin and central line (linea alba) into the peritoneal cavity.
7. Withdraw the plunger of the syringe.

RATIONALE

1. Avoid shock and drop in body temperature by prewarming fluid. Prepare all equipment in advance of procedure to ensure efficient administration.
2. To present the correct area for administration and encourage the viscera to gravitate away from site, thereby avoiding puncture during the procedure.
3. Reduce the risk of infection by clipping the hair, allowing a wide margin around the umbilicus.
4. To prevent risk of infection.
5. To desensitise the area prior to administration of fluid.

6. Ensure asepsis is maintained and introduction is efficient and smooth.

7. To check that a blood vessel has not been punctured by accident. If blood appears in the hub of the syringe, withdraw and start again. If urine or gut contents appear in the syringe, the bladder or intestine may have been punctured—withdraw and start again.

8. Introduce prewarmed fluid into the peritoneal cavity.
9. Withdraw the needle and syringe, putting gentle pressure over the injection site.

10. Remove drapes and dry area. Allow the patient to regain sternal recumbency, reassure and replace in kennel.

11. Record fluid administration details.
12. Dispose of equipment safely and appropriately.

8. If any resistance is felt, stop and restart the procedure from point 6.
9. Clean, swift removal of the needle to prevent any discomfort. Pressure to prevent leakage of body fluid.

10. Resume normal position as soon as possible to restore equilibrium. It is important to ensure the patient is comfortable before placing it back in the kennel.

11. To ensure accurate monitoring.
12. It is essential to dispose of equipment correctly to avoid contamination and accidents.

PROCEDURE: PREPARATION OF EQUIPMENT FOR INTRAVENOUS FLUID ADMINISTRATION

ACTION

1. Wash hands and wear disposable gloves.

2. Select correct equipment for intravenous fluid administration: clippers, surgical scrub solution, swabs, tapes, blade, intravenous catheter, heparinised saline, three-way tap or bung, fluid bag, infusion set, kick bowl, drip stand (Fig 4.3).

3. Check the expiry date on the fluid bag, look for any damage to the outside of the bag or for any artefacts within the fluid.

4. Remove the fluid bag from its outer covering and identify the correct outlet port. Hang the fluid bag on a drip stand.

5. Remove the infusion set from its outer coverings and switch off the flow control.

6. Remove the cover from the infusion spike and introduce the spike into the fluid bag carefully.

7. Squeeze the fluid chamber so that it fills by one-third.

8. Remove the cap from the end of the infusion line, taking care not to touch a non-sterile surface.

9. Open the flow control and allow the fluid to travel down the infusion set in a controlled manner, removing all air bubbles.

10. Switch off the flow control and replace the cap.

RATIONALE

1. It is essential to maintain levels of asepsis to avoid contamination and infection.

2. All equipment must be selected before the patient is restrained, to ensure that the procedure is performed efficiently and thoroughly.

3. Any sign of damage, abnormality or expiry date passed indicates that the sterility of the product cannot be guaranteed, therefore it would be unsafe to use.

4. Careful handling to reduce the risk of contamination. Use of a drip stand facilitates handling.

5. Switching off the flow control will prevent loss of fluid prior to connection to bag.

6. Careful handling will avoid puncture of the fluid bag with the spike, thereby avoiding contamination and fluid loss.

7. To aid control of fluid during infusion and prevent air bubbles.

8. It is important to maintain sterility at all times.

9. No air bubbles should enter the circulation and excess fluid loss from the fluid bag should be avoided.

10. To prevent leakage and maintain sterility.

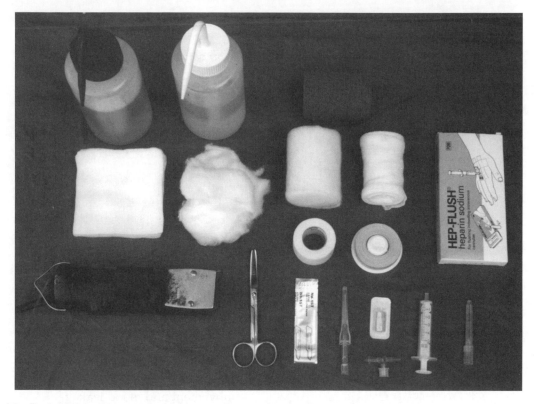

Figure 4.3 Equipment for intravenous access.

11. Dispose of equipment safely and appropriately.	11. It is essential to dispose of equipment correctly to avoid any clutter and reduce the risk of contamination and accidents.

PROCEDURE: INTRAVENOUS ACCESS TO THE CEPHALIC VEIN AND ADMINISTRATION OF FLUID THERAPY

ACTION

1. Select equipment and prepared fluid infusion. Prewarm the fluid to body temperature.

2. Assistant to restrain the patient in sternal recumbency, in the correct manner to allow access to the cephalic vein.

3. Wearing gloves, clip and prepare the site aseptically using surgical scrub and surgical spirit.

4. Ask the assistant to raise the vein.

5. With gloved hands, insert the catheter tip into the vein. Once blood appears within the catheter, remove the needle and advance the catheter fully (Fig. 4.4).

RATIONALE

1. Prepare equipment in advance of restraining the patient. Maintain body temperature and minimise discomfort by prewarming the fluid.

2. Firm handling will keep the patient at ease and reduce the risk of any accident.

3. This will help to prevent infection.

4. This dilates the vein, making it easier to see.

5. The needle is removed to prevent accidental puncture of the vein further along the lumen.

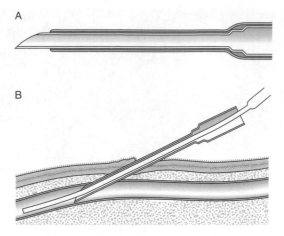

Figure 4.4 Intravenous catheters and venepuncture: A, 'over the needle' cannula; B, 'through the needle' cannula.

6. Ask the assistant to release the pressure over the vein. Place a bung or three-way tap to close over the end of the catheter.
7. Dry the area and secure the catheter to the leg with tapes.

8. Flush the catheter with a small amount of heparinised saline.
9. Remove the cap from the infusion set and attach the infusion tube to the intravenous catheter. Secure the infusion tube to the patient's leg with tapes. Bandage if necessary.
10. Open the fluid flow control.

11. Adjust the fluid control to the drip rate required for the patient. Syringe drivers and infusion pumps may be used to facilitate the delivery of the calculated drip rate.
12. Record fluid type and drip rate on the hospital card.

13. To prevent self-mutilation by the patient, bandage the area and apply an Elizabethan collar as necessary.
14. Dispose of equipment safely and appropriately.

6. To avoid excess blood loss.

7. It is important to dry the area to ensure that any tape adheres to the leg and holds the catheter in place, thus preventing movement and blood leakage.
8. To ensure patency of the catheter and prevent blood clot formation within it.
9. To ensure that the fluid infusion tube remains in place if the patient moves. Movement could cause it to become dislodged, resulting in blood loss.
10. To assess if the fluid is flowing freely. If the drip is not flowing, assess the reason and deal with it appropriately.
11. It is essential to control the rate of delivery of the fluid replacement to avoid over- or under-infusion.

12. This is to ensure accurate monitoring and clear communication between all veterinary personnel.
13. If patient mutilates area there is a risk of blood loss, sepsis and thrombosis.

14. It is essential that all items are disposed of correctly to avoid contamination and accidents.

PROCEDURE: INTRAVENOUS ACCESS TO THE SAPHENOUS VEIN AND ADMINISTRATION OF FLUID THERAPY

ACTION	RATIONALE
1. Select equipment and prepared fluid infusion. Prewarm the fluid to body temperature.	1. Prepare equipment in advance of restraining the patient. Maintain body temperature and minimise discomfort by prewarming the fluid.
2. Ask the assistant to restrain the patient in lateral recumbency, in the correct manner to allow access to the saphenous vein. Two assistants may be required to maintain the patient in the required position.	2. Firm handling will keep the patient at ease and reduce the risk of any accident. As the patient will need to be in lateral recumbency, a second assistant would be required to extend the hindlimb.
3. Wearing gloves, clip and prepare the site aseptically using surgical scrub and surgical spirit.	3. This will help to prevent infection.
4. Ask the assistant to raise the vein.	4. This dilates the vein, making it easier to see.
5. With gloved hands, insert the catheter tip into the vein. Once blood appears within the catheter, remove the needle and advance the catheter fully.	5. The needle is removed to prevent accidental puncture of the vein further along the lumen.
6. Ask the assistant to release the pressure over the vein. Place a bung or three-way tap to close over the end of the catheter.	6. To avoid excess blood loss.
7. Dry the area and secure the catheter to the leg with tapes.	7. It is important to dry the area to ensure that any tape adheres to the leg and holds the catheter in place, thus preventing movement and blood leakage.
8. Flush the catheter with a small amount of heparinised saline.	8. To ensure patency of the catheter and prevent blood clot formation within it.
9. Remove the cap from the infusion set and attach the infusion tube to the intravenous catheter. Secure the infusion tube to the patient's leg with tapes. Bandage if necessary.	9. To ensure that the fluid infusion tube remains in place if the patient moves. Movement could cause it to become dislodged resulting in blood loss.
10. Open the fluid flow control.	10. To assess if the fluid is flowing freely. If the drip is not flowing, assess the reason and deal with it appropriately.
11. Adjust the fluid control to the drip rate required for the patient. Syringe drivers and infusion pumps may be used to facilitate the delivery of the calculated drip rate.	11. It is essential to control the rate of delivery of the fluid replacement to avoid over- or underinfusion.
12. Record fluid type and drip rate on the hospital card.	12. To ensure accurate monitoring.
13. To prevent self-mutilation by the patient, bandage the area and apply an Elizabethan collar as necessary.	13. If patient mutilates area there is a risk of blood loss, sepsis and thrombosis.

ACTION	RATIONALE
14. Dispose of equipment safely and appropriately.	14. It is essential that all items are disposed of correctly to avoid contamination and accidents.

PROCEDURE: INTRAVENOUS ACCESS TO THE JUGULAR VEIN AND ADMINISTRATION OF FLUID THERAPY

ACTION

1. Select equipment and prepared fluid infusion. Prewarm fluid to body temperature.

2. Ask the assistant to restrain the patient in the correct manner to provide access to the jugular vein (see Ch. 1). Two assistants may be required to maintain the patient in the required position.

3. Wearing gloves, clip and prepare the site aseptically using surgical scrub and surgical spirit.

4. The vein will be raised by the operator by applying pressure at the base of the neck (see Ch. 1).

5. With gloved hands insert the catheter tip into the vein. Once blood appears in the catheter, remove the needle and advance the catheter fully.

6. Ask the assistant to release the pressure on the vein. Place a bung or three-way tap to close over the end of the catheter.

7. Dry the area and secure the catheter to the skin with the aid of adhesive tapes and bandage or suture in place.

8. Flush the catheter with a small amount of heparinised saline.

9. Remove the cap from the infusion set and attach the infusion tube to the intravenous catheter. Secure the infusion tube to the patient's neck with tapes. Bandage if necessary.

10. Open the fluid flow control.

11. Adjust the fluid control to the drip rate required for the patient. Syringe drivers and infusion pumps may be used to facilitate the delivery of the calculated drip rate.

RATIONALE

1. Prepare all equipment in advance of restraining the patient. Maintain body temperature and minimise discomfort by prewarming the fluid.

2. Firm handling will keep the patient at ease and reduce the risk of any accident.

3. This will help to prevent infection.

4. This dilates the vein, making it easier to see.

5. The needle is removed to prevent accidental puncture of the vein further along the lumen.

6. To avoid excess blood loss.

7. It is important to dry the area to ensure that any tape adheres to the skin holding the catheter in place. Accidental movement or displacement of the catheter from the jugular vein must be avoided, as blood loss could be considerable.

8. This maintains the patency of the catheter and prevents blood clot formation within it.

9. To ensure that the fluid infusion tube remains in place if the patient moves, thereby preventing dislodgement and blood loss.

10. To assess if the fluid is flowing freely. If the drip is not flowing, assess the reason and deal with it appropriately.

11. It is essential to control the rate of delivery of the fluid replacement to avoid over- or underinfusion.

12. Record fluid type and drip rate on the hospital card.

13. To prevent self-mutilation by the patient, bandage the area and apply an Elizabethan collar as necessary.

14. Dispose of equipment safely and appropriately.

12. This is to ensure accurate monitoring and clear communication between all veterinary personnel.

13. If the patient mutilates the area there is a risk of blood loss, sepsis and thrombosis.

14. It is essential that all items are disposed of correctly to avoid contamination and accidents.

PROCEDURE: CALCULATION OF FLUID DEFICIT AND MAINTENANCE REQUIREMENTS

Example. 20 kg dog that has been off food and water for 3 days and has been vomiting four times a day for the last 2 days.

Fluid choice. Colloid to replace or expand plasma volume, e.g Haemaccel or Gelofusine, followed by a crystalloid to replace remainder of deficit, e.g. 0.9% NaCl or Hartmann's solution, crystalloid to meet maintenance requirements, e.g. 0.18% NaCl + 4% dextrose.

ACTION

1. Calculate insensible losses × 3 days (25 ml/kg/24 h × 20 kg × 3) = 1500 ml.

2. Calculate sensible losses × 3 days (25 ml/kg/24 h × 20 kg × 1) = 500 ml.

3. Calculate loss from vomiting four times a day for 2 days (4 ml/kg/vomit × 20 × 4 × 2) = 640 ml.

4. Calculate total fluid deficit (all of the above factors added together) = 2640 ml, of which ECF deficit is 880 ml and 220 ml represents plasma volume.

5. This volume should be replaced over 24 hours, with half of the replacement being administered over 6–8 hours.

6. Meet ongoing losses/maintenance requirements at 50 ml/kg/24 h × 20 kg = 1250 ml/24 h.

7. Alternatively, calculate deficit from packed cell volume/haematocrit measurement = for every 1% rise in PCV allow for fluid deficit of 10 ml/kg.

RATIONALE

1. Insensible losses (respiratory, cutaneous, faecal) will initially continue in spite of the lack of fluid intake.

2. Sensible losses (urine) will be reduced by the lack of fluid intake, therefore calculation based on 1 day instead of 3 days.

3. Fluid loss from vomit can only be estimated but does need to be taken into account when calculating the total deficit.

4. This amount has been calculated by adding all of the above factors and represents the deficit only.

5. One-twelfth of the total deficit should be replaced with a plasma substitute as one-twelfth of the body fluid represents plasma volume (Fig. 4.1).

6. While the deficit needs to be replaced, water loss will continue due to body metabolism so it is essential to meet the ongoing maintenance requirements until the patient has recovered.

7. This can only be assessed if compared with PCV reading for a normal healthy patient.

PROCEDURE: CALCULATION OF DRIP RATE

Example. Daily maintenance for a 25 kg dog to be administered over an 8 hour period.

ACTION

1. Calculate the daily maintenance fluid requirements for a 25 kg dog at 50 ml/kg bodyweight/24 h = 1250 ml/24 h.

2. The above fluid is to be given over 8 hours. Calculate the volume of fluid to be given per hour = 156 ml/h.
3. Calculate the volume of fluid to be given per minute = 2.60 ml/min.

4. The infusion set delivers 20 drops/ml. Calculate the drops per minute—52 drops per minute.
5. Calculate the drops per second = 0.8 drop per second, or approximately 1 drop per second.

RATIONALE

1. Daily fluid requirement is a total of 50 ml/kg bodyweight to allow for 25 ml/kg bodyweight/24 h sensible losses and 25 ml/kg bodyweight/24 h insensible losses. The weight of the patient is multiplied by the millilitres of fluid for a 24 h period.
2. The calculation in step 1 is based on a 24 hour period. This is to be administered over an 8 hour period. Divide 1250 ml by 8.
3. The hourly rate is 156 ml. There are 60 minutes in 1 hour, therefore divide 156 ml by 60.
4. The volume in millilitres per minute is 2.60 and the infusion set delivers 20 drops per millilitre, therefore multiply 2.6 by 20.
5. 52 drops are to be delivered over 1 minute; there are 60 seconds in 1 minute, therefore divide 52 by 60 = 0.8.

PROCEDURE: MAINTENANCE OF INTRAVENOUS FLUID THERAPY— GENERAL MAINTENANCE

ACTION

1. Ensure the infusion site is kept clean. Avoid touching the barrel of the catheter or the site of insertion.
2. Replace dressings if they become soiled.

3. Check the catheter placement for any abnormalities such as redness, heat or swelling of the area.
4. Take the patient's temperature 3–4 times a day.

5. Flush the catheter at least twice daily with a small amount of heparinised saline.

RATIONALE

1. It is essential that the area is kept clean to avoid infection. Bandage the area where possible.
2. Any soiled dressings near to the infusion site dressing could introduce infection, so the dressings must be checked and changed regularly. Antibiotic or antiseptic cream can be applied to the site of catheter insertion to reduce the risk of infection.
3. The signs of infection include perivascular leakage and thrombus. A new catheter may have to be placed.
4. An increasing body temperature could indicate infection.
5. This is to ensure patency of the catheter. If resistance is experienced, assess the viability of the catheter and replace with a new catheter if necessary.

6. Check that fluid is flowing freely and at the correct drip rate.

6. Failure of the fluid to flow could mean that the catheter has moved or become blocked or there are problems with the infusion set or pump—all of which require immediate attention. Flush the catheter and assess the patency of the infusion set. If patency is not achieved, replace faulty or damaged equipment as necessary.

7. Check the patient's demeanour.

7. If the patient shows any change in its behaviour pattern and appears to be in discomfort, examine the infusion site for any problems. Stop the infusion and consult the veterinary surgeon.

8. Allow the patient to urinate by catheterisation, taking a dog for walks or providing litter trays for cats, and provide absorbent bedding.

8. To ensure the patient remains comfortable it must be allowed to urinate while receiving fluids. The method will depend on each individual case. Remember to measure the urine voided where possible.

PROCEDURE: MAINTENANCE OF FLUID THERAPY—REPLACING/CHANGING INTRAVENOUS FLUID BAGS

ACTION

1. Select and prepare equipment: correct fluid prewarmed, check expiry date, wash hands, wear gloves and apron.
2. Remove the new fluid bag from its outer wrapping. Identify the correct fluid outlet port and remove the cover, maintaining asepsis. Hang the new fluid bag on the patient's drip stand.
3. Ask the assistant to restrain the patient.

4. Switch off flow control on the infusion set connected to patient.

5. Holding the empty fluid bag at the base, carefully remove the infusion set and immediately insert the spike into the new fluid bag, taking care not to puncture the bag or contaminate the infusion.
6. Switch on the flow control to ensure that the fluid is flowing freely, and adjust to required drip rate.

RATIONALE

1. It is essential to make sure that all equipment is ready before the procedure to ensure efficient changing of fluid bags.
2. It is essential to identify the correct site to insert the infusion set to prevent damage or contamination. Placing the fluid bag on the drip stand will facilitate easy and efficient handling.
3. This is essential to avoid movement of the patient and risk of removal or contamination of equipment.
4. The infusion must be switched off before changing the bags to prevent any air entering the infusion tube.
5. Removal and reintroduction of the infusion set to a new bag needs to be swift to reduce the likelihood of contamination. Any contamination could result in infection entering the circulatory system.
6. It may be necessary to flush the patient's catheter after a fluid change as some backflow of blood into the catheter and infusion line may occur.

7. Record all details of fluid replacement.

8. Dispose of all equipment safely and appropriately and disinfect the area.

7. It is essential to keep accurate records to prevent under- or overinfusion of the patient.

8. It is essential for all areas to remain hygienic and equipment to be disposed of correctly to prevent infection and accidents.

PROCEDURE: MAINTENANCE OF FLUID THERAPY—REMOVAL OF INTRAVENOUS FLUID THERAPY EQUIPMENT FROM PATIENT

ACTION

1. Select and prepare equipment: tapes, swab, scissors, assistant, wash hands, wear gloves and apron.

2. Ask the assistant to restrain the patient.

3. Remove all tapes and sutures and terminate the flow by switching off the flow control.

4. Gently and quickly remove the catheter while the assistant applies pressure over the vein.

5. Maintain pressure on the site of catheter removal while placing a swab over the area. Secure with adhesive tape or bandage.

6. Dispose of all equipment safely and appropriately and disinfect the area.

RATIONALE

1. It is essential to ensure all equipment is ready before starting the procedure to ensure efficient and safe removal of the catheter from the vein.

2. It is essential that the patient is made to feel safe and any movement minimised to prevent discomfort or unnecessary haemorrhage during the procedure.

3. The infusion must be switched off before removal to prevent fluid leakage and contamination.

4. Removal of the catheter should be quick and efficient to ensure minimal discomfort to the patient.

5. Pressure must be exerted to prevent haemorrhage and haematoma formation. It may be necessary to apply sutures if a cut-down technique has been used for jugular access.

6. It is essential for all areas to remain hygienic and equipment to be disposed of correctly to prevent infection.

PROCEDURE: MONITORING OF FLUID THERAPY—GENERAL GUIDELINES

ACTION

1. Baseline parameters must be recorded prior to any fluid administration.

2. Monitoring must be performed at regular intervals and recorded on a fluid administration chart.

RATIONALE

1. It is essential to know the results of baseline tests in order to compare and assess the effectiveness of fluid administration.

2. Regular results will indicate a trend, which is more useful than a one-off measurement. Accuracy and regularity are essential requirements for effective monitoring. Everything must be recorded in writing to avoid error.

3. All deviations or abnormalities must be noted immediately.

3. It is essential that any abnormalities are reported immediately to the veterinary surgeon and acted upon to avoid further deterioration of, or complications in, the patient.

PROCEDURE: MONITORING FLUID THERAPY—ESSENTIAL PARAMETERS

Indications. All patients receiving fluids (Figs 4.5, 4.6).

ACTION

1. Pulse rate, rhythm and quality including core and peripheral pulses.

2. Mucous membrane colour and feel.

3. Capillary refill time.

4. Chest auscultation/respiratory rate and depth.

5. Peripheral oedema.
6. Body temperature—core and peripheral.

7. Urine output.

8. Skin turgor.

9. Bodyweight.

10. General demeanour/clinical observation.

RATIONALE

1. To check circulatory volume is adequate for tissue perfusion and to ensure circulation is the same throughout the body.

2. Check oxygenation levels are adequate: membranes will change colour. Check level of hydration by feel: membranes may feel moist, tacky or dry.

3. To assess effectiveness of circulating fluid volume: should be 1–2 seconds.

4. Should be clear lung sounds. Check to assess for any pulmonary oedema due to overinfusion or cardiac problems.

5. This could indicate overinfusion of fluid.
6. To assess vasoconstriction/vasodilation, and to check whether patient is suffering from a systemic infection.

7. Minimum output = 1 ml/kg/h. To assess renal function and associated circulatory volume. Less than 1 ml/kg/h could indicate renal problems due to insufficient circulatory volume.

8. To assess pliability of skin. Tenting can indicate dehydration.

9. To assess any change over a period of hours/days. Marked increase could indicate overinfusion.

10. Any sign of distress or discomfort could indicate a problem.

Patient I.D.

Clinical history

Species and breed

Age   Sex   Weight

Veterinary surgeon

Veterinary nurse

Monitor and record every .... daily

Date and time	T	P	R	MM CRT	Demeanour	Fluid type	Drip rate	Fluid input	Fluid/urine output	Weight	Medication	Comments

Figure 4.5 Example of a chart for monitoring patients receiving fluid therapy.

Name _____

Case number _____

Date and time	Fluid offered	Fluid intake	IV fluid	Drip rate

Figure 4.6 Example of a chart for monitoring fluid balance.

PROCEDURE: BLOOD COLLECTION FOR TRANSFUSION

Indications. Blood required for storage or by a recipient to replace acute or chronic haemorrhage; anaemia; clotting problems.

ACTION	RATIONALE
1. Select an appropriate donor.	1. Correct species and blood group.
2. Select equipment for blood collection: acid citrate/citrate dextrose blood collection bag, local anaesthetic, syringe, needle, clippers, surgical skin scrub solution, gloves, swabs, assistant.	2. Anticipation and preparation is essential for effective collection.
3. An assistant is needed to restrain the patient in a suitable position allowing access to the jugular vein. The patient is reassured throughout the procedure.	3. Firm restraint is required to make the donor feel safe and comfortable.
4. Clip a small area over the jugular vein and prepare the skin aseptically.	4. To reduce the risk of infection.
5. Local anaesthetic is infiltrated into the prepared site as instructed by the veterinary surgeon. Massage the area.	5. Local anaesthetic desensitises the area. The area is massaged to help absorption.
6. The needle attached to the donor blood bag is introduced by the veterinary surgeon into the jugular vein. Once blood flows into the donor bag the needle is advanced and held in place manually.	6. As collection is via a needle rather than a catheter, the needle needs to be held securely to prevent further puncture of the jugular vein resulting in considerable blood loss.
7. Hold the blood bag below the patient and roll it continually and gently.	7. Blood is collected by the action of gravity. The bag is rolled to ensure mixing of the acid citrate/citrate dextrose anticoagulant, thus preventing clotting.
8. Once the required volume of blood has been collected, the veterinary surgeon removes the needle and the assistant exerts pressure on the jugular puncture site.	8. To prevent further blood loss by providing back pressure, thereby arresting haemorrhage from the venepuncture site.
9. Fold over the blood collection tube to occlude it.	9. To avoid excess wastage within the tube.
10. If the blood is not to be administered immediately, store at 4–8°C for a maximum of 3 weeks. Label the bag clearly with the species and date of collection.	10. It is essential that blood products are stored correctly to avoid deterioration.
11. Dispose of equipment safely and appropriately.	11. It is essential to dispose of equipment correctly to avoid contamination and accidents.

PROCEDURE: BLOOD TRANSFUSION

Indications. Acute or chronic haemorrhage; acute or chronic anaemia; platelet and clotting problems.

ACTION

1. Select and prepare equipment: blood warmed to body temperature (if from storage), blood infusion set, adhesive tape, bandage, patient with intravenous catheter in place.

2. Remove the cover from the spike of the blood infusion set. Switch off the flow control and insert the spike into the correct port of the blood bag, taking care not to puncture the bag.

3. Squeeze both chambers of the blood infusion set to fill each with blood to one-third.

4. Remove the cap from the end of the infusion line and hold the line over kick bowl, taking care not to contaminate the tip.

5. Turn on the flow control switch to allow blood to travel down the infusion line to the tip in a controlled manner to remove all air bubbles.

6. Replace the cap on the infusion line and hang the infusion on a drip stand prior to connection to the patient.

7. Restrain the patient and ensure the patency of the catheter by flushing with a small amount of heparinised saline.

8. Remove the cap from the infusion line and attach the line to the intravenous catheter. Switch on the flow control to allow blood to flow into the patient.

9. When flowing freely, adjust the flow control to the required rate of transfusion.

10. Attach the infusion line securely to the patient by means of tapes, bandages or sutures (depending on which intravenous route has been chosen).

11. Monitor constantly for any signs of blood transfusion reaction and record details of

RATIONALE

1. Blood must be prewarmed prior to administration to maintain body temperature and cause minimal discomfort to the patient. All equipment must be prepared in advance of beginning the procedure to ensure efficient administration.

2. Puncturing the blood bag would result in a waste of blood and contamination of the bag, making it unsafe to use for transfusion.

3. The extra chamber within the blood infusion set provides a fibrin filter to collect any fibrin clots, preventing them entering the circulation.

4. It is essential to keep all items sterile.

5. To avoid risk of air embolism, all air bubbles must be removed from the infusion line before it is connected to the patient.

6. To ensure equipment remains aseptic.

7. It is essential to check the patency of the catheter before attachment to the blood infusion line to avoid unnecessary contamination or wastage of blood.

8. Connect and access patency. If not flowing freely, check equipment and reflush.

9. Rapid transfusion of blood should be avoided to prevent circulatory overload or reaction.

10. It is essential that the infusion line is secure to avoid displacement or leakage.

11. It is essential to keep accurate records and monitor constantly as any reaction to a

transfusion rate and time.

12. Dispose of equipment safely and appropriately.

blood transfusion is undesirable and requires immediate attention.

12. It is essential to dispose of all equipment correctly to avoid contamination and accidents.

PROCEDURE: MONITORING FOR BLOOD TRANSFUSION REACTIONS

Indications. All patients receiving blood transfusions.

ACTION

1. Assess baseline parameters before transfusion: temperature, pulse, respiration, mucous membrane colour, packed cell volume.
2. Continue to monitor patient parameters as above and record results.
3. Monitor the patient for any of the following signs: pyrexia, salivation, vomiting, diarrhoea, tachycardia, muscle tremors, facial oedema.
4. If any of the above signs are apparent, stop the infusion and inform the veterinary surgeon immediately.
5. Reassure the patient and make it comfortable.

RATIONALE

1. It is essential to obtain baseline parameters in order to identify any deviations from normal during the transfusion.
2. Immediate action is required if any signs of a reaction become apparent.
3. Any of these signs could indicate a transfusion reaction due to incompatibility or over-administration and requires immediate attention.
4. It is essential to stop the infusion if these signs are apparent to prevent further deterioration.
5. Patients can become disorientated and confused during a blood transfusion reaction and require reassurance to avoid undue stress.

FURTHER READING

Cooper B, Lane D R (eds) 1999 Veterinary Nursing, 2nd edn. Butterworth-Heinemann, Oxford

Houlton JEF and Taylor PM 1987 Trauma Management in the Dog and Cat. Wright, Bristol

Taylor RA and McGehee R 1995 Manual of Small Animal Postoperative Care. Williams and Wilkins, Baltimore

5

Provision of nutritional support

C. Bowden

Introduction

All animals must receive a balanced diet to maintain optimum levels of health. When an animal is ill, it may not want to eat or may not be able to eat, leading to deficiencies of certain vital nutrients and energy. These deficiencies will seriously slow down the rate of recovery and impair the healing process. Failure to consider some method of nutritional support may compromise the patient's chances of recovery.

When nursing the sick animal, consideration must be given to certain factors that differ from those in the healthy animal:

1. *Energy requirements.* A healthy animal needs energy for basic metabolism and for exercise. A sick animal will use much less energy in exercise but disease and stress increase the normal energy requirements.
2. *Type of food.* Sick animals often have a reduced desire to eat and thought must be given as to palatability and how to tempt them to eat. If the animal does eat, it may only eat small quantities, giving rise to the need to supply energy-dense food. In addition, the consistency must be considered in relation to the route of administration.
3. *Route of administration.* Nutritional support can be given by the enteral route, making use of the gastrointestinal tract, or by the parenteral route, providing nutrients intravenously. In some cases a patient may not be able to use part of the gastrointestinal tract, e.g. the oral cavity, and steps must be taken to bypass it using some form of feeding tube.

This chapter considers all these factors and describes in detail the techniques involved in placing feeding tubes and the nursing care needed to maintain them.

ENTERAL FEEDING

This is the administration of nutritional support using the gastrointestinal tract.

PROCEDURE: CALCULATION OF ENERGY NEEDS

ACTION

1. Calculate daily resting energy requirement (RER) for over 5 kg bodyweight:

   RER = (30 × kg) + 70 kcal.

   For example, to find the RER for a 10 kg dog:

   RER = (30 × 10) + 70
   = 300 + 70
   = 370 kcal/day.

2. Calculate daily RER for 5 kg bodyweight and under:

   RER = (60 × kg) + 70 kcal.

   For example, to find RER for a 3 kg cat:

   RER = (60 × 3) + 70
   = 180 + 70
   = 250 kcal/day.

3. Calculate illness energy requirement (IER) in relation to daily RER:
   - Hospitalised/cage rest = 1.2 × RER.
   - Surgery/trauma = 1.3–1.5 × RER.
   - Cancer/sepsis = 1.7 × RER.
   - Burns = 2 × RER.

RATIONALE

1. Kilocalories (kcal) is the measurement of energy value required to meet the metabolic needs of all patients. The RER is based on the metabolic energy needs of a patient at rest, including processes such as respiration, circulation and kidney function. Age, bodyweight and composition, and activity may affect it.

2. Animals under 5 kg have a faster metabolic rate, so require more energy per kg bodyweight compared with that needed by animals over 5 kg. This also applies to neonates, where the metabolic rate is greater than that of adults.

3. Illness and disease factors must be taken into account when feeding patients artificially. Stress and disease processes require an increase in energy to meet metabolic needs and counteract weight loss. The factors shown should be multiplied by the RER to give the kcal/day requirements.

PROCEDURE: CALCULATION OF FOOD QUANTITIES TO BE ADMINISTERED

ACTION

1. Calculate quantity of kcal to be fed to a hospitalised 10 kg dog.

   For example, a 10 kg dog requires 370 kcal/day at rest:

   = 370 (RER) × 1.2 (IER) for
   hospitalised patient
   = 444 kcal/day.

RATIONALE

1. It is essential to ascertain the energy requirement in kilocalories (kcal) before calculating the quantity of food in millilitres (ml).

2. Calculate the quantity of food in ml to be fed for a 10 kg hospitalised dog; food value 1.5 kcal/ml.

For example, the dog requires 444 kcal/day:

$$= 444 \text{ kcal} \div 1.5 \text{ kcal/ml}$$
$$= 296 \text{ ml/day}.$$

3. Divide quantity in ml into equal feeds to be administered throughout the day:
   - $296 \div 6 = 50$ ml per feed.
   - $296 \div 8 = 37$ ml per feed.
   - $296 \div 10 = 29$ ml per feed.

2. For artificial feeding it is important to choose a food that is energy dense, i.e. a small volume contains a large number of kcal. This will reduce the volume given, providing easier and more efficient administration.

3. Always divide the food quantity into equal workable amounts, depending on the method of artificial feeding. Consider the time available for feeding and each patient's needs. Avoid excessive quantities in single feeds to prevent discomfort, regurgitation or vomiting. Avoid small quantities that necessitate excessive handling and discomfort to the patient. Larger tubes, such as gastrotomy tubes, allow for larger quantities to be administered at each feed: calculations can be adjusted accordingly.

PROCEDURE: SELECTION OF FOOD FOR ENTERAL FEEDING

Indications. Aim to select a food with high-calorie density (at least 1 kcal/ml).

ACTION

1. Concentrated tinned food, e.g. recovery and convalescent diets.

2. Semi-solid foods.

3. Liquid complete foods.

RATIONALE

1. Forced feeding by hand, or for syringe and gastrotomy tube feeding. Not always easily liquidised, therefore unsuitable for smaller-bore tubes.

2. Syringe and all tube feeding. May require further liquidising for smaller-bore tubes to prevent blockage by food particles.

3. Suitable for syringe feeding, naso-oesophageal tube feeding, nasogastric and pharyngostomy tubes.

PROCEDURE: FORCED FEEDING—PLACING FOOD IN THE MOUTH

Indications. General inappetence due to change in environment, stress, underlying disease.

Food choice. Any proprietary complete balanced tinned food or energy-dense food; food of a high aroma is desirable.

ACTION

1. Select and prepare equipment: check expiry date of food, prewarm food, wash hands, damp swabs, towel, wear gloves and apron.

RATIONALE

1. Ensure all equipment is selected and prepared before beginning the procedure to allow for efficient administration.

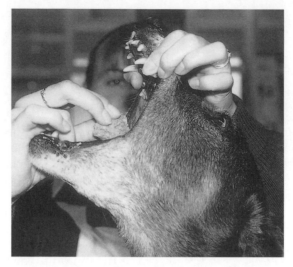

Figure 5.1 Placing food by hand directly into the oral cavity may encourage animals to begin eating after a period of illness or major surgery. Adapted, with permission, from *Veterinary Nursing*, p. 397, 2nd edn, by Lane and Cooper (1994). Butterworth Heinemann, UK.

2. Reassure the patient and ask the assistant to restrain the patient, holding the head in a normal position.

3. Take a small quantity of food. Open the patients mouth and place some food on the back of the tongue (Fig. 5.1).

4. Allow the patient to swallow and lick its lips, reassuring it throughout the procedure.
5. Repeat until the required amount of food has been administered.

6. Once all food has been administered, clean the patient's mouth with damp swabs and dry the area.
7. Record food administration and repeat at required intervals.
8. Dispose of equipment safely and appropriately.
9. Any food in tins must be covered and stored at 4–8°C between feeds.

2. Kind but firm handling will ensure the animal feels secure. Keeping the head in a normal position will reduce the risk of aspiration pneumonia.
3. Wear gloves to ensure hygiene is maintained. If the patient resents the procedure in any way, stop and offer reassurance before recommencing.
4. Encourage the patient to swallow by externally massaging the ventral pharynx.
5. If the patient becomes distressed before all the food has been administered, stop the procedure and allow the patient to calm down fully before starting again.
6. The mouth must be free of any food debris to discourage bacterial growth.
7. It is essential to keep accurate records of food administration to prevent any error.
8. This is essential to avoid contamination.

9. Food must be stored according to the manufacturer's instructions to avoid any loss of nutrients and subsequent deterioration of food quality.

PROCEDURE: FORCED FEEDING—BY SYRINGE

Indications. General inappetence due to underlying disease.

Food choice. Food of high calorific value, liquid consistency or easy to liquidise and feed with a syringe, e.g. proprietary convalescent foods.

ACTION

1. Select and prepare equipment: calculate energy requirements and food quantity; prewarmed food, catheter tip syringe, towel, assistant, wash hands, wear gloves and apron.
2. Measure correct volume of food into syringe.

3. Request assistance to hold the patient.
4. Support the patient's nose and mouth, keeping the head in a normal position.

5. Introduce the syringe into the mouth between the upper and lower premolars above the surface of the tongue.
6. Applying gentle pressure to the syringe, introduce approximately 10 ml of food into the mouth and allow the patient to swallow. Stroke the ventral aspect of the pharynx to encourage swallowing.
7. Continue with administration until the required volume has been delivered.

8. Clean and dry the patient's mouth thoroughly and replace the patient in its kennel.
9. Record food administered.

10. Dispose of equipment safely and appropriately. Clean and disinfect surface areas.

RATIONALE

1. It is essential to select and prepare all equipment before beginning the procedure to ensure efficient administration.

2. Accurately measure volume required based on calculation of energy/kcal needed.
3. Ensure the patient feels safe.
4. Firm but effective handling will ensure food is delivered safely. Keeping the head in a normal position will reduce the risk of aspiration pneumonia.
5. This area is the most suitable to aid administration and control food intake.

6. Avoid giving food quickly or in one bolus as this may cause choking. Allow the patient to swallow and breath between administrations.

7. Only continue if the patient is taking the food well and swallowing between administrations. If the patient gets distressed or fails to swallow, stop immediately.

8. Always ensure the mouth is free of any food debris and is dry, to discourage bacterial growth.
9. Accurate record-keeping is essential to avoid error.
10. It is essential to dispose of equipment correctly to avoid contamination.

PROCEDURE: NASO-OESOPHAGEAL AND NASOGASTRIC TUBE PLACEMENT AND TUBE FEEDING

Indications. Generally short-term tube feeding where there is failure to stimulate voluntary eating or a physical inability to eat. Use liquid foods only.

ACTION

1. Select and prepare equipment: naso-oesophageal or nasogastric tubes, water-soluble lubricant, speculum, pen torch, gloves, tissue glue or suture equipment, swabs, syringe and water, food prewarmed to room temperature, wash hands, wear gloves and apron.
2. Request an assistant to restrain the patient, supporting its head in a normal position. The patient will be conscious or mildly sedated.
3. Measure the distance from the external nares to the seventh rib space for a naso-oesophageal tube, and from the external nares to the tenth rib space for a nasogastric tube (Fig. 5.2). Mark the position on the tube.

RATIONALE

1. It is essential to prepare equipment before beginning the procedure to ensure efficient administration. Always prewarm food to at least room temperature as cold food can induce vomiting.

2. Firm handling makes the patient feel safe and facilitates the procedure. General anaesthesia is not normally used for placement of these tubes.
3. It is important to measure the distance before the procedure to check placement is correct.

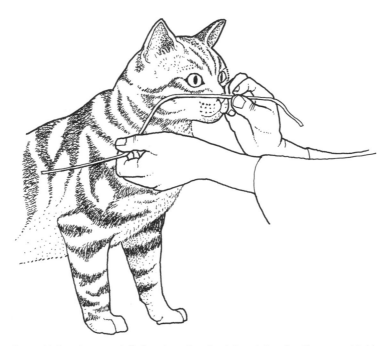

Figure 5.2 Naso-oesophageal tube placement. Before inserting the tube, determine the correct tubing length by measuring and marking the tube distance from the cat's mouth to the seventh or eighth rib (eighth or ninth rib for dogs).

4. Local anaesthetic gel or spray can be applied to the internal aspect of the nares (This is not necessary if the patient is anaesthetised.)
5. Lubricate the tip of the tube with water-soluble lubricant (avoid the use of petroleum jelly on silicone tubes).
6. The tube is introduced into the nasal cavity and advanced down the pharynx and oesophagus. In the case of a nasogastric tube, the tube is advanced to the caudal oesophagus.
7. Check for correct positioning by observing any coughing and by the introduction of up to 5 ml of water followed by auscultation for borborygmi. Once in place, occlude the end of the tube with a suitable bung.

8. Secure the exterior part of the tube to the patient's head with the aid of tissue glue or sutures over the nose and between the eyes.
9. Food may now be administered to the conscious patient (Fig. 5.3). If feeding is not to take place immediately, occlude the end of the tube with a bung and apply an Elizabethan collar.
10. Measure the correct volume of prewarmed food into a syringe, as calculated previously.

11. Remove the bung from the feeding tube and flush the tube with 3–10 ml of water.

12. Administer the food slowly (do not exceed 50 ml/kg/feed)

13. Flush tube with a further 5–10 ml water.

14. Replace the bung in the feeding tube.

15. Clean around the tube insertion site.

4. Local anaesthetic agents can be used to desensitise the nasal mucous membrane, reducing any discomfort.
5. This will allow for easy passage of the tube and minimal discomfort for the patient. Petroleum jelly reacts with silicone.
6. Nasogastric tube placement is preferred in some cases. The placement is more caudal than that of a naso-oesophageal tube, which reduces the risk of gastric reflux.
7. It is essential to ensure that the tube is placed correctly to prevent inhalation of food. Coughing and lack of borborygmi could indicate that the tube is in the trachea: the tube should be repositioned. The end of the tube must be occluded once in place to prevent excessive air being swallowed.
8. The remainder of the tube must be secured to prevent displacement.
9. It is essential to prevent patient interference, tube displacement and swallowing of air if the patient is not to be fed immediately.
10. It is important that the food quantity/energy requirements are calculated before the procedure, facilitating easy measurement at this point.
11. Flushing the tube will ensure it is patent. If resistance is experienced, repeat the procedure (carbonated water may be used in cases where food and mucus may be blocking the tube).
12. Rapid administration can lead to discomfort, regurgitation and vomiting and should therefore be avoided.
13. Water must be flushed after the food to ensure the tube is clear of any particles.
14. The bung must be replaced to prevent any leakage of fluid or food and prevent air being ingested.
15. It is essential to keep the tube insertion site clean. An antibiotic or antiseptic cream may be applied to the area to help moisturise it and to prevent infection.

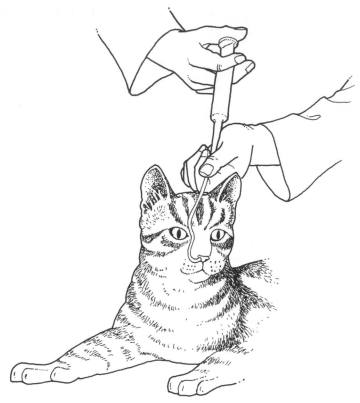

Figure 5.3 Naso-oesophageal tube feeding. Attach a syringe and instil 3 ml of water. Slowly administer food. After administration, flush with water to prevent blockage. Cap or cover tube opening. Adapted, with permission, from *Veterinary Nursing*, p. 602, 2nd edn, by Lane and Cooper (1994). Butterworth Heinemann, UK.

16. Apply an Elizabethan collar to the patient and return the patient to the kennel.
17. Follow the same feeding regimen for repeat feeds. Record all administration details.
18. Store any remaining food according to the manufacturer's instructions and dispose of all other equipment safely and appropriately.

16. Patient interference must be avoided to prevent displacement of the tube.
17. It is essential to keep accurate records to avoid any error in administration.
18. It is essential that any food is stored hygienically and equipment is disposed of correctly to avoid contamination.

PROCEDURE: PHARYNGOSTOMY TUBE PLACEMENT AND TUBE FEEDING

Indications. Short-term feeding where there is underlying disease or injury cranial to the pharynx. Used liquid diets or liquidised tinned food.

ACTION

1. Select and prepare equipment: pharyngostomy tube, clippers, surgical skin scrub solution, forceps, gloves, minor surgical kit and suture equipment, swabs, syringe and water, prewarmed food, wash hands, wear gloves and apron.

RATIONALE

1. It is essential to prepare equipment before beginning the procedure to ensure efficient administration. Food should be warmed to at least room temperature as cold food can induce vomiting.

2. The patient will be anaesthetised or sedated. Position in right lateral recumbency with the pharynx slightly elevated.

3. Measure the distance from the external nares to approximately the tenth rib space and mark the position on the tube.

4. Clip an area of approximately 6 cm × 6 cm lateral to and caudal to the angle of the jaw and prepare the skin aseptically. Drape the area.

5. The veterinary surgeon then places the pharyngostomy tube surgically (this may be aided by a specially designed introducer).

6. Correct positioning of the tube is checked by the introduction of 2–3 ml of water. Respiratory and gastric sounds are monitored. Once confirmed, occlude the end of the tube.

7. The tube is then sutured to the skin at the insertion site. Remove drapes and cover the tube with a sterile dressing and bandage (Fig. 5.4).

8. As placement is performed under general anaesthetic, do not administer food until the patient is fully conscious. Once conscious, request an assistant to restrain the patient in sternal recumbency, reassuring it throughout the procedure.

9. Measure the correct volume of prewarmed food into a syringe, as calculated previously.

10. Remove the bung from the feeding tube and flush the tube with 3–10 ml of water.

2. Correct positioning is essential to aid correct placement of the tube.

3. It is important to measure the distance before the procedure to check that the placement is correct.

4. It is essential to provide asepsis for surgical procedures.

5. This will allow for easy passage of the tube and minimal discomfort for the patient.

6. It is essential to ensure that the tube is placed correctly to prevent inhalation of food. The end of the tube must be occluded, once in place, to prevent excessive air travelling down the tube.

7. The remainder of the tube must be secured to prevent displacement, and a bandage placed over it to prevent patient interference.

8. Food must not be administered in the unconscious patient because of the absence of, or reduced, swallow and cough reflexes.

9. It is important that the food quantity/energy requirements are calculated before the procedure, facilitating easy measurement at this point.

10. Flushing the tube will ensure it is patent. If resistance is experienced, repeat the

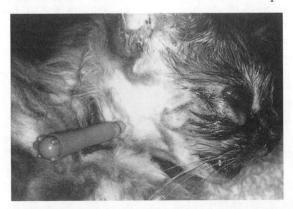

Figure 5.4 A pharyngostomy tube (placed under general anaesthesia) in a cat with a fractured jaw. Adapted, with permission, from *Veterinary Nursing*, 2nd edn, by Lane and Cooper (1994). Butterworth Heinemann, UK.

11. Administer the food slowly: do not exceed 50 ml/kg/feed.

12. Flush tube with a further 5–10 ml water.

13. Replace the bung in the feeding tube.

14. Clean around the tube insertion site.

15. Apply a dressing and light bandage to the area, being careful not to occlude the airway by excessive pressure. An Elizabethan collar may be used in some cases.

16. Repeat the procedure as required and record all food administration details.

17. Store any remaining food according to the manufacturer's instructions and dispose of all other equipment safely and appropriately.

procedure (carbonated water may be used in cases where food and mucus may be blocking the tube).

11. Rapid administration can lead to discomfort, regurgitation and vomiting and should therefore be avoided.

12. Water must be flushed after the food to ensure the tube is clear of any particles.

13. The bung must be replaced to prevent any leakage of fluid or food and prevent air being ingested.

14. It is essential to keep the tube insertion site clean. An antibiotic or antiseptic cream may be applied to the area to help moisturise it and prevent infection, as directed by the veterinary surgeon.

15. Patient interference must be avoided to prevent displacement of the tube.

16. It is essential to record accurately to prevent an error in administration.

17. It is essential that any food is stored hygienically and equipment is disposed of correctly to avoid contamination.

PROCEDURE: GASTROTOMY TUBE PLACEMENT AND TUBE FEEDING

Indications. Preferred method for longer-term feeding, underlying disease, surgery or trauma to the oesophagus. The tube can be left in place for several months; use liquidised foods.

ACTION

1. Select equipment: gastrotomy (mushroom-tipped) catheter, stylet and introducing equipment, clippers, surgical skin scrub solution, forceps, gloves, minor surgical kit and suture equipment, swabs, prewarmed food, wash hands, wear gloves and apron.

2. The patient will be anaesthetised. Position in right lateral recumbency. The tube may also be placed during a midline laparotomy; if so, the patient will be in dorsal recumbency.

3. Clip an area of approximately 15 cm × 15 cm on the lateral aspect of the patient, midway between the dorsal and ventral body surfaces and caudal to the costal arch. Prepare skin aseptically and drape the area.

RATIONALE

1. It is essential to prepare equipment before beginning the procedure to ensure efficient administration. Food should be warmed to at least room temperature as cold food can induce vomiting.

2. As the placement of this tube requires surgical intervention, a general anaesthetic is required. Correct positioning of the patient is essential to facilitate efficient preparation and tube placement.

3. It is essential to provide asepsis for surgical procedures, thereby reducing the risk of infection.

4. The veterinary surgeon places the gastrotomy tube surgically. This can be facilitated by a specially designed introducer or with the aid of an endoscope (percutaneous endoscopic gastrotomy, PEG).

5. Correct placing of the tube is checked by the introduction of 2–3 ml of water. Gastric sounds are monitored. Once confirmed, occlude the end of the tube.

6. The exterior part of the tube is secured to the patient's body wall by means of a suture or tissue glue. Remove drapes (Fig. 5.5).

7. As placement is performed under general anaesthetic, it is not advisable to administer food until the patient has regained consciousness. Once fully conscious, request an assistant to restrain the patient in sternal recumbency, reassuring it throughout the procedure. Apply a dressing and an abdominal bandage to cover the tube until food is administered.

4. This will allow for easy passage of the tube and minimal discomfort for the patient.

5. It is essential to ensure that the tube is placed correctly in the stomach and not between the visceral and parietal layers of the peritoneum. The end of the tube must be occluded, once in place, to prevent excessive air being ingested.

6. The remainder of the tube must be secured to prevent displacement.

7. Food must not be administered in the unconscious patient because of the inability to swallow or cough if gastric reflux occurs.

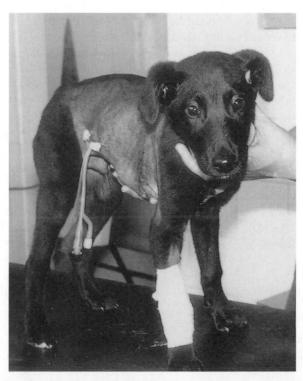

Figure 5.5   A gastrotomy tube in a 12-week-old puppy after removal of an oesophageal foreign body. Partial thickness oesophageal damage necessitated tube placement. Tube feeding (including all water requirements) was maintained for 5 days. Antibiotics were also given. Adopted, with permission, from *Veterinary Nursing*, 2nd edn, by Lane and Cooper (1994). Butterworth Heinemann, UK.

8. When ready to feed the patient, measure the correct volume of prewarmed food into a syringe, as calculated previously.

8. It is important that the food quantity/energy requirements are calculated before the procedure, facilitating easy measurement at this point.

9. Remove the bung from the feeding tube and flush the tube with 3–10 ml of water.

9. Flushing the tube will ensure it is patent. If resistance is experienced, repeat the procedure (carbonated water may be used in cases where food and mucus may be blocking the tube).

10. Administer the food slowly, as calculated previously. Larger quantities of food can be administered by this route; do not exceed 50 ml/kg/feed.

10. Rapid administration can lead to discomfort and vomiting and should therefore be avoided.

11. Flush the tube with a further 5–10 ml of water.

11. Water must be flushed after the food to ensure the tube is clear of any particles.

12. Replace the bung in the feeding tube.

12. The bung must be replaced to prevent any leakage of fluid or food and prevent air being ingested.

13. Clean around the tube insertion site.

13. It is essential to keep the tube insertion site clean. An antibiotic or antiseptic cream may be applied to the area to help moisturise it and to prevent infection, as directed by the veterinary surgeon.

14. Apply a dressing and an abdominal bandage to the area. Also apply an Elizabethan collar.

14. Patient interference must be avoided to prevent displacement of the tube.

15. Repeat the feeding regimen as required and record administration details.

15. It is essential to record accurately to prevent any error in administration.

16. Store any remaining food according to the manufacturer's instructions and dispose of all other equipment safely and appropriately.

16. It is essential that any food is stored hygienically and equipment is disposed of correctly to avoid contamination.

PROCEDURE: MAINTENANCE OF FEEDING TUBES

ACTION

1. Ensure tube and insertion site are clean and dry at all times.

RATIONALE

1. As the food being administered contains the ideal constituents for the growth of microorganisms, it is essential to remove any food leakage from the tube and surrounding area and to keep the area dry to prevent infection. Antiseptic and antibiotic creams may be applied to the skin at the tube insertion site under the direction of the veterinary surgeon.

2. Check the position and condition of the tube at least twice daily.

2. It is important to check tube position for signs of movement or displacement. The tube should also be checked for cracks or damage.

3. Flush the tube before and after administration of fluids.

3. Always flush the tube with water before the administration of food to ensure that the tube is not blocked. Always listen for any coughing or lack of borborygmi indicating that the tube has moved. If in doubt, do not continue and inform the veterinary surgeon. Always flush after feeding to ensure no food particles remain within the tube and cause a blockage later.

4. Ensure the tube remains occluded when not in use.

4. It is essential to occlude the tube when not in use to prevent unnecessary ingestion of air, leading to discomfort and distension in the patient.

5. Keep the tube area covered and free from patient interference.

5. It is essential to prevent patient interference, which may cause tube displacement. In the case of pharyngostomy and gastrotomy tubes it is advisable to cover with dressings and bandages.

6. Flush the mouth regularly with water and dry afterwards.

6. As any form of tube feeding excludes the mouth, it is essential to flush the mouth with water regularly to improve the patient's comfort.

7. When the tube is to be removed, remove all tapes and sutures. Pull the tube out gently but quickly while an assistant exerts pressure on the exit site. Sutures may be placed if necessary.

7. Tube removal is indicated if there are problems or if the animal begins to eat sufficient food voluntarily. Gastrotomy tubes should be left in place for at least 5 days to ensure adhesion of the stomach to the body wall. The procedure needs to be quick and efficient to produce minimal discomfort and reduce risk of aspiration of air or stomach contents.

8. Dispose of all equipment and disinfect the area.

8. It is essential to maintain a clean environment at all times, thereby reducing risk of infection.

PROCEDURE: MONITORING TECHNIQUES FOR ENTERAL FEEDING—GENERAL

ACTION

1. Baseline parameters must be recorded before any enteral feeding.

2. Monitoring must be performed at regular intervals and recorded on the feeding chart.

RATIONALE

1. It is essential to know the results of baseline tests in order to compare and assess the effectiveness of enteral feeding.

2. Regular results will indicate a trend, which is more useful than a one-off measurement. Accuracy and regularity are essential requirements for effective monitoring. Everything must be recorded in writing to avoid error.

Patient I.D.

Clinical history

Species and breed

Age | Sex | Weight

Veterinary surgeon

Veterinary nurse

Monitor and record every .... intervals daily

Date and time	T	P	R	MM CRT	Demeanour	Food administration	Type and rate	Food input	Fluid/urine output	Weight	Medication	Comments

A

Figure 5.6 A, B Examples of charts used for monitoring patients undergoing enteral feeding.

Small animal nutrition sheet

Client name	Admission date	Veterinary surgeon
Patient name	Age	
Sex	Weight	Veterinary nurse

Condition

emaciated	☐	....
underweight	☐	....
correct for breed	☐	Medical/surgical problems
overweight	☐	1. 3.
grossly obese	☐	2. 4.

Resting energy requirement (RER)

RER kcal/day: **Dogs** >5 kg = 30 x kg + 70
Cats/dogs 5 kg and under = 60 x kg + 70

Illness energy requirement (IER)

Cage rest/hospitalisation	1.2	× RER	☐
Post surgery/trauma	1.3–1.5	× RER	☐
Sepsis/cancer	1.7	× RER	☐
Head trauma/major burn	2	× RER	☐

RER =	kcal/day

IER = RER × ....

IER =	kcal/day

Dietary recommendations

Protein	☐	Fat	☐
Fibre	☐	Other	☐

Selected food ....

Calorific density ....

Amount to feed daily = $\dfrac{\text{IER}}{\text{Calorific density}}$ **OR**

Amount =	ml/day
Amount =	g/day

Food dosage and route

DAY 1

DAY 2

DAY 3

Plan

Continue diet for: 2 weeks   Post surgery
2–4 weeks   Trauma
4–12 weeks   Head trauma/burns
months   Chronic disease/neoplasia

Continue ....diet   for .... weeks

B

3. All deviations or abnormalities must be noted immediately.

3. It is essential that any abnormalities are reported immediately to the veterinary surgeon and acted upon to avoid further deterioration or complications for the patient.

PROCEDURE: MONITORING ENTERAL FEEDING—ESSENTIAL PARAMETERS

Indications. All patients receiving enteral nutrition (Fig. 5.6).

ACTION	RATIONALE
1. Temperature, pulse and respiration.	1. To identify infection or inflammation.
2. Bodyweight—measure daily.	2. To identify any large fluctuations that may indicate fluid imbalance.
3. Plasma glucose concentration— daily until stable.	3. To monitor blood glucose levels.
4. Urine output.	4. Minimum output = 1 ml/kg/h. To assess renal function and associated circulatory volume. Less than 1 ml/kg/h could indicate renal problems due to insufficient circulatory volume.
5. Urine glucose—every 6 hours until stable.	5. To identify hyperglycaemia.
6. General demeanour/clinical observation.	6. Any sign of distress or discomfort could indicate a problem.

PARENTERAL FEEDING

This is the administration of nutritional support by the intravenous route.

PROCEDURE: CALCULATION OF NUTRITION REQUIREMENTS AND SUGGESTED FEEDING REGIMEN

ACTION	RATIONALE
1. 10 kg patient with a septic condition requires 630 kcal/day.	1. RER × IER.
2. 4 g of protein are required per 100 kcal/ day = 25 g protein/day.	2. 630 kcal/day × 4 g protein/100 kcal.
3. 8.5% amino acid solution (AAS) available = 294 ml/day of 8.5% AAS.	3. 8.5% solution = 8.5 g in 100 ml. 25 g protein/day × 100 ÷ 8.5 = 294 ml.
4. 100% glucose provides 3.4 metabolisable kcal/g, therefore 50% solution = 1.7 kcal/g.	4. 100% solution = 100 g in 100 ml 50% solution = 50 g/100 ml (half of 100) 3.4 kcal/g in 100% 1.7 kcal/g in 50%.
5. 630 kcal energy are required = 370 ml/day of 50% glucose.	5. 630 kcal ÷ 1.7 kcal of 50% glucose solution = 370 ml.

6. The patient's energy needs can be met by feeding 370 ml of a glucose solution and 294 ml of an amino acid solution daily.
7. Electrolyte requirements are supplied by the amino acid solution.

8. Vitamin B complex should be given daily.
9. Continuous feeding may be achieved at an approximate rate of 30 ml/h.
10. The rate should start at 10 ml in the first hour, 20 ml in the second hour; 30 ml in third and subsequent hours. At completion of feeding the rate should decrease in a similar manner.

6. This will meet the patient's maintenance and illness requirements.

7. Further electrolyte solutions are unnecessary unless otherwise indicated by plasma electrolyte concentrations.
8. To meet maintenance requirements.
9. To meet total energy requirement over 24 hours.
10. It is essential to avoid rapid increases or decreases during parenteral feeding as this may cause hyperglycaemia, uraemia and shock.

PROCEDURE: INTRAVENOUS ACCESS TO JUGULAR VEIN AND ADMINISTRATION OF PARENTERAL NUTRITION

Indications. Where a patient cannot be fed enterally due to gastrointestinal disease, hepatitis, pancreatitis or intestinal obstruction. Such conditions require complete bowel rest.

Food choice. Proprietary solutions containing amino acids, glucose and lipids.

ACTION

1. Select and prepare equipment: intravenous jugular catheter, clippers, surgical skin scrub solution, prewarmed parenteral feeding solution and infusion set, suture equipment, local anaesthetic, bandage, wash hands, wear gloves and apron.
2. Ask an assistant to hold the patient in the correct manner allowing intravenous access to the jugular vein. Two assistants may be required to maintain the patient in the required position.
3. Wearing gloves, clip and prepare the site aseptically using surgical scrub and surgical spirit.
4. The assistant will raise the vein.
5. With gloved hands, insert the catheter tip into the vein. Once blood appears in the catheter, remove the needle and advance the catheter fully.
6. Ask the assistant to release the pressure on the vein and place a bung or three-way tap to occlude the end of the catheter.

RATIONALE

1. It is essential that equipment is prepared before beginning the procedure to ensure efficient administration.

2. Prewarm food for parenteral administration to prevent discomfort during administration and a subsequent drop in body temperature. Firm handling will keep the patient at ease and reduce the risk of any accident.
3. This will help to prevent infection.

4. To visualise the site.
5. The needle is removed to prevent accidental puncture of the vein further along the lumen.

6. To avoid excessive blood loss.

7. Dry the area and secure the catheter to the skin with the aid of adhesive tape or suture in place.

7. It is important to dry the area to ensure any tape adhesive sticks to the skin and holds the catheter in place. It is essential to avoid accidental movement or displacement of the catheter from the jugular vein, as blood loss could be considerable.

8. Flush the catheter with a small amount of heparinised saline.

8. This is to ensure patency of the catheter and prevent blood clot formation.

9. Remove cap from parenteral infusion set and attach infusion line to intravenous catheter. Secure infusion tube to neck region, bandage if necessary.

9. To ensure the parenteral food infusion line remains in place if the patient moves, thereby preventing dislodgement and blood loss.

10. Provide correct infusion of parenteral fluid in relation to the calculation of fluid and calorie requirements. Check that the fluid is flowing freely.

10. If the infusion is not flowing freely, look for the reason and deal with it appropriately.

11. Adjust the fluid control to the drip rate required for the patient. Syringe drivers and infusion pumps may be used to facilitate the delivery of the calculated flow rate.

11. It is essential to control the delivery of fluid replacement rate to avoid over- or under-infusion.

12. If the administration is not continuous, remove the parenteral infusion line and occlude the jugular catheter with a three-way tap. Flush the catheter with heparinised saline every 4 hours.

12. It is not always necessary to provide continuous parenteral fluids. Where feeding is intermittent, the catheter must be sealed and maintained aseptically.

13. Keep the catheter site clean and dry at all times.

13. As parenteral feeding solutions are composed of amino acids and glucose they provide the perfect environment for the growth of microorganisms, so a strict aseptic technique is essential.

14. Record the parenteral fluid administration rate on the hospital card. Repeat administration at required intervals.

14. This is to ensure accurate monitoring and clear communication to all veterinary personnel.

15. Prevent self-mutilation by the patient, bandage the area and apply an Elizabethan collar as necessary.

15. If the patient mutilates the area there is a risk of blood loss, sepsis and thrombosis.

16. Dispose of equipment safely and appropriately.

16. It is essential that all items are disposed of correctly to avoid contamination and accidents.

PROCEDURE: MONITORING TECHNIQUES FOR PARENTERAL FEEDING—GENERAL

ACTION

1. Baseline parameters must be recorded before any parenteral feeding.

2. Monitoring must be performed at regular intervals and recorded on the feeding chart.

3. All deviations or abnormalities must be noted immediately.

RATIONALE

1. It is essential to know the results of baseline tests in order to compare and assess the effectiveness of parenteral feeding.

2. Regular results will indicate a trend, which is more useful than a one-off measurement. Accuracy and regularity are essential requirements for effective monitoring. Everything must be recorded in writing to avoid error.

3. It is essential that any abnormalities are reported immediately to the veterinary surgeon and acted upon to avoid further deterioration of, or complications, to the patient.

PROCEDURE: MONITORING PARENTERAL FEEDING—ESSENTIAL PARAMETERS

Indications. All patients receiving parenteral nutrition. Administration of amino acids and glucose via intravenous routes require strict monitoring and aseptic technique due to an increased risk of infection (Fig. 5.6).

ACTION

1. Temperature, pulse and respiration.
2. Bodyweight—measured daily.

3. White blood cell count—twice weekly.
4. Plasma glucose concentration—taken daily until stable.
5. Plasma electrolytes.
6. Urine output.

7. Urine glucose—every 6 hours until stable.
8. Blood urea—as needed, particularly if it becomes elevated.
9. General demeanour/clinical observation.

RATIONALE

1. To identify infection or inflammation.
2. To identify any large fluctuations that may indicate food and fluid imbalance.
3. To identify infection or inflammation.
4. To control blood glucose levels and feeding regimens.
5. To identify any deviations.
6. Less than 1 ml/kg/h would indicate inadequate renal perfusion due to insufficient circulatory volume.
7. To identify hyperglycaemia.
8. Large increases suggest too-rapid administration of amino acids.
9. Any sign of distress or discomfort could indicate a problem.

FURTHER READING

Agar S 2001 Small Animal Nutrition. Butterworth-Heinemann, Oxford

Cooper B, Lane D R (eds) 1999 Veterinary Nursing, 2nd edn. Butterworth-Heinemann, Oxford

Houlton JEF and Taylor PM 1987 Trauma Management in the Dog and Cat. Wright, Bristol

Lewis, Morris and Hand 1987 Small Animal Clinical Nutrition, 3rd edn. Morris Marks, Topeka, KS

Taylor RA and McGehee R 1995 Manual of Small Animal Postoperative Care. Williams and Wilkins, Baltimore

6

Anaesthetic procedures

P. Millard

Introduction

Anaesthesia may be defined as the production of a reversible state of insensitivity. By using certain drugs designed to have an effect on the nervous system, anaesthesia may be general, i.e. the animal is unconscious and the entire nervous system is rendered insensitive to stimuli, or local, i.e. a small area is rendered insensitive to stimuli. Anaesthesia is used for the welfare of the animal, as it is obviously unpleasant for painful procedures to be performed on a fully sentient animal. It may also be used as a means of restraint, e.g. when using X-rays or if examining an aggressive animal; and, when properly managed, anaesthesia may significantly increase the chances of an animal's survival from an operation.

Local anaesthesia is most commonly used in large animal practice; however, it may be used in small animal practice for superficial surgery such as stitching a small skin wound, to aid diagnosis and in some cases to reduce the depth of general anaesthesia by desensitising a particular small area under treatment.

General anaesthesia is now a routine procedure in small animal practice and its use is becoming more common in exotic species (see Ch. 12). It can be achieved by the use of injectable agents, for which very little specific equipment is needed, or by the use of inhalational agents, i.e. gases or volatile liquids. The administration of inhalational agents requires the use of some expensive and complicated equipment and it is usually the job of the veterinary nurse to set up and maintain this equipment and to monitor the level of anaesthesia in the patient. It is vital that the veterinary nurse has a thorough understanding of the anaesthetic process if the patient is to survive the procedure and make a complete recovery.

This chapter describes all the procedures involved in preparing the anaesthetic equipment and in caring for the patient preoperatively, during the operation and postoperatively. It also describes the different types of circuits in common veterinary usage.

THE ANAESTHETIC MACHINE

Anaesthetic machines are designed to deliver accurate amounts of carrier gases and volatile liquids in a vapour form to the patient to produce anaesthesia (Fig. 6.1). Table 6.1 describes the parts of the anaesthetic machine.

PROCEDURE: CHECKING THE ANAESTHETIC MACHINE BEFORE USE

ACTION

1. Turn on the **spare** oxygen cylinder and check that it is full. It should read 137 bar.

RATIONALE

1. The contents of the spare cylinder must be noted to ensure a constant supply of oxygen throughout the anaesthetic.

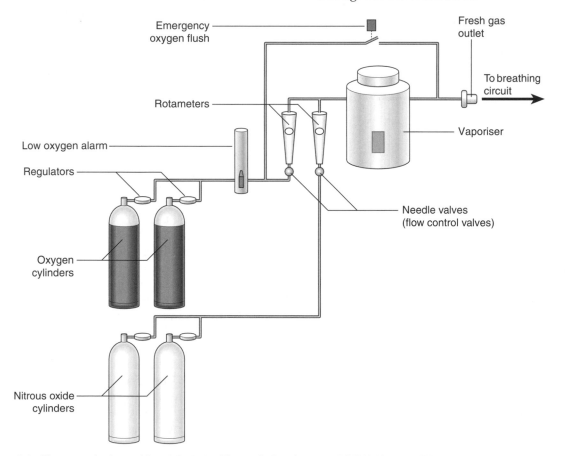

Figure 6.1 The anaesthetic machine. Adapted, with permission, from the *BSAVA Manual of Veterinary Nursing*, edited by M. Moore (1999). BSAVA, Gloucester.

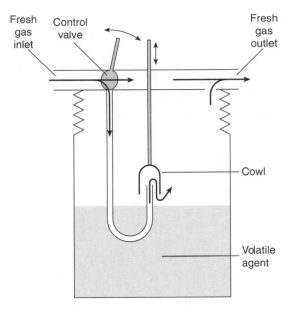

Figure 6.2 Boyle's bottle vaporiser. Adapted, with permission, from the *BSAVA Manual of Veterinary Nursing*, edited by M. Moore (1999). BSAVA, Gloucester.

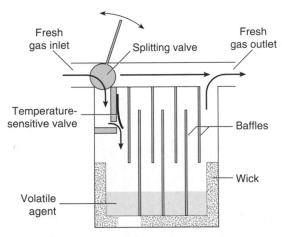

Figure 6.3 Tec and Penlon type vaporisers. Adapted, with permission, from the *BSAVA Manual of Veterinary Nursing*, edited by M. Moore (1999). BSAVA, Gloucester.

2. Turn the cylinder off and label it as full.

3. Turn on the **in-use** cylinder, check the contents and replace if necessary. Label it as in-use.

4. Repeat the process for the nitrous oxide cylinders.

2. If the current cylinder and the spare cylinder are both on, they will empty at the same time.

3. If the pressure reading is in the red area of the scale, the cylinder should be changed.

4. The spare, full cylinder should read 44 bar.

Table 6.1 Parts of the anaesthetic machine

Component	Description	Function
Gas supply	Oxygen cylinders are black with a white collar. Nitrous oxide cylinders are blue. Smaller cylinders, such as E and F, can be incorporated into the anaesthetic machine. Larger cylinders, J and G, may be kept separate and gas supply to the anaesthetic machine is through pipes in the wall	Supplies fresh oxygen and nitrous oxide to the patient
Pressure reducing valve or regulator	Usually incorporated into the yolk and is therefore impossible to identify	Reduces the pressure of the gas leaving the cylinder to ensure a constant flow to the anaesthetic machine regardless of the pressure changes within the cylinder. It provides a safe operating pressure for the machine
Pressure gauge	Usually attached to the anaesthetic machine. As the pressure in the cylinder falls, so does the pressure reading, indicating the amount of gas remaining in the tank. When using nitrous oxide, no pressure change will be seen until the cylinder is almost empty because the pressure does not fall until all the liquid has evaporated. This is not a reliable method for measuring the cylinder content of nitrous oxide: the cylinder should be weighed instead	Indicates the pressure of gas being delivered. It will read zero when the tank is empty or when the tank is switched off and the gas in the pipe evacuated
Flowmeters or rotameters	Consist of a tapered, glass tube with the flow rate written on it and either a glass ball or bobbin in the tube. Provided that the ball or bobbin can rotate freely within the tube, it will give an accurate reading of the gas flow rate A bobbin must be read from the top, a ball from the middle. Flowmeters are gas-specific and control knobs are usually colour coded: they should never be overtightened as the valve seat is easily damaged	Control and measure the flow of gas in litres per minute
Vaporisers: uncalibrated	The Boyle's bottle (Fig. 6.2) is an example of an uncalibrated vaporiser: while output can be varied, it fluctuates with temperature and gas flow changes	Deliver concentrations of volatile anaesthetic, in a vapour form, to the patient
Vaporisers: calibrated	The Tec and Penlon vaporisers (Fig. 6.3) are calibrated. They remain accurate despite temperature and gas flow changes. They are agent-specific	Deliver a known concentration of anaesthetic vapour to the patient
Back bar	Flowmeters and vaporisers can be attached to the backbar in series. This allows more than one volatile agent to be available. The 'Selectatec' manifold allows swift attachment or removal of Tec 3 and 4 vaporisers	Supports the flowmeters and vaporisers
Common gas outlet	Location varies between anaesthetic machines	Connects anaesthetic circuits, ventilators or oxygen supply devices to the machine
Oxygen flush valve	Oxygen reaches this valve swiftly, bypassing the vaporiser. High flow rates are produced. The valve may be locked open on some cases, by rotating it 90°	Provides oxygen in emergency situations and purges anaesthetic from the circuit before disconnection to minimise pollution
Low oxygen alarm	An alarm sounds, or in some cases a light flashes, when oxygen levels become dangerously low	Warns the anaesthetist of low oxygen levels

5. Check for leaking gas while turning on the cylinders.
6. Open and close the flowmeter valves.

7. Check the low oxygen alarm by turning the oxygen cylinder off and pressing the oxygen flush valve. Turn the oxygen back on.

8. Check that the correct vaporiser is fitted and that it is full.

9. Connect the correct circuit, having checked it carefully for faults.

10. Connect scavenging. Switch active systems on.

5. A faulty bodock seal can lead to gas leaks.

6. Ensure that the ball or bobbin can move and rotate freely in its cylinder.

7. The alarm should sound as the oxygen pressure falls to a dangerously low level. The flow of fresh gas through the oxygen flush valve is also confirmed.

8. The control valve should move freely. If more than one vaporiser is fitted, check each one, then ensure that only one of them is left on.

9. Leaks may result from disconnected inner tubes in coaxial circuits or from leaking reservoir bags.

10. Anaesthetic machines must not be used without some form of scavenging system.

PROCEDURE: SHUTTING DOWN THE ANAESTHETIC MACHINE

ACTION

1. Check contents of gas cylinders and remove any empty ones. Replace them with full cylinders.
2. Open the oxygen flowmeter and allow to flow at 2 l/min. Close the nitrous oxide cylinder and turn on the nitrous oxide flowmeter until the flow indicator has fallen to 0. Close the flowmeter control.
3. Turn the oxygen cylinder off and press the oxygen flush valve until no pressure reads on the pressure gauge.
4. Wipe the anaesthetic machine with disinfectant.

RATIONALE

1. To ensure that the machine is ready for the next use.

2. This will flush all nitrous oxide from the pipes. Any gas in the pipes could register when the flowmeter is switched on, implying that the cylinder is open.

3. All oxygen must be flushed from the pipes for the same reason as in step 2.

4. This minimises the risk of contamination.

PATIENT PREPARATION

PROCEDURE: PRE-ANAESTHETIC INSTRUCTIONS

ACTION

1. No food to be given for 12 hours before surgery.

2. Cats should be kept inside overnight with a litter tray until ready to go to the practice the next morning.
3. Dogs should be walked before admittance.

4. Cats must be brought to the surgery in a secure cage or basket. Dogs must wear a secure collar and a lead.
5. The client is given a time to arrive at the surgery.

RATIONALE

1. Animals that are not fasted may vomit as a result of the anaesthetic drugs. This may lead to fatal aspiration, as the swallowing reflex is reduced or lost during anaesthesia.
2. This prevents the cat from disappearing before being taken to the practice.

3. This allows the pet to urinate and defecate before going into a kennel.
4. To minimise the risk of escape.

5. This allows the nursing team to plan the surgery list and allow time for each patient to be admitted.

PROCEDURE: ADMITTING THE PATIENT

ACTION

1. Check that the patient is included on the operating list and confirm the procedure.
2. Take the client and pet into a consulting room.
3. Weigh the patient.

4. Obtain a complete history (Table 6.2).

5. Obtain a signature on the consent form (Fig. 6.4).

6. Obtain a contact phone number for the duration of the patient's stay.

7. Identify any lumps to be removed (if relevant).
8. Transfer the patient to a kennel, making sure the animal cannot escape on the way.

RATIONALE

1. A consent form should have been prepared if the patient is booked in for surgery.
2. This is more professional than dealing with the client in a busy waiting room.
3. The weight is essential for accurate administration of premedicant and induction drugs.
4. An accurate history is vital in order to evaluate the patient's anaesthetic risk.
5. The owner or agent of the patient must read, understand and sign the consent form. They must be over the age of 18 years.
6. It is vital to be able to contact the owner or an agent of the owner in the event of an emergency.
7. This will save time searching for them later.
8. It is best to ask the owner to leave before a dog is taken through so that the dog accompanies you more willingly.

Table 6.2 Questions to ask when obtaining a history

Question	Significance
1. How old is the pet?	This should be on the client records but should be checked: an older pet is a greater anaesthetic risk
2. When did the animal last eat?	If food has been consumed within 12 hours of surgery, there is an increased risk of vomiting during the anaesthetic
3. Has the animal had any previous illnesses and, if so, what treatment was given?	Client records should supplement this information; any condition involving the major body systems may increase the anaesthetic risk
4. Has the animal shown signs of any of the following in the past 24 hours: coughing, sneezing, vomiting, diarrhoea, anorexia; if so, how frequently and has the animal recovered?	The patient may be an increased anaesthetic risk due to dehydration, fever or electrolyte imbalance. It may also introduce pathogens to the environment
5. How well does the patient tolerate exercise?	Poor exercise tolerance may indicate cardiovascular or respiratory problems
6. Is the animal on any medication: if so, has it had any today?	Some drugs may alter the affects of the anaesthetic
7. Is there any history of allergies or drug reactions?	Prolonged recovery from a previous anaesthetic or anaphylactic reactions to any medication should be noted
8. When was the patient last vaccinated?	Up-to-date vaccinations should prevent the spread of contagious diseases
9. Is the patient entire or has it been spayed/castrated: if an entire female, is the animal in season or pregnant?	Particularly significant if the patient is in for ovariohysterectomy, as surgery time may be prolonged and there may be an increased risk of haemorrhage
10. Has the owner noticed any of the following: abnormal bleeding, bruising, fainting, seizures, dysuria, tenesmus?	The presence of any of these may indicate a serious illness

PROCEDURE: PRE-ANAESTHETIC CHECK—CARRIED OUT BY THE VETERINARY SURGEON

ACTION

1. Assess the function of the cardiovascular system using auscultation of the heart and palpation of the pulse. (For normal values see Table 2.1, p. 32.)
2. Assess the function of the respiratory system.
3. Palpate the abdomen.
4. Palpate superficial lymph nodes.
5. Take the body temperature (see Table 2.1, p. 32).
6. Check teeth, claws, ears, skin, coat, anal glands.
7. Check the sex of patients in for neutering.
8. Identify a cryptorchid patient before castration.

RATIONALE

1. The cardiovascular system is affected by anaesthesia. Note the heart rate and rhythm, abnormal heart or lung sounds, pulse rate and presence of a pulse deficit.
2. This is also affected by anaesthesia. Note the rate and any signs of dyspnoea.
3. This may detect the presence of an enlarged liver or abnormally small kidneys, either of which may lead to inefficient excretion of anaesthetic agents.
4. Enlarged lymph nodes may indicate the presence of infection, allergy or neoplasia.
5. Note any temperature outside the normal range.
6. The owner may wish to have any disorders corrected while the patient is anaesthetised.
7. It is far better to discover a mistake before surgery.
8. The owner can be informed of an increased fee in advance.

Name:

Address:

Contact telephone number today:

Species: Dog/Cat/Rabbit/Rodent/Bird/Reptile/Other

Pet's name: Breed: Age:

Sex: Male/Female Neutered: YES/NO Weight:

Insured: YES/NO Company: Microchipped: YES/NO

Vaccinated: YES/NO Wormed: YES/NO Treated for fleas: YES/NO

Procedure:

Pre-anaesthetic blood screen: YES/NO

Check teeth: YES/NO

Check claws: YES/NO

Any other comments:

Estimate:

I understand that payment is due at the time the animal is discharged.

Method of payment: Cash/Cheque/Credit/Debit card

I hereby give permission for the administration of an anaesthetic to the above animal and to the surgical procedure on this form, together with any other procedure that might prove necessary.

I understand that anaesthetic techniques and surgical procedures involve some risk to the animal.

I have read and understood the above statement: YES/NO

Signature of owner or authorised agent: Date:

Figure 6.4 An example of a consent form.

9. Assess pain, if relevant, before the administration of a premedicant.

10. Administer a premedicant.

9. Most premedicants contain an analgesic, which may mask signs of pain in conditions such as lameness, rendering further physical examination useless.

10. The premedicant may be administered by subcutaneous, intramuscular or intravenous injection, depending on the type of drug, speed of onset required and status of the patient (Table 6.3).

STAGES OF ANAESTHESIA

Anaesthesia is defined as a reversible state of unconsciousness. It may be considered to occur in two stages: induction and maintenance.

Induction

During the induction period, the patient passes from consciousness into unconsciousness. During this time the risk of cardiac arrest is increased and the whole process may be unpleasant for the patient. The signs displayed during induction or stage I of anaesthesia are described in Table 6.4. A smooth induction passes swiftly through stages I and II and the signs may be missed. However, when induction is via a mask or where a premedicant has not been administered, the signs are more obvious.

Induction may be carried out by intravenous or intramuscular injection, using one of the induction agents described in Table 6.5, or by using a mask and inhalation anaesthetic agent. The advantages and disadvantages of each method are discussed in Table 6.6.

Maintenance

During this period, the state of unconsciousness is maintained by the use of drugs, which may be given intravenously, intramuscularly or by the inhalational route. Inhalational agents are delivered to the patient by means of an endotracheal tube connected to an anaesthetic circuit and machine. The common inhalation agents are described in Table 6.7.

PROCEDURE: TO INTUBATE A PATIENT

After induction, an endotracheal tube (a breathing tube) may be placed in the patient's airway (intubation). This tube conducts anaesthetic gases and oxygen from the anaesthetic machine to the trachea and lungs, bypassing the nasal passages and pharynx. The patient must be sufficiently anaesthetised in order to carry out intubation. This is indicated by the following signs:

- The jaw is relaxed.
- The tongue can be held with no resistance.

- There is no gagging or swallowing reflex on introduction of the tube.

Equipment required. Selection of suitably sized cuffed tubes, lubricant to facilitate intubation, laryngoscope, local anaesthetic spray to prevent laryngeal spasm in cats, syringe or cuff inflator, stylet to aid difficult intubations, gauze bandage to tie tube in place.

Table 6.3 Common premedicant drugs

Premedicant	Family	Use	Warnings
Atropine	Anticholinergic	Traditionally used to counteract the hypersalivation caused when using ether. Used during dentistry to reduce salivation. Used to treat bradycardia during anaesthetic emergencies	
Acepromazine	Sedative/ataractic: phenothiazine	Calms the patient prior to induction. Used with opiate analgesics to produce neuroleptanalgesia	May cause seizures: avoid using in patients suffering from epilepsy or undergoing myelography. Boxers are very sensitive to the effects of acepromazine: use with caution at very low dose rates
Diazepam	Sedative/ataractic: benzodiazepine	Calms the patient prior to induction. Used as a premedicant for sick patients and to treat seizures. Can be combined with pethidine or morphine for optimum results	May not always cause sedation in animals: may cause excitement in fit, healthy dogs
Xylazine	Sedative: α_2-agonist	May be used on its own as a sedative for minor procedures. Can be used as a premedicant. Reduces the required dose of intravenous induction agent by 80%	α_2-Agonists have a profound effect on the cardiovascular system of dogs and cats. They cause extreme bradycardia. Use caution when using prior to intravenous induction agents: they increase the delay between injection of an intravenous agent and its effects being seen
Medetomidine	Sedative: α_2-agonist	As for xylazine. Atipamezole is the licensed reversal agent	As above
Pethidine Morphine Buprenorphine	Analgesic: opiod	Produce pain relief. If given prior to surgery, are more effective and lead to increased postsurgical analgesia	
Butorphanol	Analgesic	As above	
Carprofen	Analgesic	As above	

Table 6.4 Stages of anaesthesia

Stage	Signs	Suitable for
I: Voluntary excitement	Fear, apprehension, resists induction Becomes disorientated Increased pulse rate Increased respiratory rate Breath holding may occur Dilated pupil Possible salivation, vocalisation, defecation, urination All reflexes present, possibly exaggerated	Lasts from induction until the patient is unconscious
II: Involuntary excitement	Hyperactive cranial nerve activity Dilated pupil with eye central, then rotating ventromedially Swift pedal reflex Respiration irregular and gasping, then becoming regular	Begins with unconsciousness and lasts until breathing becomes rhythmic
III: Surgical anaesthesia	*Plane I* Deep, regular respiration Slight cardiovascular depression Swift pedal reflex Palpebral reflex slows Corneal reflex swift Eye rotated ventromedially Third eyelid moves across the corneal surface	Superficial skin surgery: wound suture, minor lumpectomy
	Plane II Heart rate and blood pressure slightly reduced Respiratory rate may be increased or decreased Pedal reflex slows then becomes absent Palpebral reflex slows then may become absent Corneal reflex continues Eye remains rotated ventromedially Marked muscle relaxation	Most surgery except laparotomy and thoracotomy
IV: Overdosage	*Plane III* Progressive respiratory failure Weak, thready pulse Eyeball central with dry corneal surface Pupils dilated Cyanosis Prolonged capillary refill time Accessory respiratory muscle activity leads to agonal gasping	To be avoided: may lead to prolonged recovery time. Can also cause cardiopulmonary depression, which in turn leads to poor organ perfusion. This can cause postoperative organ failure and ultimately result in cardiac arrest

Table 6.5 Common induction agents

Induction agent	Effects and use	Warnings
Pentobarbitone	A medium-acting barbiturate Slow onset of action Longer duration of anaesthesia Used to control status epilepticus At higher doses, used for humane euthanasia Produces approximately 30 minutes anaesthesia	Perivascular injection can cause severe skin reaction Recovery can take up to 18 hours in dogs, 72 hours in cats Excitement is sometimes seen on induction because the drug is slow to cross the blood–brain barrier It should be used with caution in weak or toxaemic patients
Thiopentone	A short-acting barbiturate 2.5% concentration available for small animals in a crystalline form made up with sterile water Recovery is mostly through redistribution of the drug into the patient's fat and not through metabolism Produces approximately 20 minutes anaesthesia	Perivascular injection can result in severe skin slough Reconstituted solution should be discarded after 24 hours Prolonged recovery in sight-hounds due to their limited fat stores It is cumulative and therefore cannot be used as a maintenance agent It should not be used in animals under 3 months of age
Methohexitone	A short-acting barbiturate Rapidly metabolised, therefore not as cumulative as thiopentone: small boluses may be administered as required to maintain anaesthesia Twice as potent as thiopentone Produces approximately 10 minutes anaesthesia	Perivascular injection can cause irritation A brief period of apnoea follows induction Reconstituted solution must be discarded after 24 hours Excitement is seen on recovery in patients that have not been premedicated
Alphaxalone and alphadolone	These two steroids are combined to form Saffan Can be given by intramuscular injection Licensed for cats, goats and ferrets Suitable for use in many exotic species Produces approximately 10 minutes anaesthesia	The steroids are contained in the solvent Cremophor EL, which causes severe anaphylaxis in dogs Causes histamine release in cats, which can lead to swelling of paws and ears Laryngeal oedema may occur in some cats Unsuitable for patients suffering from renal or hepatic abnormalities
Ketamine	A dissociative agent Produces mild anaesthesia with profound analgesia Combined with α_2-agonists, opiod analgesics and benzodiazepines to produce anaesthesia in cats, dogs, rabbits and small rodents Combined with α_2-agonists to induce horses	
Propofol	A substituted phenol Produces rapid induction when injected intravenously Rapidly metabolised in the liver and therefore not as cumulative as thiopentone: further increments may be administered as required to maintain anaesthesia Sight-hounds recover more quickly than when given thiopentone Produces approximately 15–20 minutes anaesthesia	Severe muscle twitches are sometimes seen after prolonged use A brief period of apnoea and a fall in blood pressure may be seen on induction Vials should be discarded once opened

Table 6.6 Methods of induction

Method	Advantages	Disadvantages
Mask induction A tightly fitting black rubber/clear plastic mask is placed on the animal's face; 100% oxygen is administered for 2–3 minutes to allow the patient to adjust to the mask. The anaesthetic concentration is then gradually introduced until it is 3–4%	The patient's airway is not damaged Induction is smooth when patients are depressed or heavily sedated Used for administering oxygen and inhalation agents when endotracheal intubation is not possible Useful for birds and small mammals	May be very distressing for the patient Masks increase the mechanical deadspace Atmospheric pollution is a significant hazard Airway obstruction can occur
Chamber induction The conscious patient is placed inside the chamber, which should be large enough for the animal to lie with its neck extended. Oxygen and the anaesthetic agent at a concentration of 4–5% is then delivered via an air inlet. The patient is removed when it loses its ability to stand	Induction chambers are useful for small mammals Ideal for uncooperative patients	Only suitable for small patients Risk of vomiting Cardiopulmonary function cannot be monitored Risk of atmospheric pollution
Intravenous induction The induction agent is injected into the cephalic vein over a 10–15 seconds period, as a 'bolus'; half the calculated dose is administered. If the patient is not sufficiently anaesthetised to allow intubation after 15–30 seconds a second dose is administered (one-fourth of the calculated dose). This is repeated until the required depth is reached	Smooth, rapid induction The induction agent can be given to effect so minimal quantities are used Most induction drugs can only be given intravenously	Patients must be well restrained Risk of perivascular injection, particularly with thiopental sodium
Intramuscular induction This method can only be used with certain drugs, such as ketamine/xylazine mixtures, neuroleptanalgesics and opiates. Recovery is usually prolonged	Technically easier than intravenous injection Useful in fractious patients when intravenous access is not possible	The patient is given the induction agent according to weight Cannot dose to effect so easily Slower onset

Table 6.7 Common inhalation agents

Inhalation agent	Properties	Effects and use	Warnings
Halothane	Relatively low solubility Colourless, volatile liquid Decomposed by light Contains the preservative thymol	Fairly rapid induction and recovery Modest muscle relaxation Poor analgesic	Sensitises the heart to adrenaline (epinephrine) and therefore may cause dysrhythmias Fall in cardiac output and subsequent hypotension Respiratory depression Lowered body temperature Up to 20% may be metabolised by the liver following retention in fat stores Thymol may cause the vaporiser settings to stick
Isoflurane	Very low solubility Colourless, volatile liquid No preservatives are required	Even more rapid induction and recovery Good muscle relaxation Poor analgesic Inhalation of choice for patients with cardiac, liver or kidney disease, and neonatal and geriatric patients	Little effect on cardiac output Respiratory depression Less than 0.2% may be metabolised by the liver due to the low fat solubility of isoflurane
Enflurane	Very similar to isoflurane	Very similar to isoflurane	Marked respiratory depression Induces seizure-like muscle spasms and should be avoided in epileptic patients
Methoxyflurane	High solubility Preservatives required	Slow induction and recovery Good muscle relaxation Considerable analgesia	Decreases cardiac output Marked respiratory depression Over 50% is metabolised by the liver and excreted through the kidneys Must not be used in patients given flunixin—it will lead to severe renal damage

ACTION

1. Select several endotracheal tubes of varying sizes and measure the required length against the patient's head and neck.
2. Inflate the cuff and check for excessive wear and the patency of the tube.

3. Lubricate the tube with sterile lubricant.

4. Restrain the patient in lateral or ventral recumbency.
5. Ask an assistant to extend the neck and hold the patient's head so that the nose is pointing upwards (Fig. 6.5).
6. Hold the upper jaw stationary while the tongue is pulled out and down so that it lies between the lower canines. Pull the lower jaw downwards by pulling the tongue down until the epiglottis can be clearly seen.
7. Using the selected tube, push the soft palate away dorsally if necessary. Push the epiglottis down with the tip of the tube and then insert the tube between the vocal folds into the trachea (Fig. 6.7).
8. If intubating a cat, spray a topical local anaesthetic on to the larynx and introduce the tube during inhalation, at which point the vocal folds are open.
9. In cats and brachycephalic breeds of dog, a laryngoscope is sometimes used to assist intubation.
10. The tube must not be introduced too far or endobronchial intubation may occur (Fig. 6.8).
11. Once the tube is inserted, confirm correct placement in the trachea (rather than the oesophagus) by ventilating the patient with 100% oxygen and applying pressure to the reservoir bag. Observe the movements of the chest wall.
12. Inflate the cuff of the tube just enough to prevent oxygen escaping around the cuff.

RATIONALE

1. This will enable the veterinary surgeon to select the one best suited for the patient and avoid excessive mechanical deadspace.
2. Rubber tubing can perish over time, causing malfunction of the cuff. If the cuff does not inflate, the anaesthetic gases may leak around it during anaesthesia and fluid and debris may be inhaled. Patency is essential for the delivery of oxygen and anaesthetic gases.
3. This allows smooth, atraumatic introduction of the tube.

6. In this position the visibility of the anatomy of the pharynx is maximised (Fig. 6.6).

7. The soft palate sometimes obscures the view of the epiglottis, which in turn covers the opening into the trachea.

8. The larynx of a cat is very sensitive so local anaesthetic is used to desensitise it, preventing laryngospasm.

9. The smooth blade of the handle enables the operator to move the epiglottis aside and the light source illuminates the pharyngeal area.
10. This results in the ventilation of only one lung.
11. Oesophageal intubation results in oxygen and anaesthetic gas being delivered to the stomach rather than the lungs. The stomach will inflate and the patient is unlikely to remain anaesthetised.

12. Overinflation can damage the tracheal mucosa or cause occlusion of the tube. Underinflation may enable the patient to breathe around the tube and foreign material may pass into the trachea.

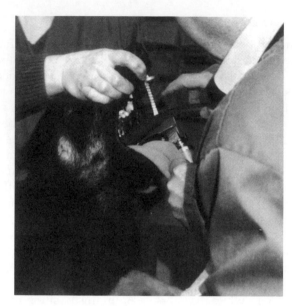

Figure 6.5 Position of an animal for intubation. Reproduced, with permission, from *Small Animal Anaesthesia* by McKelvey et al (1999). Mosby, UK.

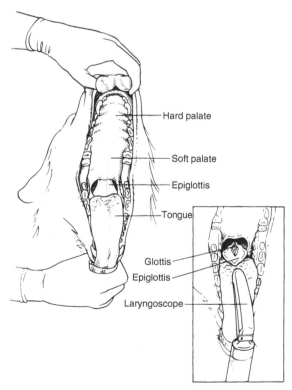

Figure 6.6 Anatomy of the pharynx. Inset: When the epiglottis is depressed, the glottis is exposed. The endotracheal tube is advanced through the glottis. Reproduced, with permission, from *Small Animal Anaesthesia* by McKelvey et al (1999). Mosby, UK.

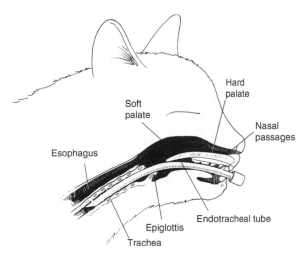

Figure 6.7   Intubation of a cat. The anatomy is illustrated. Reproduced, with permission, from *Small Animal Anaesthesia* by McKelvey et al (1999). Mosby, UK.

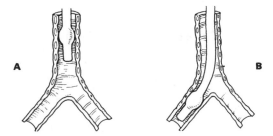

Figure 6.8   Placement of an endotracheal tube in the trachea: A, correct placement; B, endobronchial intubation (incorrect). Reproduced, with permission, from *Small Animal Anaesthesia* by McKelvey et al (1999). Mosby, UK.

13. To avoid accidental extubation, secure the tube in place using a piece of gauze bandage. This is tied around the end of the tube over the plastic connector, then secured over the mandible or the top of the patient's head with a quick-release bow.

13. The plastic connector will support the tube, preventing it from collapse when the tie is pulled tight. A quick-release fastening such as a bow is used for easy removal in an emergency.

PROCEDURE: TO REMOVE THE ENDOTRACHEAL TUBE—EXTUBATION

ACTION

1. Untie the piece of gauze bandage holding the endotracheal tube in place.

2. Deflate the cuff.

3. In dogs, the tube is left in place until the swallowing or gag reflex returns.

4. Cats should be extubated before the swallowing reflex returns. Signs of impending arousal include tail, limb or head movements or an active palpebral reflex.

RATIONALE

1. This is usually untied before signs of arousal are seen so the tube can be removed quickly when swallowing occurs.

2. Deflation of the cuff is essential, as an inflated cuff can easily damage the tracheal mucosa. After oral surgery, the cuff may be left partially inflated to dislodge debris and blood in the proximal trachea as the tube is withdrawn.

3. The swallowing reflex helps protect the animal from aspiration in the event of vomiting.

4. Delayed extubation may lead to laryngospasm.

PROCEDURE: CARE OF ENDOTRACHEAL TUBES

Care and maintenance of endotracheal tubes depends on the type of material of which the tube is made.

ACTION

1. Rinse the tubes in running water.

2. Soak in a detergent solution.
3. Scrub the tubes inside and out, using specialist brushes.
4. Thorough rinsing is essential.

5. Dry thoroughly and check for patency, cuff inflation and general wear. Discard any faulty tubes.
6. The method of sterilisation will depend on the type of material: red tubes should be sterilised using ethylene oxide but must be aired for at least 48 hours before use; polysiloxane tubes can be autoclaved.
7. Store the tubes in a dry, cool environment away from direct sunlight.

RATIONALE

1. Any debris and fluid that would otherwise deactivate the use of a detergent will be removed.
2. This will soften any residual debris.
3. All debris and mucus will be removed.

4. All traces of detergent must be removed to prevent chemical or ischaemic tracheitis.
5. This ensures that no animal is intubated with a faulty tube, which could compromise the anaesthetic or threaten the patient's life.
6. Heat causes red tubes to deteriorate, so they should not be autoclaved. Airing after sterilisation with ethylene oxide is essential to avoid chemical tracheitis.

7. Correct care and storage of endotracheal tubes will prolong their life.

ANAESTHETIC CIRCUITS

The anaesthetic circuit connects the patient to the anaesthetic machine. The most common circuits used today fall into two categories: rebreathing and non-rebreathing. All circuits have advantages and disadvantages, depending on the clinical situation, so it is recommended that a practice should have a range of circuits available for use.

Anaesthetic circuits have three functions:

- delivering oxygen and anaesthetic gases to the patient

- carrying carbon dioxide away from the patient
- removing potentially harmful gases from the operating theatre via a scavenging system.

CIRCUIT: JACKSON REES MODIFIED T-PIECE (NON-REBREATHING) (FIG. 6.9)

Equipment. 0.5 litre reservoir bag (open-ended if no pop-off valve), expiratory limb (corrugated tubing), inspiratory limb for fresh gas (narrow gauge plain tubing), pop-off valve (used with a closed bag).

No valves therefore little resistance to breathing.
A flow rate of 2.5–3 times the minute volume is required

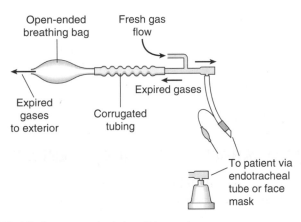

Figure 6.9 Jackson Rees modified T-piece anaesthetic breathing system.

ADVANTAGES

- Intermittent positive-pressure ventilation (IPPV) can be carried out.
- Bag movement acts as a respiratory monitor.
- Minimal apparatus deadspace and resistance.

Suitable for: small dogs (under 8 kg), cats, neonates and birds.

Flow rates: 2.5–3 × minute volume.

DISADVANTAGES

- High gas flow rates required.
- The incorporation of a pop-off valve increases resistance.
- Scavenging is difficult when an open bag is used.

CIRCUIT: MAGILL (NON-REBREATHING) (FIG. 6.10)

Equipment. 2 litre reservoir bag, corrugated tubing, expiratory (Heidbrink) valve, 2 × 'T' connectors.

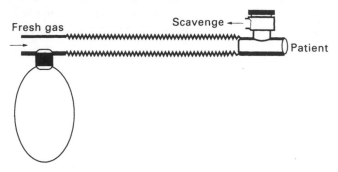

Figure 6.10 The Magill anaesthetic breathing system. Reproduced, with permission, from *Veterinary Nursing*, p. 618, 2nd edn, by Lane and Cooper (1994). Butterworth Heinemann, UK.

ADVANTAGES

- Efficient, general-purpose circuit.
- Readily maintained and sterilised.

DISADVANTAGES

- The location of the Heidbrink valve is inconvenient for scavenging and surgery around the head area.
- Cannot be used for prolonged IPPV because rebreathing will occur, causing hypercapnia.
- Offers considerable resistance and increased mechanical deadspace.

Suitable for: patients over 8 kg.

Flow rates: 1–1.5 × minute volume.

CIRCUIT: LACK AND PARALLEL LACK (NON-REBREATHING) (FIG. 6.11)

Equipment. 2 litre reservoir bag, coaxial tubing (outer inspiratory limb) or parallel corrugated tubing, expiratory valve.

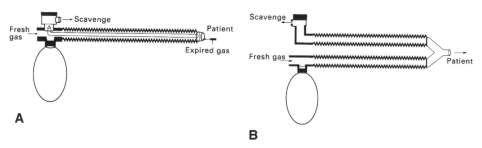

Figure 6.11 A, The Lack anaesthetic breathing system; B, the parallel Lack anaesthetic breathing system. Reproduced, with permission, from *Veterinary Nursing*, p. 618, 2nd edn, by Lane and Cooper (1994). Butterworth Heinemann, UK.

ADVANTAGES

- The valve position allows improved access to the head and to scavenging attachments.
- The length of the circuit (1.5 m) allows the anaesthetic machine to be positioned away from the patient.
- Lightweight, exerting less drag than the Magill circuit.

Suitable for: patients weighing 10–60 kg.

Flow rates: 1–1.5 × minute volume.

DISADVANTAGES

- Cannot be used for prolonged IPPV.
- The coaxial tubing may become disconnected, causing rebreathing.

CIRCUIT: BAIN (NON-REBREATHING) (FIG. 6.12)

Equipment. 2 litre reservoir bag, coaxial tubing (inner respiratory limb), expiratory valve.

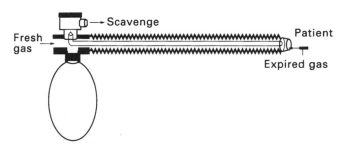

Figure 6.12 The Bain anaesthetic breathing system. Reproduced, with permission, from *Veterinary Nursing*, p. 619, 2nd edn, by Lane and Cooper (1994). Butterworth Heinemann, UK.

ADVANTAGES

- Can be used for continuous IPPV.
- The length of the circuit (1.8 m) improves access to the patient.
- The expired air passing through the outer tubing warms the inspired air, so conserving patient temperature.
- Low drag and reduced mechanical deadspace.

Suitable for: patients weighing 8–30 kg.

Flow rates: 2.5–3 × minute volume.

DISADVANTAGES

- Inner limb disconnection could cause rebreathing. This can be checked by plugging the end with a syringe while oxygen is flowing: the flowmeter indicator will fall if the tubing is connected.
- High flow rates are required.

CIRCUIT: TO AND FRO (REBREATHING) (FIG. 6.13)

Equipment. 2 litre rebreathing bag, Waters' canister containing soda lime, fresh gas inflow, expiratory valve.

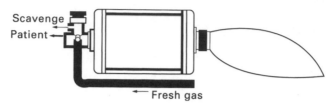

Figure 6.13 Horizontal to and fro anaesthetic breathing system. Reproduced, with permission, from Veterinary Nursing, p. 617, 2nd edn, by Lane and Cooper (1994). Butterworth Heinemann, UK.

ADVANTAGES

- Greater heat conservation (although hyperthermia may occur with prolonged use).
- Bidirectional flow improves the removal of carbon dioxide.
- As there is a low circuit volume, denitrogenation is achieved rapidly and gas concentrations can be altered quickly.
- High gas efficiency.
- IPPV can be carried out.
- Inexpensive (compared with a circle system)

Suitable for: patients weighing over 15 kg.

Flow rates: there is no circuit factor for the to and fro system and minute volume is not required. The flow rate is 10 ml × kg per minute.

DISADVANTAGES

- Channelling may occur if the soda lime does not completely fill the canister.
- Mechanical deadspace increases during surgery as the soda lime is exhausted.
- Bronchiolitis may occur as a result of aspiration of alkaline dust from the soda lime. This can be minimised by placing a gauze filter at the patient end of the canister.
- Sited close to the patient, which may be inconvenient during head surgery.
- Bulky and can cause considerable drag on the tubing.
- Cannot use nitrous oxide in the mixture.

CIRCUIT: CIRCLE SYSTEM (REBREATHING) (FIG. 6.14)

Equipment. Fresh gas inflow inlet, inspiratory and expiratory one-way valves (unidirectional), 'Y' connector to patient, pressure relief valve incorporating scavenging equipment, rebreathing bag, soda lime canister.

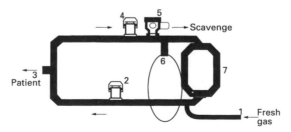

Figure 6.14 Circle anaesthetic breathing system. Reproduced, with permission, from *Veterinary Nursing*, p. 616, 2nd edn, by Lane and Cooper (1994). Butterworth Heinemann, UK.

ADVANTAGES

- Mechanical deadspace remains unchanged during surgery.
- Bronchiolitis is unlikely because the soda lime canister is much further away from the patient.
- High gas efficiency.
- IPPV can be carried out.
- Less circuit inertia than with the to and fro system.

Suitable for: patients weighing over 15 kg.

Flow rates: there is no circuit factor for the circle system and minute volume is not required.
The flow rate is 10 ml × kg per minute.

DISADVANTAGES

- Expensive.
- High resistance.
- Cannot use nitrous oxide.
- Complex, bulky and difficult to clean.

PROCEDURE: REPLACING SODA LIME

Soda lime is used to absorb the carbon dioxide formed in rebreathing circuits such as the circle system and the to and fro system. It consists of:

- 80% sodium hydroxide ('soda')
- 18% calcium hydroxide ('lime')
- silicates—help to bind the soda lime and reduce the formation of irritant dust.

- pH indicators—change colour as the soda lime becomes exhausted (either pink to white or white to lilac).

ACTION

1. Put on protective clothing, including gloves, apron and goggles. A mask may also be used.

2. Follow the manufacturer's instructions when filling the canister in a circle system.
3. The soda lime canister must be filled completely: do not try to save soda lime by partial filling.

4. Compact the soda lime tightly in the Waters' canister of the to and fro circuit.

RATIONALE

1. Soda lime is caustic and must be handled with caution. A mask will reduce inhalation of dust.
2. Circle systems vary: some canisters are designed to be used once only.
3. The removal of carbon dioxide depends on the exhaled air being in close contact with the soda lime during the expiratory pause. If there is insufficient soda lime, the exhaled air will pass straight through the canister.
4. Exhaled gas may pass over the top of the soda lime (channelling) if it does not completely fill the canister. This may result in hypercapnia.

CALCULATING ANAESTHETIC GAS FLOW RATES

An accurate flow rate should be calculated for each anaesthetic procedure to prevent hypoxia and hypercapnia and to ensure that the patient remains anaesthetised. Several factors must be taken into account when calculating flow rates, including the patient's tidal volume and respiratory rate and the circuit being used:

- *Respiratory rate* is the number of breaths taken per minute.
- *Tidal volume* is the amount of gas passing into and out of the lungs in each respiratory cycle. It is estimated as follows:

  Cats/small dogs = 15 ml/kg
  Medium/large dogs = 10 ml/kg.

- *Minute volume* is the amount of gas passing into and out of the lungs in 1 minute and is calculated from the tidal volume and respiratory rate of the patient:

  minute volume (ml/kg) = tidal volume × respiratory rate.

(Approximately 200 ml/kg/min using an average tidal volume of 10 ml/kg and an average respiratory rate of 20 breaths per minute.)

- *Circuit factors*—the factor by which the minute volume must be increased in order to prevent rebreathing (Table 6.8). These values are used to calculate the correct settings for the anaesthetic machine in relation to the particular patient.

1. Calculating the maintenance flow rate of anaesthetic gas to the patient

The formula is:

Bodyweight (kg) × tidal volume (ml) × respiratory rate (no. of breaths/min) × circuit factor = gas flow rate (ml/min).

Example:

The gas flow rate for a 30 kg labrador with a respiratory rate of 20 breaths/min on a Magill circuit would be calculated as follows:

30 kg × 10 ml × 20 breaths/min × 1–1.5 = 6000–9000 ml (6–9 litres)/min.

2. Combining gases

When nitrous oxide is used in a circuit, the amount of oxygen delivered to the patient is limited by the fact that in order to prevent hypoxia oxygen levels must **never** drop below 33% of the total inspired gas. Nitrous oxide is most effective as an analgesic when used at 66%. When calculating flow rates, a 2 : 1 ratio of nitrous oxide : oxygen is required.

Example:

A 12 kg spaniel with a respiratory rate of 20 breaths/min is connected to a parallel Lack circuit. Nitrous oxide is to be used. The formula is:

Table 6.8 Circuit factors

Type of circuit	Circuit factor
Jackson Rees modified T-piece (Ayr's)	2.5–3 × minute volume
Bain	2.5–3 × minute volume
Magill	1–1.5 × minute volume
Lack	1–1.5 × minute volume
To and fro—closed	No circuit factor: calculate flow rates using 10 ml/kg/min
Circle—closed	No circuit factor: calculate flow rates using 10 ml/kg/min
To and fro—partial rebreathing	No circuit factor: calculate flow rates using 25 ml/kg/min
Circle—partial rebreathing	No circuit factor: calculate flow rates using 25 ml/kg/min

Bodyweight (kg) × tidal volume (ml) × respiratory rate (breaths/min) × circuit factor = gas flow rate.

12 kg × 10 ml × 20 breaths/min × 1–1.5 = 2400–3600 ml (2.4–3.6 litres)/min

2400–3600 ml ÷ 3 = 800–1200 ml oxygen

800–1200 ml × 2 = 1600 ml–2400 ml nitrous oxide.

3. Circle and to and fro Circuits

A patient on either of these circuits is rebreathing the same gas continually so very low gas flow rates are required. Neither of these circuits has a circuit factor so the calculation of flow rate using the circuits as closed systems uses 10 ml/kg/min as the minimum oxygen requirement for an animal (Table 6.8). Flow rates of 25–50 ml/kg/min are recommended if using the circuits as partial rebreathing systems.

4. Induction

As a general rule, higher flow rates are used during induction. This is particularly important if a mask or induction chamber is being used, as a higher flow rate enables the gas and anaesthetic to saturate the anaesthetic circuit and dilute the patient's exhaled gases.

5. Recovery

Gas flow rates are increased at the end of an anaesthetic, once the vaporiser is turned off, in order to flush exhaled gas from the circuit.

Note: Monitoring anaesthesia. It is vital that the status of the central nervous and cardiopulmonary systems is monitored throughout anaesthesia at 5 minute intervals. All data should be recorded on anaesthetic monitoring records. In order to minimise cardiopulmonary depression, the animal should be maintained at a depth of anaesthesia that just prevents a response to surgery. Signs indicating the depth of anaesthesia are illustrated in Table 6.4. These should be used in conjunction with accurate monitoring using methods described in Tables 6.9–6.13.

Table 6.9 Methods of monitoring the patient during anaesthesia

Method	Used to measure	Description
Palpation of superficial arteries	Heart rate and rhythm Pulse quality	The arteries used in an anaesthetised animal are the femoral, lingual, facial, digital and coccygeal. Use of the peripheral arteries is recommended because they will be the first to indicate developing hypotension
Palpation of the apex beat	Heart rate and rhythm	Used in small mammals or when peripheral pulses are not palpable owing to hypotension
Auscultation	Heart rate and rhythm, myocardial contractility and valve action	Oesophageal stethoscopes are recommended because they remain in place throughout anaesthesia; the tip is positioned next to the heart
Electrocardiography	Heart rate and rhythm	ECGs demonstrate the electrical activity of the heart and show arrhythmias. They give no indication of cardiac output
Cardiac monitor	Heart rate	A simplified ECG that gives an audible bleep when it registers an 'R' wave
Pulsoximetry	Pulse rate and haemoglobin levels	The device is attached across the tongue and measures arterial oxygen saturation
Blood pressure monitors	Blood pressure	An inflatable cuff is placed on a limb proximal to the site of a distal artery. The cuff abolishes arterial blood flow distal to the cuff. As the cuff is deflated the returning blood flow is detected
Mucous membranes	Hypotension, perfusion, vasoconstriction, cyanosis, hypercapnia	Mucous membrane colour should be salmon pink and can be assessed by looking at the gingiva, conjunctiva, anus, vagina or penis
Capillary refill time (CRT)	Hypovolaemic shock, cardiovascular depression	A mucous membrane is blanched: the time taken to return to normal is the CRT
Respiratory monitors	Respiratory rate	Detect the difference between the inspired (cool) air and expired (warm) air. They do not register respiratory depth
Apnoea alert monitors	Apnoea	An alarm is triggered after a period of apnoea. The trigger period can be set by the operator
Temperature	Hypothermia	Feeling the patient's extremities and taking the rectal temperature will give an indication regarding peripheral circulation
Pedal reflex	Depth of anaesthesia	This reflex is caused by pinching in between the digits. It is usually lost by Stage III, Plane II
Palpebral reflex	Depth of anaesthesia	The eyelids will blink when the medial canthus is touched. It is usually lost during Stage III, Plane II
Corneal reflex	Anaesthetic overdose	The cornea is very sensitive and should only be tested as a last resort. If absent, anaesthetic overdose has occurred
Blood loss	Hypotension	Calculate the weight of a dry swab. The amount of blood loss can be calculated by weighing the blood-soaked swabs and subtracting their dry weight: 1 g = 1 ml
Saliva and tears	Anaesthetic depth	As anaesthetic depth increases, these secretions slow until they are absent

Table 6.10 Changes in respiratory pattern seen during anaesthesia

Term	Definition	Cause	Action
Bradypnoea	Below normal respiratory rate	Effects of the anaesthetic drugs Anaesthesia too deep	Lighten anaesthesia
Tachypnoea	Above normal respiratory rate	Anaesthetic insufficient Awareness of pain	Deepen anaesthesia Administer analgesics
Dyspnoea	Difficulty breathing	Obstruction in the thorax Obstruction of the anaesthetic circuit	Check that the patient has a patent airway Check circuit is attached: watch the bag for respiratory movements
Apnoea	Absence of respiration	Effects of some induction agents such as propofol, thiopentone and methohexitone Respiratory arrest	Check that the patient's airway is patent: check tube positioning and for blockage Perform IPPV with 100% oxygen at a rate of 20–30 breaths per minute

Table 6.11 Changes in heart rate seen during anaesthesia

Term	Definition	Cause	Action
Bradycardia	Heart rate lower than normal	Effects of drugs such as medetomidine and acepromazine Increasing depth of anaesthesia Illness	Monitor closely Lighten anaesthesia Administer atipamezole if necessary
Tachycardia	Heart rate higher than normal	Effects of drugs such as atropine and ketamine Insufficient anaesthesia Decreasing depth of anaesthesia	Monitor closely Deepen anaesthesia
No heart rate		Cardiac arrest	Thoracic massage at a rate of 60–80 compressions per minute Apply a compression bandage around the chest to increase venous return to the heart

Table 6.12 Changes in pulse rate seen during anaesthesia

Pulse	Cause	Action
Increased rate	Stress Pain Light anaesthesia Pyrexia Hypoxia Hypercapnia	Premedicate with ataractics such as acepromazine Administer analgesics Deepen anaesthesia Administer antipyretics Check oxygen flow rates Check that no rebreathing is occurring
Decreased rate	Anaesthesia too deep Systemic illness Effects of anaesthetic drugs such as medetomidine	Lighten anaesthesia Administer atipamezole if necessary
Weak, thready	Poor circulation: possible hypovolaemic shock Administration of α_2-agonists Peripheral venous constriction	Administer fluid therapy
Strong, jerky	Congenital heart defects: patent ductus arteriosus, pulmonary/aortic stenosis Malfunction of heart valves	Monitor closely

Table 6.13 Changes in the colour of mucous membranes seen during anaesthesia

Colour	Cause	Action
Pale	Hypovolaemic shock Hypotension Anaemia Haemorrhage	Administer fluid therapy
Cyanotic	Respiratory obstruction Cardiac arrest Administration of nitrous oxide with little or no oxygen	Check airway, breathing, circulation. Remove obstruction. Perform IPPV and thoracic massage as required Administer 100% oxygen
Icteric	Hepatic abnormalities	Monitor closely
Brick red	Carbon monoxide poisoning Toxaemia	Administer 100% oxygen

PATIENT RECOVERY

Once surgery has been completed, switch off the vaporiser and nitrous oxide.
Run 100% oxygen through to prevent hypoxia if nitrous oxide has been used.
The circuit should be flushed with oxygen before final disconnection
to avoid atmospheric pollution.

It is essential to monitor the patient closely throughout the recovery period: postoperative mortality occurs when attention relaxes. The patient should be placed in a warm, quiet, accessible kennel with emergency equipment close to hand. The length of time taken to recover depends on various factors, including:

- age of the patient
- health of the patient
- anaesthetic agent given
- length of the anaesthetic
- environmental and body temperatures.

PROCEDURE: CARE OF THE PATIENT DURING RECOVERY

ACTION

1. Monitor vital signs.

2. Keep the patient calm.

3. Keep orifices and surgical sites clean and dry.
4. Keep the patient warm.
5. Administer postoperative medication.

6. Prevent patient interference with wounds.

7. Assess the patient for postoperative discomfort.

RATIONALE

1. A change can be detected swiftly and acted upon immediately.

2. Excitement on recovery causes increased blood pressure, which may dislodge clots and cause haemorrhage.

3. To minimise the risk of contamination.
4. Hypothermia will delay recovery.
5. Analgesics should be administered before recovery begins, to maximise their effect.

6. Apply dressings, bandages or an Elizabethan collar as necessary.

7. If there are any signs of pain, such as vocalisation, panting, abnormal posture, dilated pupils or tachycardia, inform the veterinary surgeon immediately.

8. Monitor fluid and nutritional intake.

8. If the patient is on intravenous fluids, maintain at the given rate. Otherwise allow access to water and give a small amount of a recovery diet.

9. Allow the patient the opportunity to urinate and defecate.

9. Urinary catheterisation may be indicated if prolonged recovery is expected.

10. Discharge the animal.

10. This should only occur once the veterinary surgeon is satisfied that the patient has fully recovered.

PROCEDURE: DISCHARGING A PATIENT

ACTION

1. Make sure that all drugs, instructions and invoices are prepared in advance.

2. Take the client into a consulting room.

3. Give directions regarding feeding, exercise, medication, care of dressings, care of wounds, follow-up appointments, stitch removal and possible complications.

4. Make any follow-up appointments and take payment (if not already carried out).

5. Return the pet to its owner, making sure wounds are clean and no catheters are left in place.

RATIONALE

1. The reception staff can take payment and make follow-up appointments while the owner is waiting for a veterinary nurse or veterinary surgeon to speak to them.

2. This ensures privacy and minimal distraction.

3. Directions should be given verbally and backed up with written instructions to which the owner can refer at home.

4. The client should take this opportunity to ask any questions.

5. This should be the last step because the client will not take in any information once reunited with their pet!

ANAESTHETIC EMERGENCIES

An anaesthetic emergency is anything that poses a threat to the patient's life. Constant monitoring is essential to detect the early warning signs of a potential emergency, such as a gradual decrease in respiratory rate prior to respiratory arrest.

The outcome of an emergency depends on:

- correct preparation of an emergency kit
- early observation of warning signs
- correct assessment of the problem
- prompt action.

Table 6.14 describes the contents of an anaesthetic emergency kit, which should be regularly checked for out-of-date drugs and restocked. It should be kept near the theatre and be readily available. Table 6.15 lists possible emergencies and the action to be taken.

Table 6.14 Contents of an anaesthetic emergency kit

Contents	Reason	Indication
Adrenaline (epinephrine) 0.05–0.1 mg/kg	Increases the heart rate and the force of the contraction (therefore increasing cardiac output)	Cardiac arrest. Unresponsive hypotension
Atropine 0.02–0.05 mg/kg	Vagolytic	Bradycardia
Doxapram 5–10 mg/kg	Respiratory and central nervous system stimulant	Apnoea Respiratory arrest
Dobutamine 1–5 µg/kg/min	Increases the force of cardiac contractions	Hypotension
Lidocaine (lignocaine) Dogs 1–6 mg/kg Cats 0.25–1.0 mg/kg	Antidysrhythmic	Ventricular premature contractions and ventricular tachycardia
Naloxone 0.01–0.02 mg/kg	Narcotic antagonist	Reverse accidental overdose of Small Animal Immobilon, pethidine, fentanyl, morphine, etorphine
Dexamethasone 1–2 mg/kg	Anti-inflammatory	Treatment of shock
Atipamezole Dogs 0.05–0.2 mg/kg Cats 0.5 mg/kg	α_2-agonist antagonist	Reverse accidental overdose of medetomidine, xylazine and detomidine
Sodium bicarbonate 1.0 mmol/kg	Alkalitic	Treatment of metabolic acidosis
Tracheostomy tube	To perform emergency tracheostomy	Laryngeal/oropharyngeal obstruction
Syringes and needles	To administer drugs	
Intravenous catheters, giving set, tape	To administer intravenous fluids	Hypovolaemic shock
Swabs, surgical kit, dressing materials	To perform cardiac massage	Cardiac arrest

Table 6.15 Anaesthetic emergencies

Emergency	Signs	Action
Apnoea	Absence of breathing Irregular gasping with twitching neck muscles Spasmodic diaphragm contractions Dilated pupils Cyanosis No movement of reservoir bag	Administer 100% oxygen by IPPV Give respiratory stimulants (may have side-effects)
Airway obstruction	Non-productive respiratory effort Inspiratory snoring Cyanosis Eventual cardiac arrest	Locate and remove the obstruction If not possible, perform emergency tracheostomy Intubate and administer 100% oxygen by IPPV
Cardiac arrest	Agonal breathing Possibly respiratory arrest No femoral pulse Dilated pupils	Start cardiopulmonary resuscitation (CPR) (see Ch. 9)
Bradycardia	Very slow heart rate	Administer 100% oxygen Give vagolytic drugs such as atropine
Haemorrhage	Blood at surgical site Tachycardia Pale mucous membranes Increased CRT Weak, thready pulse	Administer fluid therapy: plasma volume expanders
Hypothermia	Cold extremities Low body temperature Bradycardia Pale mucous membranes Cardiac arrest	Minimise surgical time Keep patient as dry as possible Irrigate exposed viscera with warmed fluids Increase operating room temperature Insulate the patient to prevent further heat loss
Hypotension	Increased CRT Pale mucous membranes Weak pulse	Administer fluid therapy Give adrenaline (epinephrine) or dobutamine

SPECIALISED TECHNIQUES

Local anaesthesia

In practice, local anaesthetics are most commonly used in large animal work, but they may be used in small animal practice for the following:

- superficial surgery
- to facilitate certain procedures
- during surgery to reduce the depth of general anaesthesia
- as a means of diagnosis.

Local anaesthetics work by blocking local nerve transmission to the area, thus reducing sensation. Table 6.16 describes the local anaesthetic techniques in common use.

Muscle relaxation

Many drugs, including general anaesthetics, produce muscle relaxation to a certain degree; however, at times absolute relaxation is required and specific neuromuscular blocking agents are used. These act directly on the neuromuscular junction and stop the transmission of motor nerve impulses to striated muscle. They have no effect on smooth or cardiac muscle. They do not cross the blood–brain barrier and so do not alter consciousness. Neuromuscular blocking agents will eliminate some of the obvious signs of inadequate anaesthesia, such as movement, eye position and cranial nerve reflexes, so care must be taken to ensure that the depth of anaesthesia is appropriate to the procedure being undertaken.

Other signs of inadequate anaesthesia that are not affected by neuromuscular blocking agents include:

- mydriasis
- lacrimation
- salivation
- tachycardia
- hypertension.

When a muscle relaxant is used, the respiratory muscles are blocked and the patient is unable to breathe normally. Some means of supporting ventilation, such as IPPV, must be available and the patient should be intubated and connected to an anaesthetic machine.

The indications for the use of muscle relaxants are listed in Table 6.17; the common muscle relaxants are described in Table 6.18.

Table 6.16 Local anaesthetic techniques

Technique	Description	Use
Surface	Gels, ointments, sprays and drops, which are applied to the skin or mucous membranes	Drops can be applied to the eye to facilitate ocular examination Gel can be applied to urinary catheters and endotracheal tubes to facilitate placement Ointment can be applied to the skin prior to intravenous catheterisation Spray can be applied to the larynx in cats to prevent laryngeal spasm on endotracheal intubation
Infiltration	Injection of local anaesthetic along the line of surgical incision	Facilitates the suture of small skin wounds
Regional: perineural	Local anaesthetic is injected around the major nerves, which provide sensation to the operation site	Diagnosis of lameness by performing a nerve block Cornual nerve block used for disbudding calves
Regional: intravenous	A tourniquet is placed around a limb and local anaesthetic is injected intravenously, distal to the tourniquet. Results in good analgesia of the distal limb. Effective after 5 minutes and lasts until the tourniquet is removed	Surgery on the feet of cattle Occasionally used in limb surgery in dogs
Spinal: epidural	Local anaesthetic is injected into the space between the dura mater and the periosteum lining the spinal cord. It blocks nerves as they leave the spinal canal, resulting in loss of motor and sensory function	Used to provide muscle relaxation and pain relief during pelvic limb orthopaedic procedures and providing analgesia to the anus and perineum

Table 6.17 Indications for the use of muscle relaxants

Use	Description
Thoracic surgery	The intercostal muscles are thoroughly relaxed, minimising damage by rib retractors, which leads to less postsurgical pain. Access into the surgical site is made easier
Ophthalmic surgery	Muscle relaxants keep the eye in a central position throughout general anaesthesia, making corneal surgery possible
	There are no eye reflexes to disturb delicate eye surgery being carried out
High-risk cases	The amount of general anaesthetic required is reduced when muscle relaxants are used, which in turn reduces the degree of cardiovascular depression
Oesophageal foreign bodies	The striated muscle of the oesophagus of the dog is completely relaxed, which makes the removal of an oesophageal foreign body easier
Orthopaedic surgery	Reduction of dislocations is eased when muscle relaxants have been administered

Table 6.18 Common muscle relaxants

Drug	Effects	Warnings
Depolarising		
Suxamethonium	Very short acting	Evidence of muscle pain on recovery
Non-depolarising		
Pancuronium	Long duration of action	Causes modest tachycardia
		Cumulative so cannot be topped up
Vercuronium	Intermediate duration of action (20–30 minutes) Non-cumulative Has little cardiovascular effect	
Atracurium	Rapid onset Intermediate duration of action (30–40 minutes) Breaks down spontaneously in the body, can therefore be used in animals with poor liver and kidney function	Inactivated by thiopentone and other alkaline solutions, so thoroughly flush catheters before administration

CONTROL OF POLLUTION—SCAVENGING

Anaesthetic gases must be scavenged from the anaesthetic system to avoid atmospheric pollution and potential damage to in-contact theatre personnel. Disorders such as malignancies, abortion and infertility, and liver damage have been linked to exposure to the gases. Under the COSHH (Control of Substances Hazardous to Health) regulations, an employer must assess the risk of exposure and take appropriate action to protect employees.

Scavenging can be achieved in two ways: active scavenging and passive scavenging. In both cases a scavenge tube is connected to the expiratory valve, pressure relief valve or expiratory limb of an anaesthetic circuit to conduct waste gases away from the theatre to a safe site.

Active scavenging

Gas is drawn along the scavenge tube by negative pressure generated by an extractor fan. An air-brake receiver prevents the fan exerting negative pressure on the anaesthetic circuit and it also allows several systems to be scavenged from one extraction unit.

Passive scavenging

Passive systems either direct the gas into an activated charcoal canister or pass it straight to the air outside the building through ducts in the wall. These systems rely on the combined effects of gas flowing into the anaesthetic circuit, expiratory effort and elastic recoil from the reservoir bag to propel the gas along the tubing. The scavenge tube must not be excessively long or it will offer too much resistance to expiration. Activated charcoal canisters do not absorb nitrous oxide. They must be weighed frequently in order to assess when they are saturated.

FURTHER READING

Cooper B, Lane DR (eds) 1999 Veterinary Nursing, 2nd edn. Butterworth-Heinemann, Oxford.

McKelvey D, Hollingshead KW 1994 Small Animal Anaesthesia. Mosby, London

Moore M (ed.) 1999 Manual of Veterinary Nursing. BSAVA, Gloucester

Simpson G (ed.) 1991 Practical Veterinary Nursing. BSAVA, Gloucester

7

Theatre practice
P. Millard

Introduction

The management and maintenance of the theatre environment is of prime importance in a situation where patients, already weakened by their existing condition, are further subjected to procedures that may be painful, bewildering and traumatic.

The main focus in running an efficient operating theatre is on maintaining a good aseptic technique. This must be applied not only to the more obvious care of instruments, preparation of the surgical site and to scrubbing-up techniques, but also to the daily routine of maintaining the hygiene of the theatre and associated preparation areas and to the personal hygiene of all who work in the area. It takes very little upset in any of the procedures to compromise asepsis and introduce infection, which could in turn lead to wound breakdown, systemic infection, reduced surgical success rate and inevitably an effect on the reputation of the practice.

It is usually the responsibility of the veterinary nurse to organise all matters concerned with the operating theatre and its efficient function and it is to the nurse and her management routines that the veterinary surgeon will turn if things go wrong.

STERILISATION

Sterilisation can be defined as the process by which instruments and drapes are rendered aseptic (or sterile) by the destruction or removal of all microorganisms, including spores. This can be achieved by various methods, including:

- heat sterilisation: hot-air oven, autoclave
- cold sterilisation: ethylene oxide, radiation.

Boiling cannot be considered to be a method of sterilisation because it does not reach a high enough temperature to destroy bacterial spores.

Chemical solutions based on chlorhexidine or gluteraldehyde will kill bacteria if items are soaked in them. It may be used for surgical equipment that cannot be sterilised using any other method; however, it should only really be considered to be a method of disinfection.

Hot-air oven

Hot-air ovens produce a dry heat. Microorganisms are more resistant to dry heat so high working temperatures are required for a long period of time (Table 7.1). Long cooling periods are also required and the very high temperatures may damage metal items. A safety device should be fitted to the door to prevent accidental opening before the oven is cool. Care should be taken not to overload the oven, as air will be unable to circulate freely.

Use is limited by the long period of time required for sterilisation and cooling; however, hot-air ovens are useful for items damaged by moist heat, such as glassware, powders, oils and sharp cutting instruments.

Autoclave

This is the most common method of sterilisation used in veterinary practice. In normal circumstances, water cannot reach temperatures greater than 100°C (boiling point) before producing steam. If water is boiled under pressure, the boiling point is raised so the temperature of the steam is greater. This steam produces heat, which penetrates to the innermost layer of the packs. The moisture increases the permeability of the heat. Care should be taken to avoid overloading or blocking the inlet and outlet valves. Items to be autoclaved should be free from grease and protein in order to achieve effective penetration of steam.

The majority of autoclaves designed for modern veterinary practice incorporate a drying cycle. Steam is exhausted and replaced by filtered air which heat-dries the packs (Table 7.2).

Table 7.1 Hot-air ovens: working temperature and time ratios

Item	Temperature (°C)	Time (min)
Glassware and non-cutting instruments	180	60
Powders and oils	160	120
Sharp, cutting instruments	150	180

Table 7.2 Autoclaves: working temperature, time and pressure ratios

Pressure (kg/cm^2)	Pressure (p.s.i.)	Temperature (°C)	Time (min)
1.2	15	121	12
1.4	20	126	10
2	30	134	3.5

PROCEDURE: USE OF THE ETHYLENE OXIDE STERILISER

ACTION	RATIONALE
1. Place individually packed items into a polythene liner bag.	1. Liner bags are supplied with the steriliser.
2. Place a scored ampoule containing ethylene oxide liquid inside the liner bag and seal the bag with a metal twist tie.	2. The bag must be sealed in order to keep the gas circulating around the contents.
3. Put the liner bag into the steriliser unit.	
4. Snap the ampoule from outside the bag to release the gas.	4. To minimise exposure to gas.
5. Close and lock the door to the steriliser unit and turn the ventilator on.	5. Accidental opening of the unit can be prevented if the unit is locked.
6. After 12 hours turn on the pump.	6. This aerates the unit before it is safe for the operator to open.
7. Two hours after aerating, remove sterilised items.	7. This will ensure that any toxic gas has been removed.
8. Store items for a further 24 hours in a well-ventilated room.	8. This ensures that all the ethylene oxide has dissipated.

Autoclaves are used for sterilising instruments, drapes, gowns, swabs and some rubber or plastic items.

Ethylene oxide

Ethylene oxide gas sterilises by inactivating the DNA in the cells of the pathogen, thus preventing their replication. It is, however, toxic, irritant to tissues and very inflammable. In order to comply with COSHH regulations manufacturer's instructions **must** be followed. The steriliser, a plastic container fitted with a ventilation system, should be located in a well-ventilated area, such as a fume cupboard away from working areas. Room temperature must be kept at a minimum of 20°C during the cycle.

Sterilisation by ethylene oxide is suitable for anaesthetic tubing, endotracheal tubes, fibre-optic equipment, optical instruments, plastic items such as catheters and syringes, high-speed drills and battery-operated drills. Everyday items such as instruments, gowns and drapes may also be sterilised in this manner but the length of the cycle restricts its use.

Radiation

Sterilisation is achieved using gamma irradiation. It can only be carried out under controlled industrial conditions. Many pre-packaged items used in practice, such as needles, syringes and catheters, are sterilised in this way.

Monitoring the efficacy of sterilisation

It is essential that the effectiveness of any sterilisation method be constantly monitored to ensure that all microorganisms, including bacterial spores, are destroyed. Different sterilisation methods require different working conditions in terms of time and temperature. It is also important to choose the correct method of monitoring efficacy of sterilisation (Table 7.3).

Packing materials for sterilisation

There are a number of different packing materials available for the preparation of items to be sterilised. Selection will depend largely on the method of sterilisation but factors such as cost and personal preference may also be taken into account (Table 7.4).

Table 7.3 Methods of monitoring the efficacy of sterilisation

Method	Description	Use
Chemical indicator strips	Paper strips that change colour when the correct temperature and time have been reached. They are placed in the centre of the pack prior to sterilisation	Autoclave: select the correct strip for the cycle Ethylene oxide
Browne's tubes	Small glass tubes filled with an orange liquid that turns green when the correct temperature is reached and maintained for the correct time	Autoclave Hot-air oven
Bowie–Dick indicator tape	A beige tape impregnated with chemical stripes that change to black when the correct temperature has been reached (121°C). It does not indicate whether the pack has been exposed for the correct time, therefore it is not a reliable method	Autoclave
Ethylene oxide tape	As above, only the tape is green with lines that change to red on exposure to ethylene oxide	Ethylene oxide
Spore strips	Strips of paper impregnated with spores (usually *Bacillus stearothermophilius*) are placed in the load. After sterilisation, they are cultured for 72 hours. Provided that sterilisation has been achieved, no growth will be visible. This is an accurate method, although the delay in obtaining the results is a major disadvantage	Autoclave Ethylene oxide Hot-air oven

Table 7.4 Packing materials for sterilisation

Packing material	Advantage	Disadvantage	Method of sterilisation
Self-seal pouches	Easy to pack Clear front to view contents Paper back with sterilisation indicator Ideal for individual instruments	Puncture by heavy or sharp instruments (double packing will prevent puncturing but increase the cost)	Autoclave Ethylene oxide
Nylon film	Cheap May be reused Sealed with Bowie–Dick tape	Repeated use leads to brittleness and can cause tiny holes that can go unnoticed	Autoclave
Polythene bags supplied by ethylene oxide manufacturers	Easy to pack Strong	Overpacking can lead to poor gas circulation	Ethylene oxide
Linen drapes	Conforming Used to pack surgical equipment Strong Reusable	Permeable to moisture Require laundering Liable to wear	Autoclave (with a drying cycle) Ethylene oxide (if not too tightly packed)
Paper drapes	Water-repellent Disposable Used to pack surgical equipment	Non-conforming Can tear easily	Autoclave (with a drying cycle) Ethylene oxide (if not too tightly packed)
Metal tins	Long-lasting Useful for gowns, drapes, swabs, instruments Cannot be punctured	Expensive to buy Require a large autoclave Often multiuse, which may lead to contamination of contents	Autoclave (with a drying cycle) Hot-air oven
Cardboard cartons	Reusable Cannot be punctured easily Sturdy Useful for specialised kits	Expensive to buy Bulky to store	Autoclave (with a drying cycle)

PROCEDURE: PACKING AN ITEM FOR STERILISATION

ACTION

1. Select the appropriate packaging material for the method of sterilisation to be used.

2. Select the correct size of packaging for the item to be sterilised.

3. Label the pack with the contents.

4. Write the date on the pack.

5. Write the name of the person preparing the pack on the pack label.

RATIONALE

1. A packaging material that is non-permeable to steam would not be suitable for an autoclave.

2. Some methods of packaging, such as self-seal pouches, can be costly to use so do not choose too large a pouch.

3. This will save opening incorrect packs, which would then require re-sterilisation.

4. Sterilised items should be repackaged and sterilised again if not used within 3 months.

5. This allows any problems with the packing to be traced.

MAINTAINING THE THEATRE ENVIRONMENT

It is vital to have a strict cleaning regimen in the operating theatre and preparation room to maintain a high standard of asepsis. Both daily and weekly cleaning procedures are essential. In addition to this there are some general rules for maintaining asepsis in the theatre (Table 7.5).

PROCEDURE: DAILY CLEANING ROUTINE

ACTION

1. Damp dust all surfaces and equipment using dilute disinfectant.
2. Wipe the table and surfaces with dilute disinfectant between patients. Clean the floor if it is soiled.
3. Remove used instruments, drapes, etc. after each procedure.
4. At the end of the day, vacuum to remove debris and hair.

RATIONALE

1. Using a dry cloth would merely move dust around the room.
2. This prevents cross-contamination from one patient to the next.

3. To avoid contaminating the next surgical site.
4. Fine particles will be collected more efficiently using a vacuum.

Table 7.5 Maintaining an aseptic theatre

Action	Rationale
1. The least number of people should be present and movement kept to a minimum	1. Any movement will increase the risk of wound contamination by airborne particles
2. Personnel must wear the correct theatre attire at all times	2. This will avoid contamination from clothing, skin and hair
3. Clip and disinfect the patient away from the theatre	3. Hair and debris would contaminate the theatre
4. Use a new set of instruments for each surgical procedure	4. Cross-contamination between patients must be avoided
5. Carry out 'clean' operations before contaminated procedures	5. Contamination from high-risk procedures should then not occur
6. Discard any instrument that becomes contaminated	6. The remaining surgical instruments must remain aseptic
7. If asepsis is broken by any member of the surgical team it must be rectified	7. Further contamination can then be avoided

5. All waste material and soiled equipment must be removed.
6. All surfaces, including lights and sinks, must be thoroughly cleaned using dilute disinfectant.

5. The warm operating theatre is an ideal breeding ground for microorganisms.
6. Contaminated dust particles will settle on all surfaces and must be removed.

PROCEDURE: WEEKLY CLEANING ROUTINE

ACTION

1. Remove all portable equipment from the operating theatre.

2. Clean the equipment, including the castors.

3. Scrub the ceiling, walls, floor and all fixtures thoroughly using a disinfectant with detergent properties.
4. Use cleaning utensils that are specifically designed for the operating theatre. They should be sterilised or washed in a washing machine after use.

RATIONALE

1. Dirt and debris quickly build up in less accessible areas such as those behind equipment.
2. Castors soon fail to run smoothly if they are not cleaned regularly.
3. Detergent will remove any organic matter, which could otherwise inactivate the disinfectant.
4. This will minimise cross-contamination from other areas of the veterinary practice.

The surgical scrub

The surgical scrub is performed to reduce the levels of both resident and transient microbes on the hands. The hands come into the closest contact with the surgical site and, although sterile gloves may be worn, these cannot be relied on entirely as they may be punctured before surgery is complete.

The correct equipment should be prepared in advance so the complete process from scrubbing to gowning and gloving can be carried out in an aseptic manner. The equipment required is as follows:

- sink with elbow, knee or foot controls
- cleansing agent dispenser

- disposable nail file or orange stick
- sterile scrubbing brush
- sterile towels
- sterile gown
- sterile gloves.

Ideally, a general handwashing procedure is carried out at the beginning of the day. A full surgical scrub is then carried out, lasting up to 10 minutes, before the first surgical procedure; a shorter scrub may then be carried out between subsequent procedures provided there has been no major contamination of the hands.

Before beginning any handwashing procedure, all jewellery and watches must be removed. Nails should be short and free from varnish.

PROCEDURE: GENERAL HANDWASHING ROUTINE

ACTION

1. Turn on the water and adjust to a warm temperature.
2. Allow the water to wash over the hands and drain from the wrists to the fingertips.

RATIONALE

2. This will remove any gross contamination.

3. Clean the fingernails with an orange stick or nail file.

4. Apply plain soap and massage into the hands, from the wrists to the fingertips, in a circular motion, including the backs of the hands.

5. Rinse, allowing the water to drain from the fingertips. Repeat step 4.

6. Turn off the water.

7. Dry hands thoroughly with paper towels.

3. Once this has been carried out each day it may be omitted from further washing procedures.

4. It is important to remove all traces of dirt because these may inactivate the antiseptic solution used in the surgical scrub.

5. Repeating the washing procedure will ensure the removal of any residual organic matter.

6. The hands must not touch the tap so if the elbow, foot or knee cannot operate it, an assistant may be required. If this is not possible, a paper towel may be used and then discarded.

7. Air hand-dryers are unsuitable because they spread microorganisms around the environment. Reusable towels are unsuitable because they harbour microorganisms.

PROCEDURE: SURGICAL SCRUB (FIG. 7.1)

ACTION

1. Turn on the tap to produce a gentle stream and adjust the temperature.

2. Keeping forearms higher than the elbows at all times, wet the arms and hands and apply plain soap.

3. Work the soap into a lather and spread over the hands and arms to 5 cm above the elbow.

4. With the fingers under the stream, clean the nails with a file or orange stick.

5. Repeat step 3 using a surgical scrub solution.

6. Take a sterile brush, moisten it under the stream and apply the surgical scrub solution.

7. Scrub the nails using a straight stroke.

8. Starting with the little finger, scrub each of the four planes of each finger in straight strokes.

9. Clean the palm of the hand and back of the hand using a circular motion.

10. Scrub to 5 cm above the elbow using a circular motion.

RATIONALE

1. A gentle stream will minimise splashing.

2. It is important to keep the hands above the elbows to allow any water to run away from the scrubbed area, avoiding recontamination.

3. Any surface dirt and grease will be removed.

4. Discard the file by dropping it into the sink.

7. Make sure the bristles of the brush clean under the nails.

8. Include the interdigital spaces.

9. Care must be taken not to overscrub the back of the hand because the skin is more delicate and therefore more susceptible to trauma.

10. Maintain a lather at all times, adding water and scrub solution as necessary.

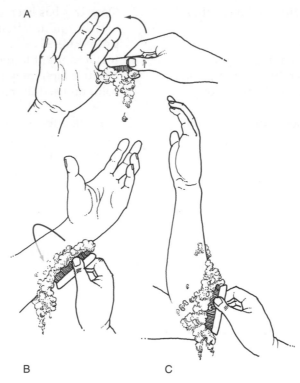

Figure 7.1 The surgical scrub sequence. A, Starting with the little finger and working across to the thumb, scrub each surface of each digit. B, Scrub the forearm, again scrubbing the entire circumference. C, Scrub elbow area to 5 cm (2 inches) above the elbow, including all surfaces.

11. If using two brushes, discard the first brush into the sink and take the second brush with the scrubbed hand. If not, rinse the brush and add scrub solution before transferring to the other hand.
12. Repeat the process for the remaining hand and forearm.
13. Maintaining the hands above the elbows, rinse both hands thoroughly and allow the water to drain into the sink.
14. Wash the hands and arms again, using surgical scrub solution, but this time do not include the elbows.
15. Rinse, then dry hands using a sterile towel (see following procedure).

11. Once one hand is scrubbed, it must not become recontaminated or the procedure will have to be repeated.

12. Use the same method to ensure that no part of the skin is missed.
13. Avoid getting water on to clothing because this may lead to strike-through.
14. This ensures that the hands do not come into contact with any area that has not been scrubbed.
15. Hold hands above the elbows with palms facing the chest. Do not allow the hands to touch each other.

PROCEDURE: DRYING HANDS AFTER THE SURGICAL SCRUB (FIG. 7.2)

ACTION

1. Stand clear of any surfaces and pick up the corner of the towel with the left hand.
2. Allow the towel to unfold without shaking it.

3. Let the towel fall over the palm of the right hand and use the first quarter to dry the fingers, palm and back of the left hand. Dry each finger separately and ensure the interdigital areas are included.
4. Using the second quarter of the towel, dry the left forearm and elbow.

5. With the dry left hand, pick up the towel by the fourth quarter, which is hanging free, and drape it over the palm of the left hand.
6. Dry the right fingers, palm and back of the hand with the fourth quarter, and the arm and elbow with the third quarter.

RATIONALE

1. Avoid touching any surface with the sterile towel or scrubbed hands.
2. Shaking the towel will increase the risk of it touching a surface and will also circulate airborne microbes.
3. The right hand is used to support the towel and dry the left hand, taking care not to touch the top side of the towel or come into contact with the left hand itself.

4. By using a separate quarter for each hand and arm, the degree of asepsis achieved is increased.
5. The procedure followed for drying the left hand is repeated for the right hand.

6. In some cases, two towels are available. In this case, use one-third of the towel for the fingers, one-third for the palm and back of the hand and the remainder for the arm and elbow. The process is repeated for the other hand with the second towel.

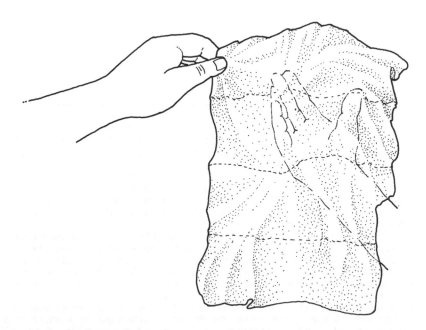

Figure 7.2 Drying the hands after the surgical scrub.

7. Discard the towel and proceed to gowning and gloving.

7. The hands must not be allowed to touch the part of the towel used to dry the arms and elbows.

Theatre attire

In order to achieve asepsis, outdoor clothing should be replaced with specific theatre attire by all the surgical team. While nothing except the surgical gown is actually sterile, the clothing acts as a barrier to microorganisms (Table 7.6).

PROCEDURE: FOLDING A SURGICAL GOWN FOR STERILISATION (FIG. 7.3)

ACTION

1. Lie the gown flat on a work surface with the inside of the gown face down.

2. Fold one side of the gown into the centre, tucking the ties in.
3. Fold the other side of the gown right across to the other side, also tucking ties in.

4. Making sure that the inside collar of the gown is on top, concertina the rest of the gown lengthways until it is the size required to fit into the sterilising pack.

Another method of folding a gown ready for sterilisation is shown in Figure 7.4.

RATIONALE

1. In this position, all creases can be removed, ties identified and sleeves straightened. The outer surface of the gown will be folded in so that, when it is put on, ungloved hands will not contaminate it.
2. Ties must be tucked in to avoid accidental contamination when gowning.
3. This enables the gown to be folded neatly into a sterile pack but it will still unfold easily when put on.
4. When gowning in an aseptic manner, the gown must be picked up by the inside shoulders and allowed to gently unfold.

Table 7.6 Theatre attire

Item	Description
Scrub suits	A top and trousers, worn only in the operating room. The top should be tucked into the trousers and the trousers should either have cuffed legs or be tucked into surgical boots. They should be changed daily, or more often if soiled. Sterilise periodically
Footwear	Shoes or boots designed to be non-slip, antistatic, comfortable and easily cleaned. Not to be worn outside the theatre. Alternatively, shoe covers may be used
Headwear	Hair can be a major source of contamination, so it should be completely covered in the operating room. There are various types of theatre hats available, some paper-based designed as single use and others lint-free machine-washable
Facemasks	Facemasks filter air from the nose and mouth but must be close fitting to avoid bacteria entering the surgical environment through the sides of the mask. They should be changed between operations
Surgical gowns	Surgical gowns are sterile and worn over the scrub suit. Ideally they should have long sleeves with cuffs. Both reusable and disposable gowns are available. Reusable gowns require the correct folding technique prior to sterilisation in order for the veterinary surgeon to put the gown on in an aseptic manner
Surgical gloves	Surgical gloves should be worn for all surgical procedures. They come prepacked in a variety of sizes and are sterile. Gloves without powder are recommended because the powder acts as a foreign body and may cause wound-healing problems

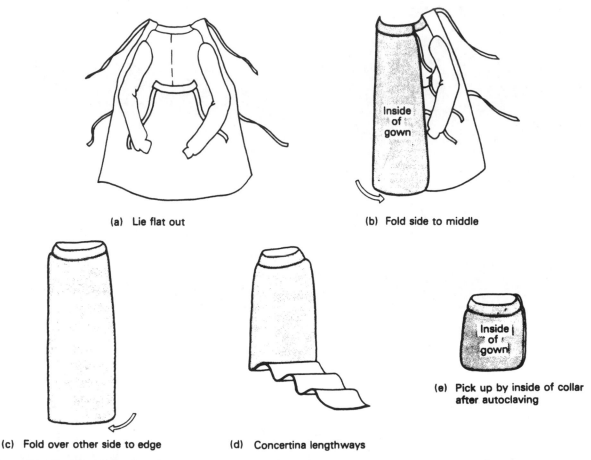

(a) Lie flat out

(b) Fold side to middle

Inside of gown

(c) Fold over other side to edge

(d) Concertina lengthways

Inside of gown

(e) Pick up by inside of collar after autoclaving

Figure 7.3 Folding a gown. Reproduced, with permission, from *Veterinary Nursing*, p. 528 and 597, 2nd edn, by Lane and Cooper (1994). Butterworth Heinemann, UK.

PROCEDURE: PUTTING ON A BACK-TYING SURGICAL GOWN (FIG. 7.5)

ACTION

1. Remove the sterile gown from its pack, hold by the shoulders and allow to gently unfold.

2. Slip one hand into each sleeve and push up to, but not through, the cuff. Arms should be opened wide but no attempt to adjust the gown over the shoulders should be made.

3. An unscrubbed assistant, touching only the inside of the back of the gown, should pull the gown over the shoulders and secure the ties at the back.

RATIONALE

1. Holding the gown correctly allows the sleeves to be clearly identified. Allowing the gown to gently unfold minimises air movement and the risk of contaminating the gown.

2. Hands should remain in the sleeves of the gown to avoid contamination. Efforts to pull the gown over the shoulders create a contamination risk.

3. The inside of the gown is no longer considered sterile and can therefore be handled.

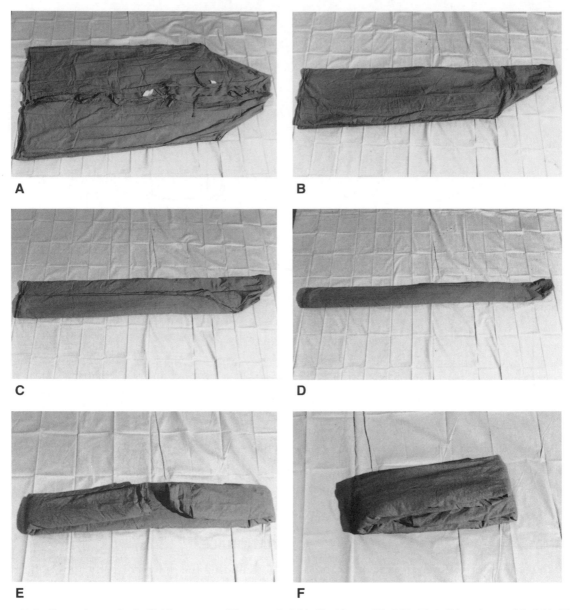

Figure 7.4 Alternative method of folding a gown. The gown is folded inside out (A), folded in half lengthways (B), folded in half lengthways again (C), and again in half lengthways (D); the top and bottom edges are folded to the middle (E); and the gown is then folded in half again (F). Reproduced, with permission, from *Veterinary Nursing*, p. 529, 2nd edn, by Lane and Cooper (1994). Butterworth Heinemann, UK.

4. With hands still inside the gown sleeves, pick up the waist ties and hold them out to the sides. The assistant grasps the ends and secures them at the back, taking care not to touch any part of the gown.

4. The back of the gown is now considered non-sterile and should not come into contact with any sterile equipment or drapes.

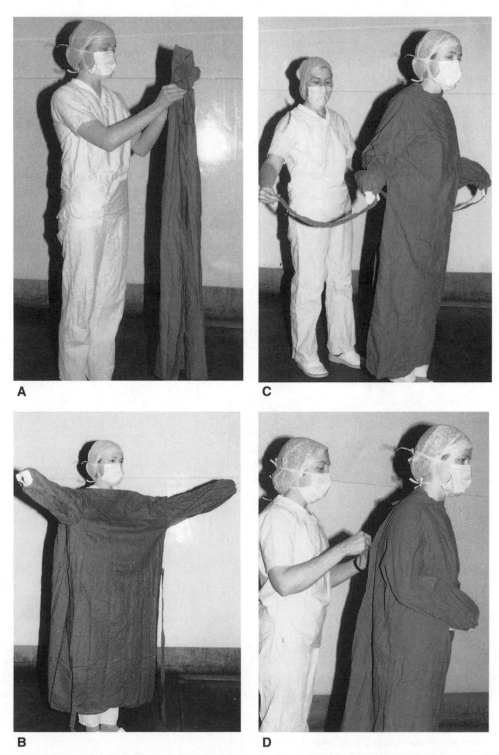

Figure 7.5A–D   Putting on a back-tying surgical gown. Reproduced, with permission, from *Veterinary Nursing*, p. 533, 2nd edn, by Lane and Cooper (1994). Butterworth Heinemann, UK.

PROCEDURE: PUTTING ON A SIDE-TYING GOWN (FIG. 7.6)

ACTION

1. Follow points 1–3 above.
2. Keeping hands within the sleeves, pass the side tie, which is attached to a paper tape, to the assistant.
3. The assistant passes the tie around the gown. Take the tie back, leaving the assistant holding the paper tape, and tie the gown at the side.

RATIONALE

2. There is no risk of contamination if the hands are kept inside the sleeves.

3. The assistant has not contaminated the gown because he or she has only held the paper tape. The gown is now sterile all the way around, not just at the front as with the previous method.

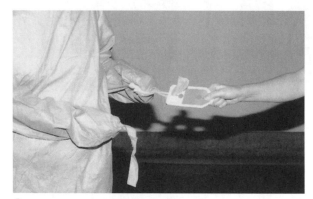

A

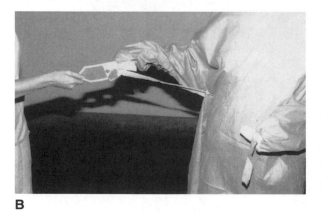

B

C

Figure 7.6A–C   Putting on a side-tying surgical gown. Reproduced, with permission, from *Veterinary Nursing*, p. 534, 2nd edn, by Lane and Cooper (1994). Butterworth Heinemann, UK.

PROCEDURE: CLOSED GLOVING (FIG. 7.7)

ACTION

1. Keeping the hands inside the sleeves of the gown, turn the glove packet so that the fingers face towards the body.

2. Pick up the right glove (which is on the left) by the rim of the cuff with the right hand.
3. Turn the hand over so that the palm is upwards with the fingers of the glove facing towards the body (Fig. 7.7C).
4. Using the left hand, grasp the other rim of the glove and pull it over the right hand until it covers the cuffs of the gown.
5. The left hand, within the sleeve of the gown, can adjust the fingers of the right glove until comfortable.
6. Pick up the left glove with the left hand and repeat the process.

RATIONALE

1. The risk of contamination is minimised because the outsides of the gloves do not have the chance to come in contact with the skin.
2. By turning the glove packet round the right glove is on the left and vice versa.
3. The glove will be in the correct position to be pulled on.
4. Both hands still remain within the sleeves of the gown to prevent contamination of the outer surface of the glove.
5. The glove must fit snugly but not too tightly.
6. At no time will the skin of the hands have come into contact with the outside of the gloves, thus minimising contamination.

PROCEDURE: OPEN GLOVING (FIG. 7.8)

ACTION

1. Push both hands through the cuffs of the gown.

2. With the pack of gloves facing forward, pick up the right glove with the left hand, touching only the inner folded-down surface of the glove.
3. Pull the glove on to the right hand, leaving the cuff folded back, and hook over the thumb.

4. Slide the gloved fingers of the right hand under the left cuff and pull on to the left hand. Hook the thumb under the folded cuff, as above.

5. The gloved fingers of the left hand are then slid under the fold of the right glove. Unhook the thumb and pull the folded part of the glove over the cuff of the gown.
6. Repeat for the left hand.

RATIONALE

1. A disadvantage of using the open method of gloving is that the gloves may be contaminated by skin contact.
2. The inside of the glove may be touched freely because it should never come into contact with other sterile items such as gown and drapes.
3. This will avoid touching of the contaminated inner surface by the gloved left hand when unfolding to cover the gown cuff.
4. Only the sterile outer surface of the glove may be touched by the gloved right hand, to avoid contamination.

5. By covering the cuff of the gown, no skin contact is possible, thereby minimising any risk of contamination.

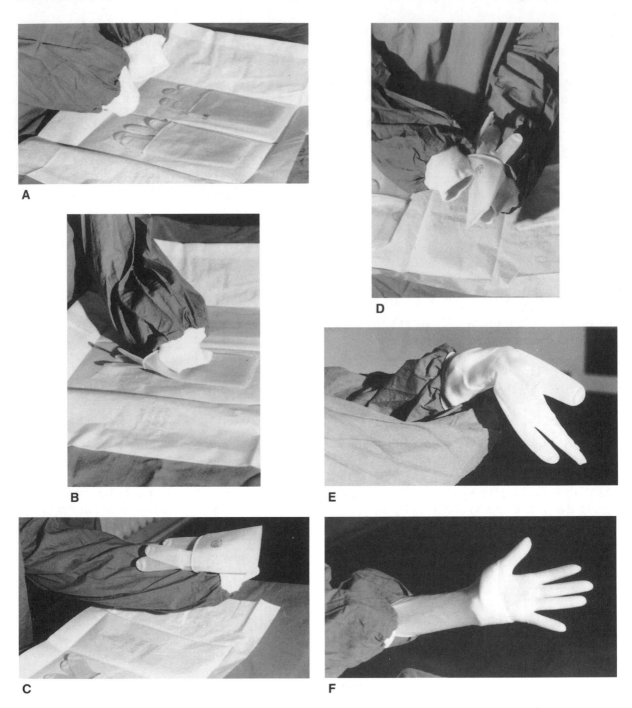

Figure 7.7A–F   Closed gloving technique. Reproduced, with permission, from *Veterinary Nursing*, p. 535, 2nd edn, by Lane and Cooper (1994). Butterworth Heinemann, UK.

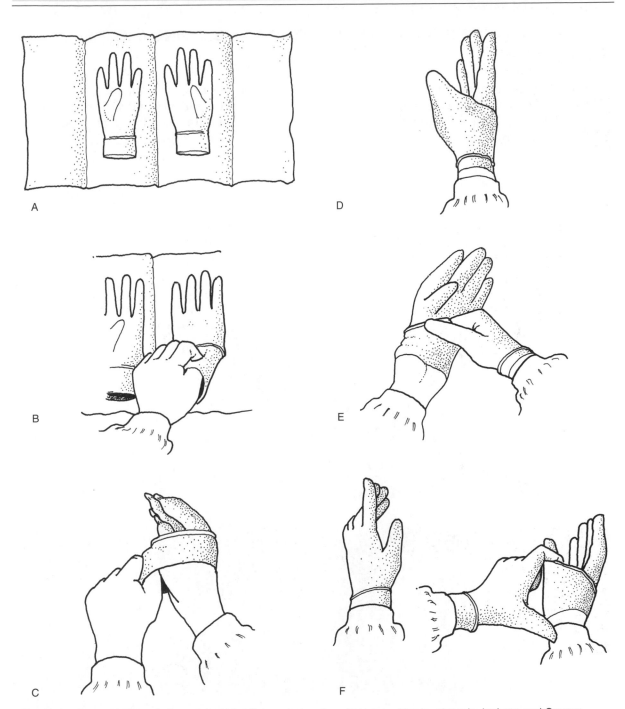

Figure 7.8 Open gloving technique. Adapted, with permission, from *Veterinary Nursing*, 1st edn, by Lane and Cooper (1994). Butterworth Heinemann, UK.

PROCEDURE: THE PLUNGE METHOD OF GLOVING (FIG. 7.9)

ACTION

1. A scrubbed assistant holds the sterile glove open while the hand is inserted, while still in the sleeve of the sterile gown. Repeat for the second hand.

RATIONALE

1. The high risk of contaminating both personnel involved is a disadvantage of this method and it is therefore rarely used in veterinary practice.

Preparation of the surgical site

The skin and coat of the patient are major sources of wound contamination because it is impossible to remove all bacteria; however, careful preparation of the surgical site will minimise the risks.

Clipping the area surrounding the surgical site is best carried out with the patient anaesthetised. If the patient is considered an anaesthetic risk, clipping the patient before induction can reduce anaesthetic time.

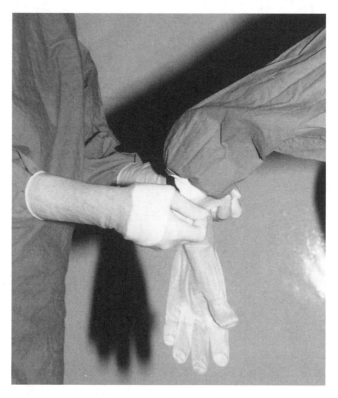

Figure 7.9 Plunge gloving method. Reproduced, with permission, from *Veterinary Nursing*, p. 536, 2nd edn, by Lane and Cooper (1994). Butterworth Heinemann, UK.

PROCEDURE: CLIPPING

ACTION

1. Ensure the clippers are clean and in good working order.
2. Clip with the grain of the hair first, then clip against the hair.

3. Clip 5–15 cm beyond the line of the incision.

4. Make sure all edges are neat.

5. If clipping around an open wound or near the eyes, apply an appropriate gel or ointment first.

RATIONALE

1. Poorly maintained clippers are more likely to nick the skin and cause irritation.
2. Removal of long, thick hair is easier with the grain. For a closer clip, cutting against the hair is most effective.
3. The surgeon will be able to extend the incision if necessary.
4. Clients will not be impressed if the clipping is untidy.
5. Tiny hairs will act as foreign bodies in an open wound and are very difficult to remove. They cause intense irritation if they get into the eye.

PROCEDURE: PREPARATION OF THE SKIN

ACTION

1. Carry out steps 2–7 in the preparation area.
2. Put on surgical gloves; they do not need to be sterile at this stage.

3. Use a chlorhexidine or povidone-iodine solution.
4. Use lint-free swabs.

5. With the 'clean' hand, select a fresh swab and pass it to the 'dirty' hand.

6. Starting at the incision site, scrub the skin, working in a circular pattern out towards the edge of the clipped area.
7. Once the edge has been reached, discard the swab, select a fresh swab with the 'clean' hand and repeat until there is no discoloration on the swab.

8. Transfer the patient to the theatre and position for surgery.
9. Wearing sterile gloves and using sterile swabs and water, repeat the scrub procedure described above.

RATIONALE

1. Contamination of the theatre is avoided.
2. This will protect the patient's skin from contamination by the nurse's hands and protect the hands from the antiseptic solutions.
3. They both have antiseptic and detergent properties.
4. They will not contaminate the site by leaving tiny particles or threads.
5. It is good practice to keep one hand 'clean' to prevent contamination of fresh swabs by the other hand, which will scrub the patient and therefore be 'dirty'.
6. By moving in a circular pattern no part of the area should be missed.

7. Care must be taken not to return a 'dirty' swab to the centre of the area. The hair at the edge of the area should be included in the scrub to remove debris and flatten hair out of the way but be careful not to make the patient too wet to avoid strike-qthrough or hypothermia.
8. The site is likely to have become contaminated in the move.
9. Sterile equipment is used to create an environment that is as aseptic as possible.

10. The final skin preparation is carried out by a member of the surgical team, again using sterile swabs, this time held by Rampley sponge-holding forceps. An alcoholic solution of skin disinfectant is applied and left to dry on the skin.

10. The alcohol solution will remove any remaining detergent and provide residual bactericidal activity. Do not apply to open wounds or mucous membranes. Do not use diathermy if an alcohol solution has been applied.

Draping the patient

Draping the patient is carried out to maintain asepsis during surgery. The entire patient must be covered, leaving just the surgical area exposed. In order to maintain asepsis, a member of the surgical team who is gowned and gloved carries out the draping (Table 7.7).

When folding a fenestrated drape, it is important to use a similar method to that for a plain drape but the fenestration should end up

Packing drapes for sterilisation

When preparing a drape for sterilisation, the aim is to ensure that all parts are sterilised evenly, and when the drape is handled by the surgical team it will unfold easily. This can be achieved by either folding the drape in a concertina fashion or folding it corner to corner. The concertina method is illustrated in Figure 7.10.

on top of the drape so it can be clearly identified in the sterilisation packaging.

PROCEDURE: DRAPING WITH FOUR PLAIN DRAPES (FIG. 7.11)

ACTION

1. Pick up the first drape and allow it to unfold away from the trolley or table.

2. Fold back the edge of the drape underneath itself. This will line the edge of the incision.

RATIONALE

1. The sterile drape must not be allowed to become contaminated by touching a non-sterile area.

2. This will produce a double layer at the edge of the draped area, protecting it from strike-through.

Table 7.7 Types of drape

Drape	Advantages	Disadvantages	Comments
Disposable	Water resistant Prepacked and folded Presterilised Will prevent strikethrough Lint-free Always in perfect condition	Expensive Less conforming Large stock required Less accurate fenestration size	Can be used under or over a cloth drape Ideal for surgery where fluid is likely to be present Can be secured with sterile spray or may be self-adhesive
Reusable	Cheaper Conforming Required size fenestration using four plain drapes	Porous, which can lead to strikethrough Labour intensive: washing and drying Become poor quality with repeated use Require an autoclave with an effective drying cycle	Secured to the skin with towel clips: if the tips puncture the cloth they are no longer sterile and must be replaced

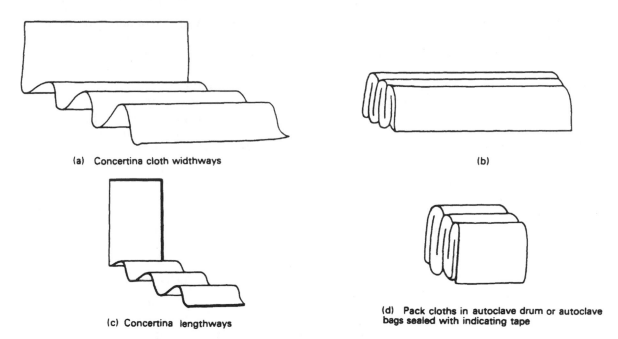

(a) Concertina cloth widthways

(b)

(c) Concertina lengthways

(d) Pack cloths in autoclave drum or autoclave bags sealed with indicating tape

Figure 7.10 Folding surgical drapes. Reproduced, with permission, from *Veterinary Nursing*, p. 530, 2nd edn, by Lane and Cooper (1994). Butterworth Heinemann, UK.

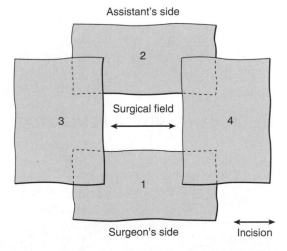

Assistant's side

2

Surgical field

3

4

1

Surgeon's side

Incision

Figure 7.11 Draping with four plain drapes. Adapted, with permission, from the *BSAVA Manual of Veterinary Nursing*, edited by M. Moore (1999). BSAVA, Gloucester.

3. With the hands inside the drape, hold the drape along the folded edge.
4. Apply the first drape on the surgeon's side.

5. Place the second drape on the opposite side to the first drape.

6. The third and fourth drapes are placed at the ends of the surgical site.
7. Apply further drapes to cover any remaining exposed areas of the patient or table.

8. Place a towel clip diagonally across each corner with one tip on each drape. Secure by picking up a small fold of skin.
9. Cover the clips with the corner of each drape.

3. This will prevent the hands from touching the patient when the drape is placed.
4. This prevents contamination of the surgeon when leaning over the patient to place the subsequent drapes.
5. The surgeon may place this drape by leaning across the patient, or the assistant may place it from his or her side.
6. They can be placed in any order.

7. It is very important to cover the patient, the entire table and the area between the surgical site and the instrument trolley.
8. Care must be taken not to contaminate the clips by piercing the drape.
9. This will stop the clips getting accidentally caught and pulled.

PROCEDURE: DRAPING A LIMB (FIG. 7.12)

ACTION

1. Cover the lower part of the limb with a bandage and hold it upright. It may either be held by an assistant or secured to a drip stand.
2. Place a plain drape over the rest of the body and the opposite limb of the patient.
3. Place a smaller drape on top of the initial drape and lower the limb.
4. Wrap the second drape around the limb and secure with a towel clip.
5. Further drapes are placed over the surgical site.

RATIONALE

1. The lower part of the limb is a source of contamination. The limb is held upright to allow further drapes to be placed.
2. This reduces the risk of contamination from the rest of the body.
3. The limb should only be in contact with the second drape.
4. The limb now has two layers covering it to avoid it contaminating the surgical area.
5. The patient should now be fully draped with only the surgical site visible.

PROCEDURE: DRAPING WITH A FENESTRATED DRAPE

ACTION

1. Pick up the drape and allow it to unfold away from the trolley or table.

2. With hands inside the drape, hold the drape along the edge.
3. Looking through the fenestration, place the drape over the surgical site.

RATIONALE

1. Avoid touching anything that will break the sterility of the drape. If asepsis is broken, discard the drape and start again with a new one.
2. The hands must not touch the patient's skin or coat.
3. If the fenestration is too large, apply further plain drapes over the top to reduce it. If the fenestration is too small, discard the drape and start again with a fresh one.

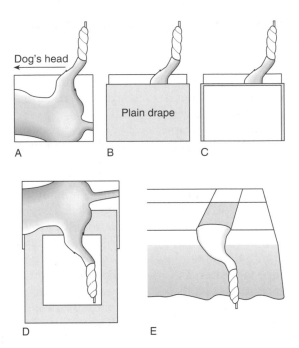

Figure 7.12 Draping a limb for surgery. A, The lower limb is bandaged and attached by tape to a transfusion stand; B, a plain drape is laid over the body and the opposite limb of the patient; C, a smaller plain drape is laid on top of this; D, the tape is then cut and the limb lowered on to the inner drape; E, the drape is carefully wrapped around the limb and secured with a towel clip. Plain drapes or a fenestrated drape is then applied over the surgical site.

4. Secure the drape with towel clips at each corner.

4. The clips cannot be concealed under the drape and are therefore more likely to get caught on instruments during surgery.

INSTRUMENTATION

Preparation of the instrument trolley

The instrument trolley can be prepared by the scrubbed nurse or by the circulating nurse using Cheatle forceps. It should be prepared immediately before use; if there is a delay in the start of surgery, the instruments must be covered with a sterile drape to minimise the risk of contamination from the environment.

The top of the instrument trolley will not be sterile. It should be covered with a waterproof sterile drape, to prevent bacterial strikethrough in the event that the trolley gets wet, followed by a cloth drape. It is common to pack instruments within a waterproof drape and cloth drape, which can then be unfolded to cover the base of the trolley. Where instruments are taken from multiuse sterilisation drums, two layers of cloth drapes are necessary.

PROCEDURE: DRAPING A TROLLEY USING CHEATLE FORCEPS

ACTION

1. Pick up the pair of Cheatle forceps, one in each hand, using the thumb and ring finger, with the tips of the forceps pointing down.
2. Using one of the forceps to steady the drape, open the other forceps and pick up the drape, keeping it folded.
3. Move away from any surfaces. With the free forceps, grasp one corner of the drape and, with arms held out in front, remove the first forceps and allow the drape to gently unfold.

4. Select the adjacent corner with the other forceps, straighten the drape and carefully pass it behind the instrument trolley so the trolley is between you and the drape.
5. Gently bring the drape towards you, covering the trolley. When the trolley is covered, release the drape before your arms drop below waist level.
6. Return the Cheatle forceps to their sterile container.

RATIONALE

1. The middle two fingers of each hand can then be used to support the forceps.

2. If the drape is allowed to unfold too soon, it is likely to touch a non-sterile surface and become contaminated.
3. It is essential to stand clear of anything that may contaminate the drape, including yourself. The drape should not be shaken to unfold it as this increases air movement and risk of contamination.
4. Draping the trolley towards you prevents contamination from your clothing because you do not have to lean over the trolley to place the drape.
5. If you allow the Cheatle forceps to drop below waist level there is an increased risk of touching a non-sterile surface.

6. While the handles of the forceps are non-sterile, the tips must remain sterile or be discarded.

PROCEDURE: LAYING OUT AN INSTRUMENT TROLLEY

ACTION

1. Identify the instruments and equipment required for the surgical procedure to be carried out.
2. Place the instruments on to the trolley in order of use from left to right.

3. Place a sterile drape over the trolley until it is ready to be used.

RATIONALE

1. Having all equipment prepared in advance can reduce surgery time and therefore anaesthetic time.
2. This enables the surgeon or scrubbed nurse to select the required instrument quickly and efficiently.
3. The risk of environmental contamination is minimised.

Assisting during surgery

Throughout a surgical procedure there should ideally be two nurses assisting: one acting as a circulating nurse the other as a scrub nurse. The circulating nurse, while in a scrub suit, is not gowned and gloved. The scrub nurse is gowned and gloved in order to assist the surgeon during the procedure. Their individual roles are as follows:

THE CIRCULATING NURSE

- Assist in the preparation of the theatre, instruments and equipment
- Adjust and tie the gowns of the surgical team
- Position the patient on the operating table
- Prepare the surgical site
- Connect equipment such as diathermy and suction
- Unwrap suture material and extra equipment required
- Record suture material and swabs used
- Assist the anaesthetist if required
- Prepare and apply postoperative dressings when necessary
- Maintain the cleanliness of the theatre in readiness for the next procedure.

THE SCRUB NURSE

- Prepare the instrument trolley
- Pass instruments to the surgeon as required
- Swabbing as required
- Removing soiled instruments or swabs from the surgical area
- Retract tissue and cut sutures when required
- Counting swabs, needles and sutures as they are used and at the end of surgery.

PROCEDURE: HANDLING AND PASSING INSTRUMENTS

ACTION

1. Identify the procedure being performed.

2. Instruments should be pressed firmly into the surgeon's hand so they are ready for use.
3. Pass ringed instruments into the palm with the points outwards and curves upwards.

4. Dissecting forceps and the scalpel are passed into a finger grip.
5. After use, clean with a swab and replace in the same position back on to the trolley.

RATIONALE

1. The surgeon's instrument requirements can then be anticipated.
2. The surgeon will not have to look away from the surgical site.
3. The instrument is then ready for use and sharp points or blades will not damage the surgical gloves.
4. The instruments are ready for use.

5. Instruments not in use should not be left to clutter the surgical site. If they are returned to the correct position on the trolley they can quickly be found next time they are required.

PROCEDURE: SWABBING

ACTION

1. Count all swabs before and during surgery.

2. Use the swabs to blot the viscera.

RATIONALE

1. It is essential to keep a record of all swabs used and a close watch on their whereabouts.
2. Do not wipe the blood away or clots, which are forming to control the haemorrhage, will be removed and bleeding may begin again.

3. Dispose of used swabs into a bowl.

4. Count all swabs before the incision is closed.

3. Do not leave them on the trolley or at the surgical site because they may dampen the drapes and allow bacterial strikethrough.
4. They should equal the total number used during the procedure. This ensures that none are accidentally left in the wound.

Care and maintenance of surgical instruments

Surgical instruments are commonly made of either chromium-plated carbon steel or stainless steel. Tungsten carbide inserts are often added to the tips of stainless steel instruments because it improves their hardness and resistance to wear. Instruments with tungsten carbide inserts are identified by their gold-coloured handles.

Good quality instruments are costly but will last for many years if they are handled correctly and maintained properly. New instruments require lubricating before use.

PROCEDURE: CLEANING AND MAINTAINING INSTRUMENTS

ACTION

1. In accordance with the COSHH regulations, protective clothing such as rubber gloves and an apron must be worn.
2. Remove instruments from the theatre as soon as surgery is complete.

3. Remove and dispose of any sharp items such as needles, scalpel blades or glass vials.
4. Remove any packaging, swabs or suture material.
5. Separate any delicate equipment.

6. Rinse the instruments in cold water to remove blood and tissue as soon as possible.

7. Soak the instruments in warm water containing a specified instrument-cleaning agent.
8. Using a small brush, scrub each instrument under running water, paying particular attention to serrations, joints and ratchets.
9. The instruments may be put into an ultrasonic cleaner after manual cleaning, then thoroughly rinsed.
10. Dry the instruments thoroughly.

11. Inspect each instrument for damage, non-alignment of the tips or jaws, stiff hinges, bent ratchets, pitting, corrosion and loose screws.

RATIONALE

1. The risk of contamination by blood or tissue from a patient with a possible zoonotic disease is minimised.
2. This minimises the risk of contaminating the fresh set of instruments prepared for the next surgical procedure.
3. These should be placed into sharps containers or glass bins as appropriate.
4. Dispose of these in the clinical waste.
5. This should be cleaned separately to avoid damage.
6. Blood allowed to dry on to the instrument will lead to pitting of the surface. Hot water should not be used because it causes coagulation of proteins.
7. Dismantle instruments and open box joints and ratchets to free all debris.
8. Debris may become trapped.

9. Ultrasonic cleaners are very efficient at removing debris that is inaccessible to manual cleaning.
10. Water left in joints and ratchets may lead to corrosion.
11. If any faults are identified, the instrument must be removed from the kit and either repaired or replaced.

12. Lubricate the instruments with a suitable instrument lubricant.

13. Package ready for sterilisation.

Surgical kits

It is common practice to have a number of surgical kits made up ready for use. Each kit should be clearly identified as to its contents so the correct instruments can be prepared for surgery. Colour-coded autoclavable plastic tape is often used to identify all the instruments belonging to the same kit. Figure 7.13 illustrates some instruments commonly found in general kits.

While surgical kits will vary according to surgeon preference, some guidelines for some general kits are set out below.

12. The life of the instruments will be prolonged, especially those with joints and ratchets.

13. Cover sharp points, identify the instrument and date the pack.

General surgical kit

- Scalpel handle
- Rat-tooth forceps
- Dressing forceps
- Mayo scissors
- Metzenbaum scissors
- 4 × large Spencer Wells artery forceps
- 4 × small Spencer Wells artery forceps
- 2 × Allis tissue forceps
- Gelpi self-retaining retractors
- Langenbeck hand-held retractors
- 4 × Backhaus towel clips
- Needle holders

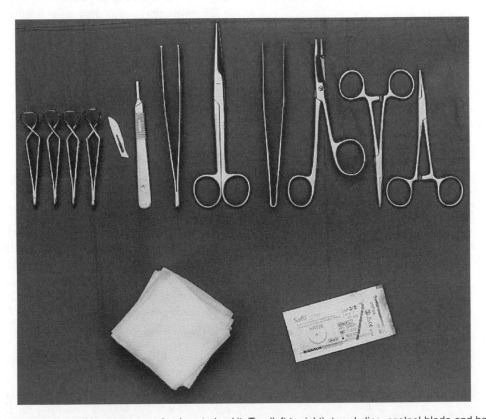

Figure 7.13 Commonly used instruments: a basic suturing kit. Top (left to right): towel clips, scalpel blade and handle, rat-tooth forceps, Mayo scissors, dressing forceps, Gillies needle holders, Spencer Wells forceps. Bottom (left to right): swabs, suture materials. Reproduced, with permission, from *Quick Reference Guide to Veterinary Surgical Kits*, p.80, by Masters and Bowden (2001). Butterworth Heinemann, UK.

This kit would be suitable for laparotomy, gastrotomy, tumour removal, ovariohysterectomy, pyometra, orchidectomy, caesarean section, hernia or rupture repair.

General eye kit

- Small scalpel handle
- Eyelid retractors
- Microcorneal forceps
- Microdissecting forceps
- Ophthalmic scissors
- Capsular forceps
- Irrigating cannula
- Iris repositor
- Castroviejo needle-holders

This kit would be suitable for enucleation, entropion or ectropion, removal of eyelid tumours, conjunctival flap, distichiasis.

Orthopaedic pinning kit

- Scalpel handle
- Rat-tooth forceps
- Dressing forceps
- Mayo scissors
- 4 × Spencer Wells artery forceps
- 4 × Mosquito artery forceps

- 2 × Allis tissue forceps
- 2 × Homann hand-held retractors
- Gelpi self-retaining retractors
- Selection of Steinemann pins
- Jacobs chuck and key
- Orthopaedic ruler
- Hacksaw and blade
- Pin cutters
- Needle holders

Care of specialist equipment

Diathermy

Diathermy is used to either cut or coagulate tissues. Unlike electrocautery, which uses an electric current to create a red-hot probe that is applied to the tissue, diathermy relies on alternating high-frequency currents to produce local heat within the tissue at the site of application. It is applied to control haemorrhage and decrease surgical time.

Monopolar or bipolar electrodes can be used to apply diathermy. Monopolar diathermy is used for cutting and coagulation and requires the patient to be 'earthed'. Bipolar diathermy allows more control over the depth and location of coagulation. It does not require the patient to be earthed and it cannot be used for cutting.

PROCEDURE: PREPARATION OF DIATHERMY EQUIPMENT

ACTION

1. Prepare the diathermy machine by placing a contact plate in a suitable position on the operating table. The plate should be connected to the diathermy machine by a wire.

2. Select the required electrodes.

3. Do not prepare the surgical site with alcohol-based surgical solution.

RATIONALE

1. This is done to 'earth' the patient. Contact gel can be applied to the plate before the patient is placed on to it. Alternatively, a rectal probe can be used. The current is transferred via the plate or probe to the ground. Electrical burns to the patient will then be avoided.

2. The cutting electrode can be a flat blade, scalpel blade or wire. A flat blade, ball electrode or dissecting forceps can be used to achieve coagulation diathermy. Dissecting forceps grasp the tissue and the current is applied by touching the forceps with the electrode.

3. Do not use any inflammable material such as alcohol in conjunction with diathermy: there is a risk of fire.

4. Follow the manufacturer's instructions regarding sterilisation, maintenance and operation of the unit.

4. Some parts, such as the handles and attachments, can usually be sterilised.

Cryosurgery

Cryosurgery is used to kill cells within a specific area with minimal damage to surrounding healthy tissue. This is achieved by the application of controlled extreme cold, which eventually destroys the cells. The cells are damaged by the effects of freezing and later die.

PROCEDURE: PREPARATION FOR CRYOSURGERY

ACTION

1. Wear protective clothing: apron, goggles and thick gloves. Avoid splashing yourself.
2. Do not touch any metal surfaces that have been cooled by liquid nitrogen.
3. Select a suitable refrigerant—generally liquid nitrogen.
4. Prepare the surgical site by clipping and cleaning the area.

5. Protect the surrounding healthy tissue.

6. Select the correct size of probe for the procedure to be carried out.

7. Apply the probe to the area and then remove it before applying it again. This cycle must be repeated for optimum effect.

8. Discuss postoperative care with the client: daily cleaning of the area is necessary; there may be skin sloughing and a slight discharge; erythema and oedema often occur in the first 24 hours; and hair-covered areas may heal with unpigmented hair.
9. Wash the probe in mild detergent, gently rubbing discoloured areas.

10. Do not use corrosive or abrasive solutions.

11. Follow manufacturer's instructions. Some probes may be sterilised.

RATIONALE

1. Liquid nitrogen can cause severe cold burns.
2. Again, severe cold burns may occur.

3. A suitable container must be used to store the liquid nitrogen.
4. Surface lesions do not require asepsis. Normal aseptic procedures should, however, be carried out for deeper lesions.
5. Apply petroleum jelly or polystyrene to protect healthy tissue from the effects of the freezing.
6. The most efficient method of applying cryosurgery is under pressure by a spray using a hollow probe.
7. Temperatures below −20°C rapidly freeze the tissues. Slow thawing occurs when the probe is removed. The patient may be required to have cryosurgery a number of times before the targeted cells are killed.

8. These points should be discussed with the owner before the start of surgery. If the patient is a show animal, the change in hair colour at the affected site could be a problem.

9. A build-up of debris, particularly on the tip of the probe, can lead to corrosive deposits building up, which damage the probe.
10. These cause thinning of the metal components.
11. Not all cryosurgery units can be sterilised.

Endoscopes

Endoscopy is the non-invasive visual examination of the interior of a body cavity. A light source is combined with a series of optical lenses and mirrors to create a delicate, expensive instrument.

Two types of endoscope are used in veterinary practice: rigid and flexible. The flexible endoscopes may be fibreoptic or video endoscopes. Fibreoptic endoscopes contain glass-fibre bundles and, although flexible, they are brittle and care must be taken not to break the individual strands.

PROCEDURE: CLEANING AN ENDOSCOPE

ACTION	RATIONALE
1. Clean the endoscope immediately after use.	1. If left covered in dirt, the endoscope will be more difficult to clean and will deteriorate owing to the presence of dried blood and mucus.
2. Never immerse an endoscope in liquid unless the manufacturer's instructions specifically state that you can. Do not autoclave or place in a hot-air oven.	2. Considerable damage will occur to the delicate control section or light connector if liquid enters them.
3. With the light source still attached, connect the water bottle and suction pump.	3. Follow manufacturer's instructions.
4. Prepare the recommended disinfectant.	4. Approximately 1 litre is required.
5. With the tip of the endoscope in the solution, aspirate by depressing the suction button.	5. This ensures that patency is maintained.
6. Clean the biopsy valve with a cotton bud and the biopsy channel with a specific cleaning brush, then clear rinse using suction.	6. This area must be cleaned thoroughly to remove any traces of tissue.
7. Disconnect the water bottle, block the water inlet and blow all the water out of the channel by depressing the water/air button.	7. Water must not be left in here as it leads to deterioration of the working parts.
8. Wipe the insertion tube with lint-free swabs dampened with disinfectant. Rinse with clear water.	8. Swabs must be lint-free to avoid leaving tiny threads.
9. Wipe the light guide tube with dampened swabs.	9. Remove any residual disinfectant.
10. Apply an alcohol solution to the ocular lens and clean carefully.	10. The alcohol will evaporate quickly without leaving smears.
11. Dry the endoscope thoroughly by hanging it up on a secure hook.	11. Any residual liquid will run downwards away from the control.
12. Store in a carrying case or cabinet.	12. This will protect the endoscope from damage.

FURTHER READING

Bowden C, Masters J 2001 Quick Reference Guide to Veterinary Surgical Kits. Butterworth-Heinemann, Oxford

Cooper B, Lane DR (eds) 1999 Veterinary Nursing, 2nd edn. Butterworth-Heinemann, Oxford

Moore M (ed.) 1999 Manual of Veterinary Nursing. BSAVA, Gloucester

Simpson G (ed.) 1991 Practical Veterinary Nursing. BSAVA, Gloucester

8

Surgical nursing procedures

T. Samuel

Introduction

After the diagnosis and treatment of a patient's condition has been completed by the veterinary surgeon it is often the task of the veterinary nurse to dress and bandage the affected area. Depending on the site and type of wound, the aim of bandaging is to cover and protect the area from contamination and the risk of infection and to prevent the patient from interfering with the wound, both of which will delay the rate of healing. Bandaging is also used to immobilise fractured or dislocated bones to reduce discomfort and accelerate healing.

Many wounds will not require bandaging and in some cases a bandage may draw the patient's attention to the area, leading to self-mutilation. This must be considered when deciding whether or not to apply a bandage. In all cases the wound must be cleaned and dressed and the patient placed under observation. At first this may be done by the nurse, and later when the patient goes home, the owner must be instructed as to how to deal with the wound and the warning signs to watch out for.

This chapter describes the steps involved in wound care and in the various types of bandage. It also covers biopsy techniques and the correct method of scaling and polishing an animal's teeth—a procedure that is often performed by the veterinary nurse.

PROCEDURE: WOUND MANAGEMENT

ACTION	RATIONALE
1. Place the animal in a comfortable position on a table.	1. If the animal feels uncomfortable it will try to escape.
2. Ask an assistant to restrain the animal so that it is relaxed but secure and the wound is accessible for treatment.	2. The assistant will be able to react quickly should the animal try to escape. The animal may resent the wound being touched.
3. Wash your hands with a surgical scrub.	3. It is important not to introduce infection into the wound.
4. Control any haemorrhage.	4. Any bleeding should be controlled, as a large loss of blood may cause shock.
5. Check for signs of shock and treat.	5. If left untreated, the animal's condition will deteriorate.
6. Assess the type of wound and treat accordingly (Table 8.1).	6. Different types of wound need different treatment, dressings and aftercare. A general anaesthetic/sedative may be needed.
7. For open wounds, fill the wound with a sterile lubricant and clip hair away from around the wound.	7. The lubricant prevents hair from contaminating the wound. The hair is clipped to allow the area to be cleaned aseptically.
8. Clean the area surrounding the wound with a surgical scrub and warm water. Clean the wound by lavage with warm, sterile saline in a 20 ml syringe with a 20 G needle. Continue until all debris has been flushed away.	8. Cleaning the wound in this way will provide enough pressure to remove contamination without damaging the cells.
9. Assess the blood supply to the wound. If necessary debride the wound by using a scalpel blade to remove necrotic tissue and restore blood supply.	9. Necrotic tissue must be removed. The area must have a good blood supply to start the healing process.
10. Close the wound if necessary (Table 8.1). Suturing techniques are covered later in this chapter.	10. First-intention wound healing occurs when the edges of the wound are held together. Second intention or granulation is the healing of an open wound.
11. Apply a light dry dressing to first-intention wounds. A secondary and tertiary layer may be applied for protection.	11. This will absorb any blood or exudate produced by the wound and protect the wound from infection, trauma and patient interference.
12. For second-intention wounds, use a moist dressing that will not dry out the wound. The use of a hydrogel applied to the wound before the primary layer is applied is recommended. Apply secondary and tertiary layers.	12. A moist dressing will provide the correct environment to promote a healthy bed for granulation and re-epithelialisation. The secondary layer absorbs any exudate and provides support. The tertiary layer acts as a protective outer layer, holding the others in place.

Table 8.1   Wound classification

Type	Comments	Treatment
Open wounds Incised	There is a break in the covering of the body surface Skin edges are clean and clearly defined. The cut edges may bleed freely. The wound will heal quickly, by first intention. Caused by sharp, cutting materials e.g. scalpel or glass	Ensure that deeper structures are not damaged before closing the wound. Hold edges together with sutures
Laceration	The wound is irregular in shape, with possible tissue loss. There may be little blood loss. Risk of infection is high. The wound will heal by second intention, with possible scarring	Assess the wound, i.e. is any skin available for closure/partial closure by suturing. Dress the wound
Puncture	Surface wound is small with a deep track running down from it. The surface wound will heal quickly, trapping bacteria and causing an abscess to form. Common causes are bites, airgun pellets and thorns	Remove the cause of the injury. The wound must be kept open to allow infection to escape and granulation tissue to develop at the bottom of the tract. Application of warm compress or poultice will encourage this
Abrasion	The epidermis has been rubbed off, exposing the dermis. Can be painful, as nerve endings are exposed. Although not serious, there is a risk of contamination	Clean and dress the wound with a moist dressing
Abscess	A collection of pus enclosed in an area of inflamed tissue. Commonly results from a puncture wound	The abscess must be lanced (unless already burst), but only when it is 'pointing'. This is the thinning of the skin, over the abscess, indicating a point that can be lanced. Placing a warm compress on the area will encourage this. Using a scalpel blade at 90°, incise the wound. Express the pus. Flush the wound with sterile saline until clear. Keep the wound open and continue to flush daily. The wound will heal by second intention
Closed wounds Contusion	The injury does not penetrate the thickness of the skin A bruise. Occurs when blood vessels are ruptured due to a blow to the skin surface. May be seen in an open wound	Arrest the internal haemorrhage by applying a cold compress
Haematoma	A collection of blood under the skin causing swelling. The wound is soft and often painless. If left, the blood will clot, contract and become 'knobbly'	Arrest the internal haemorrhage by applying a cold compress and, if possible, apply a firm dressing. Surgical intervention may be necessary to drain the haematoma
Other Types Skin graft	A portion of skin is taken from one area of the body to fill a deficit in another part. There are two types: • a *pedicle graft* involves moving the entire skin thickness to another area; this heals by first intention • a *free skin graft* moves the epidermis and part or all of the dermis; this heals by second intention	Dress according to type
Ulcer	A local excavation of the surface of an organ or tissue. An ulcer contains inflammatory exudate within a crater. This heals by second intention	Remove the cause of the injury, dress with a moist dressing if anatomically possible. Treat bacterial infections
Tumour	Any abnormal swelling in or on part of the body that has no physiological use. May be benign or malignant	Before treatment the type of tumour must be identified. Surgical intervention is often necessary

13. Ensure that the dressing is comfortable and that the patient will not interfere with it.

13. Reasons for interference include the bandage being too tight, resulting in poor circulation, pain, sutures too tight and boredom. An Elizabethan collar, topical sprays and supervised muzzling may be used.

14. Explain the aftercare of the wound and dressing to the owner.

14. Protect from wet and dirt by covering with a plastic bag. Observe for patient interference, odour, sores, discharge and slipping. Change the dressing when advised.

PROCEDURE: BANDAGING TECHNIQUES—GENERAL POINTS

ACTION

1. Prepare all equipment necessary for the type of bandage.

2. Place the animal in a comfortable position on a table.
3. Ask an assistant to restrain the animal so that it is relaxed but secure, and the area for bandaging is accessible.
4. Apply a primary dressing to any wounds.

5. Apply the bandage. Wherever possible, apply the bandage in a 'reverse wind' method.
6. Ensure that the bandage is comfortable and that the patient cannot interfere with it.

7. Explain the aftercare of the wound and dressing to the owner.

RATIONALE

1. This will save time and allow you to complete the bandage without leaving the animal.
2. If the animal feels uncomfortable it will try to escape.
3. The assistant will be able to react quickly should the animal try to escape. The animal may resent the wound being touched.
4. This layer is applied directly to the skin surface. It is necessary to ensure the correct environment to protect the wound and encourage healing. Dressings can be moist or dry.
5. This will create a more even tension.

6. Reasons for interference include the bandage being too tight, resulting in poor circulation, pain, sutures too tight, and boredom. An Elizabethan collar, topical sprays and supervised muzzling may be used.
7. Protect from wet and dirt by covering with a bag. Observe for patient interference, odour, sores, discharge and slipping. Change the dressing when advised.

Table 8.2   Bandaging techniques

Type	Indications	Comments
Robert Jones	Support and immobilisation of fore- and hindlimbs, commonly used in fractures. Reduction of pain, oedema and haemorrhage	A light, but firm cylindrical bandage
Velpeau sling	Support and immobilisation of the elbow joint after luxation or surgery	
Ehmer sling	Support and immobilisation of the hip, after reduction of a luxation	
Ear	Support and protection of the ear after trauma, or postoperatively after resection or haematoma	One or both ears can be included. Ensure that the ear position is marked
Chest	Support and protection of wounds and dressings Useful for holding chest drains in place	
Limb	Support and protection of wounds, reduction of pain, swelling and movement	Ensure toes and dewclaw are padded. Work from distal to proximal. Include the whole foot and joint above the injury
Tail	Protection of wounds from environmental trauma and/or self-mutilation	Elastoplast may be applied directly to the hair to prevent this bandage from slipping
Splint	Immobilisation of an injury below the elbow and stifle	Limited to lower limbs. Immobilisation cannot be achieved above the elbow and stifle because of the large mass of muscle that surrounds the bones. Application is often painful for the patient and therefore limited to a first aid procedure Common splints used in practice: gutter splints—made of hard plastic, lined with foam, and snap off to the correct length; Zimmer splints—made of pliable aluminium backed in a foam composite
Cast	Immobilisation of a limb	Common cast material: plaster of Paris—bandage covered in gypsum (calcium sulphate) that sets hard when water is added; polyurethane-based and thermoplastic materials—lightweight, waterproof, short drying time and more radiolucent than plaster of Paris

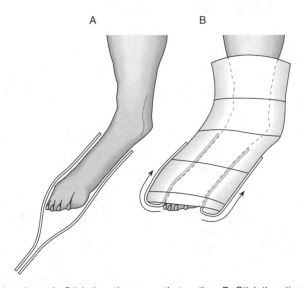

A   B

Figure 8.1   The Robert Jones bandage. A, Stick the stirrups gently together. B, Stick the stirrups to the conforming bandage.

Individual bandaging techniques (Table 8.2)

PROCEDURE: ROBERT JONES BANDAGE

ACTION	RATIONALE
1. Apply two strips of 2.5 cm wide zinc oxide tape to the cranial and caudal aspects of the lower third of the limb. Allow another 10 cm of tape to overhang the toes, and gently stick together.	1. These strips will later be included in the bandage, and form the 'stirrups' (Fig. 8.1A).
2. Apply cotton wool around the entire length of the limb. Pay particular attention to any bony prominences. Use at least three layers, depending on the size of the animal. Ensure that it is of an even thickness throughout.	2. This layer provides the support. The greater the amount of cotton wool, the more immobilised the limb becomes. Larger animals will require more layers.
3. Compress the cotton wool by bandaging it with a conforming bandage appropriate to the size of the animal. Leave two nails showing at the bottom.	3. This must be applied firmly and evenly to gain maximum support. The two nails can be used as a guide to circulation, and will also encourage the animal to use the limb to some degree.
4. Continue applying conforming bandage until sufficient tension has been created.	4. The bandage should be approximately three times the width of the animal's leg. When it is 'flicked' with your finger, it should sound like a ripe melon.
5. Separate the zinc oxide tapes from each other. Twist the tape 180° and stick to the conforming layer (Fig. 8.1B).	5. This will prevent the bandage from slipping down the limb.
6. Apply a layer of cohesive bandage over the conforming bandage.	6. This will protect the other layers.

PROCEDURE: VELPEAU SLING

ACTION	RATIONALE
1. Apply cotton wool padding to the carpal and metacarpal areas of the affected limb.	1. This area will be held in flexion, and needs to be padded for the comfort of the animal.
2. Apply conforming bandage, appropriate to the animal's size, above the carpal for several turns (Fig. 8.2A).	2. This secures the bandage.
3. Flex the elbow and shoulder and, at the same time, take the bandage over the shoulder, under the chest, medial to the other front leg and back to the carpal.	3. This will hold the shoulder and elbow in flexion against the body.
4. Flex the carpus and include this in the bandage (Fig. 8.2B). Continue up over the shoulder and under the chest as before.	4. The carpus, elbow and shoulder should now be held in flexion against the chest.
5. Continue in this manner until the whole limb is held securely.	5. The animal should not be able to move the limb, but make sure that the sling does not impede respiration.
6. Apply a layer of cohesive bandage over the conforming bandage (Fig. 8.2C).	6. This will protect the other layers.

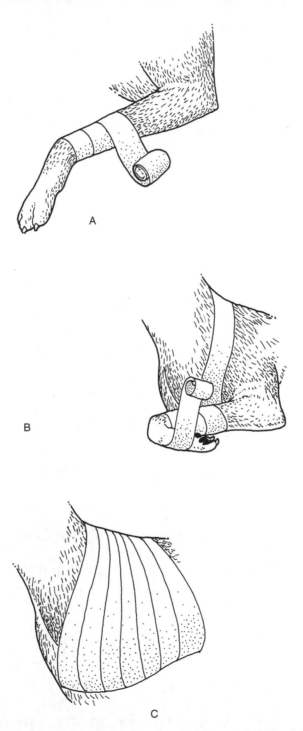

Figure 8.2 The Velpeau sling. A, Wind the conforming bandage around the carpal. B, Flex the carpus. C, Apply a layer of cohesive bandage over the top.

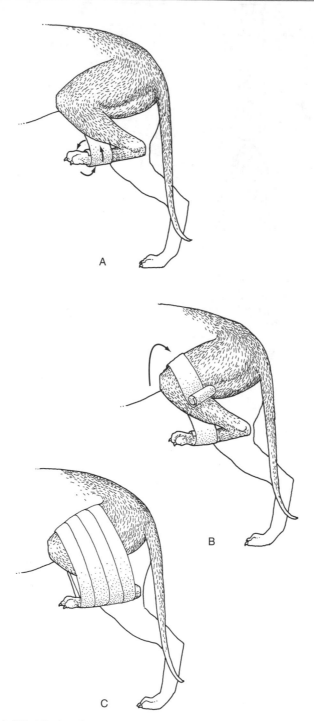

Figure 8.3 The Ehmer sling. A, Wind the bandage around the metatarsal. B, Bring the bandage over the lateral thigh. C, Apply a layer of conforming bandage.

PROCEDURE: EHMER SLING

ACTION

1. Apply cotton wool padding to the metatarsal area of the affected limb.

2. Apply conforming bandage, appropriate to the animal's size, around the padding for several turns (Fig. 8.3A). Ensure that the last bandage turn finishes on the lateral side of the metatarsal.

3. From this point, take the bandage up the medial aspect of the stifle, pad the top of the femur, and bring the bandage over to the lateral aspect of the thigh (Fig. 8.3B). The limb should be held in flexion.

4. Take the bandage down to the medial aspect of the metatarsals, and around to the lateral aspect. You are back at the starting point.

5. Continue in this manner until the whole limb is securely held.

6. Apply a layer of cohesive bandage over the conforming bandage (Fig. 8.3C).

RATIONALE

1. This is the starting point of the sling, which should be padded to provide comfort for the animal.

2. This secures the bandage.

3. This is half-way to the complete figure-of-eight that is the aim of the bandage.

4. This figure-of-eight bandage ensures that the foot is rotated inwards and the hock outwards, which in turn pushes the femoral head into the acetabulum.

5. The animal should not be able to move the limb.

6. This will protect the other layers.

PROCEDURE: EAR BANDAGE

ACTION

1. Apply cotton wool padding to the top of the head, above the ear flap. Fold the affected ear(s) up on to the padding.

2. Ensure that any wounds are dressed. Cover the ear(s) with cotton wool padding. Ensure that the padding is the same size as the ear flap.

3. Apply a layer of synthetic padding. Start at the top of the skull, run cranially around the ear that is down (if any), under the jaw, and back up to the start point.

4. Continue as above, but apply the padding caudally around the healthy ear. Ensure that the bandage is not too tight around the larynx and trachea. Continue until the ear(s) and padding are covered.

5. Apply a cohesive bandage, appropriate to the animal's size, in the same manner. Continue until the padding layer is covered.

RATIONALE

1. This will provide comfort and absorb any discharge. One or both ears can be folded on top of the head.

2. This helps to keep the bandage neat, with no pieces hanging over the face of the animal, but large enough to be effective.

3. The idea is to keep the healthy ear exposed. This is achieved by using a figure-of-eight design, winding the bandage cranially then caudally around the healthy ear (Fig. 8.4A).

4. Check that the bandage does not impede the animal's respiration.

5. This will secure and protect the other layers.

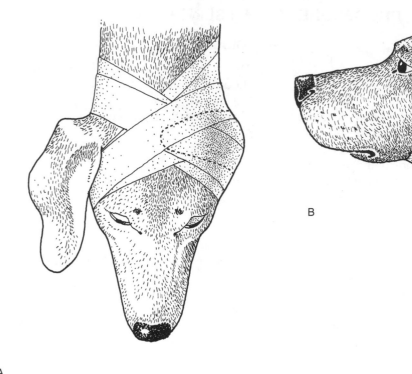

Figure 8.4 The figure-of-eight design for an ear bandage. A, Wind the bandage around the head in a figure-of-eight. B, Mark the position of the ear with an arrow.

ACTION	RATIONALE
6. Mark the direction of the bandaged ear with an arrow (Fig. 8.4B).	6. This will help when the bandage is removed. The operator will know where the earflap is and can avoid injuring it.

PROCEDURE: CHEST BANDAGE

ACTION

1. Start the bandage between the shoulder blades. Apply a layer of synthetic padding material cranially over the right lateral scapula. Bring the bandage through the front legs, caudal to the left scapula. Bring the bandage up to the start point.

2. From the start point, take the bandage caudal to the right scapula, through the front legs, cranial to the left scapula. Bring the bandage over the left lateral scapula back to the start point.

3. Continue in this manner several times, moving the end point caudally, half the width of the bandage.

RATIONALE

1. This is halfway to achieving the desired figure-of-eight bandage.

2. The figure-of-eight is complete.

3. This style ensures that the bandage does not slip backwards.

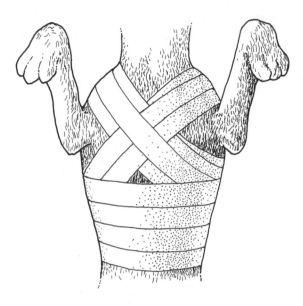

Figure 8.5 Chest bandage.

4. Wind the bandage around the chest, working caudally, until the desired size is achieved (Fig. 8.5).
5. Apply a cohesive layer, appropriate to the animal's size, in the same manner. Continue until the padding layer is covered.

4. Check at regular intervals that the bandage does not impede the animal's breathing.

5. This will secure and protect the other layers.

PROCEDURE: LIMB BANDAGE

ACTION

1. Apply cotton wool padding between the digits and pads of the affected limb (Fig. 8.6A).
2. Apply a secondary layer of synthetic padding. Start on the cranial aspect of the limb, over the toes to the caudal aspect, and return to the start (Fig. 8.6B). Turn the bandage by 90° (Fig. 8.6C) and cover the toes in a figure-of-eight. Work from distal to proximal. Overlap the bandage by half its width.
3. Continue up the limb until over the joint above the injury (Fig. 8.6D).
4. Apply a tertiary layer, again working from distal to proximal.

RATIONALE

1. This will absorb sweat and prevent the digits from rubbing together.

2. This layer is used for padding and support. It will also absorb any exudate from the wound.

3. This will provide more support for the limb and in turn hold the bandage in place.
4. This layer is used to hold the other layers in place and create an outer layer that will withstand daily wear and tear. A layer of conforming bandage followed by a cohesive layer is often used; however, the cohesive layer alone is often enough.

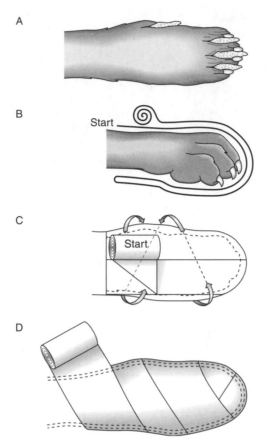

Figure 8.6 Limb bandage. A, Pad the digits and pads with cotton wool. B, Bandage over the toes. C, Twist the bandage through 90°. D, Continue winding the bandage up the limb.

PROCEDURE: TAIL BANDAGE

ACTION

1. Following the dressing, cover any wounds by placing an empty syringe case over the end of the tail. Ensure the end of the case is pierced with a hole for ventilation (Fig. 8.7).
2. Apply a layer of cohesive bandage caudally to cranially over the syringe case.

3. Continue applying the bandage, working the animal's hair into each wind.
4. Elastoplast may be applied to the top of the tail bandage.

RATIONALE

1. This will prevent further trauma to the wound should the animal want to wag its tail!

2. Cohesive bandage has more grip on the hair than conforming bandage, making it less likely to come off; however, in shorthaired dogs, Elastoplast may have to be used to hold the bandage in place.
3. This will help the bandage to stay in place.

4. This may be needed for extra grip.

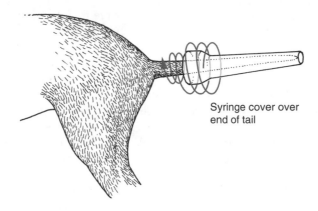

Syringe cover over
end of tail

Figure 8.7   Tail bandage.

PROCEDURE: SPLINTING A LIMB

ACTION

1. Apply two layers of synthetic padding to the affected limb. Cover the joints both above and below the injury. Pay particular attention to bony prominences.

2. Apply the splint to the limb. Ensure that it is long enough to immobilise the joints above and below the injury.
3. Hold the splint in place with adhesive tape in two or three places.
4. Apply a layer of cohesive bandage over the top.

RATIONALE

1. To stabilise the injury both joints must be included. The padding provides comfort; however, the splint must be in close contact to provide immobility. Some splints have padding attached and, when used, less additional synthetic padding is needed.
2. Many different types of splint are available.

3. This holds the splint in place.

4. This protects the splint.

PROCEDURE: CASTING USING PLASTER OF PARIS

ACTION

1. Before applying the cast ensure that the fracture has been reduced.
2. Cover the limb with tubular gauze, appropriate to the animal's size. Ensure that the joints above and below the injury are covered. Allow 2 cm of extra gauze at either end.
3. Apply a layer of synthetic padding, again leaving 2 cm at either end.
4. Unroll the plaster of Paris bandage by 10 cm and immerse in hand-hot water for a few seconds.

RATIONALE

1. Reduction is necessary for optimum healing of the site.
2. This can be applied using a metal frame. This will be folded back later to create a smooth end.

3. This is for the animal's comfort. Apply more padding to joints and bony prominences.
4. Unrolling 10 cm makes it easier to find the end of the bandage when it is wet. The drying time is shortened if warm water is used.

5. Squeeze out excess water from the bandage. Apply to the limb, working distally to proximally. Overlap the bandage by half.
6. Ensure even coverage over the joints.
7. Turn over the tubular gauze and padding at the ends. Smooth into the plaster of Paris.
8. Smooth and mould the cast into the correct shape.
9. The bandage must be completely dry before allowing the animal to bear weight on the limb.
10. Ensure that the circulation is checked regularly by using the protruding toes as a guide.

5. Leave the middle two toes protruding from the end of the cast; these can be used as a guide to circulation.
6. The cast can become weak over these points.
7. This creates a neat and tidy cast.
8. Any changes must be done before the bandage dries.
9. Drying times vary; refer to manufacturer's instructions.
10. The toes should be warm to touch. Cold toes may indicate that the cast is too tight.

Drainage systems (Table 8.3)

PROCEDURE: USE OF THE PENROSE DRAIN

ACTION

1. Clean and debride the wound.

2. Using a scalpel blade, make an incision at the top of the wound (Fig. 8.8A), working from the inside to the outside of the wound. The incision should be no wider than the width of the drain. Leave the tip of the blade protruding.
3. Using a pair of sterile artery forceps, grasp the tip of the blade. Retract the scalpel blade until the tips of the artery forceps are showing on the inside of the wound (Fig. 8.8B).

RATIONALE

1. This will reduce the risk of infection and increase the blood supply to the wound, accelerating the rate of wound healing.

3. This technique maintains the incision.

Table 8.3 Drainage systems

Type	Comments
Closed drains	No exposure to the environment. Can be active (suction) or passive (reliant on gravity)
Thoracic: water trap	Fluid or air is drawn out from the thorax by gravity. It is prevented from returning by a water trap placed at least 80 cm away from the animal. Use in non-ambulatory patients only
Thoracic: Heimlich valve	Inlet is attached securely into the animal, while the outlet is attached to a giving set and bag
Urinary catheter	Drainage of the bladder. Can be indwelling and attached to a giving set and bag
Needle and syringe	Used in many situations as a low-pressure active drain
Open drains	Exposure to the environment. All types are passive
Penrose	Broad, hollow latex tubing. Fluid passes over the surface by capillary action
Seton	Usually a sterile gauze bandage packed into an area. A 'tail' is left protruding
Sump	Similar to a Penrose drain. Air passes inside to the wound, while fluid passes over the outside Used in deep abscesses

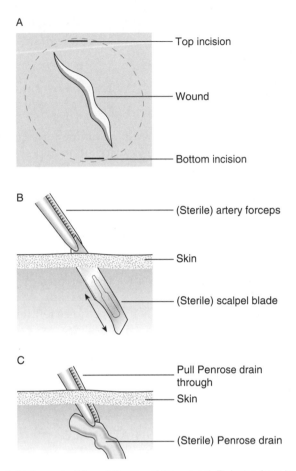

Figure 8.8 The Penrose drain. A, Make an incision at the top of the wound. B, Incise from inside to outside. C, Pull the drain through.

4. Release the blade and dispose of it safely.

5. Attach the end of the Penrose drain to the artery forceps and pull through (Fig. 8.8C). Release when 4–5 cm are showing.

6. Repeat this procedure at the base of the wound.
7. Suture the wound.
8. Suture the Penrose drain at either end, to the skin at the point of the incisions made earlier. Use two single interrupted sutures, preferably in a nylon of a different colour to the wound sutures.
9. Cut the ends of the drain so that 2–3 cm protrude.

4. This leaves the artery forceps through the incision.
5. This technique inserts the drain without the need to release, and return to the incision, thus reducing soft-tissue damage and time taken.

7. The wound is separate from the drain.
8. The sutures hold the drain in place. The different colours allow easy identification of the sutures when it comes to removing them.

9. A longer length than this increases the risk of contamination.

10. The wound can be dressed to absorb any exudate draining from the tubing. Ensure that the site is bathed and the dressing changed daily.
11. If the drain is left uncovered, advise the owner to bathe the site twice daily with salt water.
12. Advise the owner of the signs that may indicate infection and fluid build-up.
13. Prevent the animal from removing the drain.

14. When removing the drain, prepare the area aseptically.
15. Remove the sutures on the top site and pull the drain upwards until clean drain is showing.
16. Cut the drain horizontally at this point.

17. Remove the sutures at the bottom site and pull the drain through from this point.

10. This reduces the risk of contamination and keeps the drain open.

11. This removes the exudate, keeps the drain open, and reduces the risk of contamination.

12. Examine for signs of oedema, redness, pain, irritation and systemic illness.
13. Use an Elizabethan collar appropriate to the animal's size.
14. There is a risk of contamination.

15. About 5 mm of clean drain is necessary. This maintains asepsis.

16. This ensures that only 'clean' drain enters the wound.
17. The holes left will heal by granulation.

Fracture management

PROCEDURE: FIRST AID PROCEDURE IN A CASE OF A SUSPECTED FRACTURE

ACTION

1. Check the animal's airway, breathing and circulation.

2. Restrain the animal in a comfortable position. Gently examine for injuries.
3. Control haemorrhage.

4. Examine the patient for fractures. This must be done gently to prevent further injury.
5. If possible, clean any wounds and apply a sterile dressing.
6. Gently apply a splint or Robert Jones bandage to the affected limb.
7. If necessary, transport the animal to the surgery, constantly monitoring the patient's condition. Ensure that the animal is adequately restrained.

8. Treat the animal for shock.
9. Administer analgesia as directed by the veterinary surgeon.

RATIONALE

1. This must be done before checking for other injuries. The animal will die within a few minutes without oxygen.
2. An injured animal is more likely to try to escape and/or bite.
3. Loss of blood will cause the animal to go into shock.
4. Pain, swelling, loss of use, abnormal position and crepitus indicate a fracture.
5. This may not be possible if first aid treatment is not in practice.
6. This will immobilise the limb, reducing pain and further damage.
7. It is often easier to move the animal with two people. A stretcher may be necessary for large animals. If a spinal injury is suspected then always use a rigid stretcher (see Ch. 1).

9. The animal will be in pain.

Table 8.4 Methods of fracture fixation

Type	Comments
External techniques	
Splints	See Bandaging techniques
Casts	See Bandaging techniques
Robert Jones bandage	See Bandaging techniques
Internal fixation	
Intramedullary pins include:	Inserted into the medullary cavity
Steinmann pin	Straight sharpened pins. Choose the correct size, as the pin must be a snug fit
Kirschner wire/nail	As above
Rush pin	Curved pins, used in pairs
Cerclage wire	Made from stainless steel. Can be used as single sutures, in conjunction with pins or plates, or as a tension band for avulsed fractures
Bone plates and screws include:	
Venables plate	Self-tapping screws are inserted into holes in the bone
Sherman plate	Similar to the Venables plate but not as strong
Compression bone plate	A tap is used to cut a thread in the bone for the screws. This gives a stronger hold
Lag screws	Half or fully threaded screws that draw fragments back into position
External/internal fixation	
External fixator	A series of pins screwed into the bone through the skin, held in place by scaffolding on the outside
Cage rest	Limited movement of the animal. Common treatment with a fractured pelvis

10. When stable, the patient may be X-rayed to diagnose the extent of the injuries.

11. Any fractures may then be reduced and fixation performed (Table 8.4).

10. An animal suffering from shock is not a good candidate for sedation/anaesthesia. Treatment for shock is of primary importance to stabilise the patient before administering an anaesthetic.

11. There are severals methods of treatment. Choice depends on the location of the fracture.

Suturing techniques (Fig. 8.9)
PROCEDURE: SIMPLE INTERRUPTED SKIN SUTURE

ACTION

1. Ensure that the wound to be closed is aseptic and has a good blood supply.
2. Select an appropriate suture material for the wound (Table 8.5).
3. Select an appropriate type of needle holder and grasp using the thumb and ring finger.
4. Position the threaded needle at a right angle in the needle holder. Grasp the needle along two-thirds of its length.
5. Pick up a pair of rat-toothed forceps with the other hand. These should be held like a pencil.
6. Stabilise the skin on the far side of the wound with the forceps. Push the tip of the needle though the skin towards you.

RATIONALE

1. This reduces the risk of infection and increases the rate of wound healing.
2. This will depend on the type of tissue being sutured.
3. This grip aids precision in placing and using the needle.
4. This will prevent the needle from bending.

5. The forceps are used to hold the skin stable.

6. The 'bite', i.e. the distance from the skin edge to the point at which the tip of the needle enters the skin, should be equal to the skin thickness.

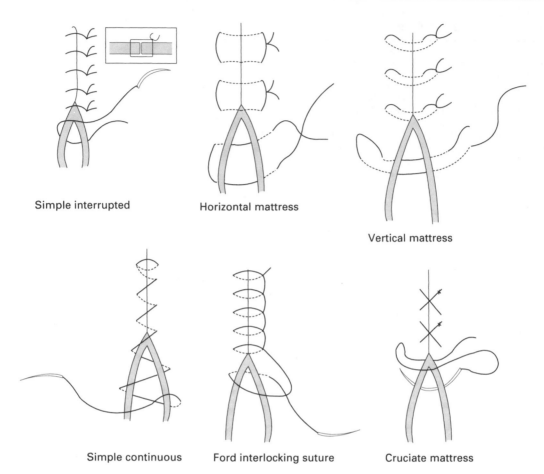

Simple interrupted   Horizontal mattress

Vertical mattress

Simple continuous   Ford interlocking suture   Cruciate mattress

Figure 8.9 Common suture patterns used in the skin. Reproduced, with permission, from *Veterinary Nursing*, p. 557, 2nd edn, by Lane and Cooper (1994). Butterworth Heinemann, UK.

Table 8.5 Suture materials

Type	Characteristics	Indications
Absorbable		
Chromic catgut	Derived from the intestines of cattle and sheep A synthetic catgut is available. A monofilament that knots well. Occasional tissue reaction Strength lasts for 14 days	Subcutaneous, subcuticular and muscle sutures
Polyglactin 910 (Vicryl)	A braided synthetic suture. High tensile strength lasting for 21 days. Totally absorbed in 70–90 days	Subcuticular, subcutaneous, muscle and mucous membrane
Polyglycolic acid (Dexon)	As polyglactin but absorption is longer. Knots can slip undone	Subcuticular, subcutaneous, muscle and mucous membrane
Polydioxanone (PDS*11)	A synthetic monofilament. High tensile strength lasting for 42 days. Causes little tissue reaction	Subcutaneous, subcuticular and muscle sutures
Non-absorbable		
Monofilament nylon (Ethilon)	Minimal tissue reaction, high tensile strength. Knots must have at least three throws for stability	Skin
Braided silk (Mersilk)	A natural suture material. Adequate tensile strength. Can attract infection. Occasional tissue reaction	Skin
Braided nylon (Nurolon)	Produced to mimic silk. Less tissue reaction, high tensile strength	Skin

7. Release the needle and skin. Regrasp the tip of the needle and pull through.
8. Stabilise the near side of the wound with the forceps. Push the needle through the underside of the skin.
9. Release the needle and skin. Regrasp the tip of the needle and pull through.
10. Tie the knot. Use a surgeon's knot on the first throw by looping the ends around each other twice. Follow with two single knots. These should be in a reef knot, not a granny knot.

11. Cut the ends of the suture as short as possible without the risk of the knot undoing.
12. Repeat the suture along the length of the wound.

7. The needle is through the far side of the wound.
8. This 'bite' should be the same size as the first.

9. The needle has now passed through both sides of the wound.
10. The knot can be tied by hand or by instrument; with practice, the latter is less time-consuming. The skin edges should be brought together so that they are just touching. The first throw should never be pulled tight, as that is done with the later throws.
11. This will help prevent the animal biting the sutures, leading to removal.
12. In a simple wound, work the stitches from left to right or right to left. If the wound is irregular, place a few sutures along the wound and fill in the spaces. This will create an even closure.

Biopsy techniques (Table 8.6)

PROCEDURE: FINE-NEEDLE ASPIRATION

ACTION

1. Place the animal in a comfortable position on a table.
2. Ask an assistant to restrain the animal so that it is relaxed and secure and the site is accessible.

RATIONALE

1. If the animal feels uncomfortable it will try to escape.
2. The assistant will be able to react quickly should the animal try to escape. The animal may resent the site being touched.

Table 8.6 Biopsy techniques

Type	Comments	Indications
Fine-needle aspirate (FNA)	Simple and quick to perform. Examination will provide information on cell type only. Can be performed on a conscious patient	Swellings, bone marrow and soft tissue
Needle core biopsy (Tru-cut)	Quick to perform. Requires special needle. More information provided than FNA. Patient may need a general anaesthetic (GA) or sedation	Swellings and organs
Punch biopsy	Quick to perform. Requires special punch. More information provided than FNA. Patient may need a GA or sedation	Skin, soft tissue and organs
Incisional (wedge)	No special equipment. A portion of the mass is surgically removed. Provides much information on type of mass. Patient will require a GA	Skin, soft tissue and organs
Trephine	Special instrument required. Removes a circular area of tissue. Patient will require a GA	Bone lesions
Excisional biopsy	Removal of entire mass or organ. Provides full information on type. Patient will require a GA	Mass or organ that can be excised completely

3. Clean the area selected for the biopsy with surgical scrub and warm water until aseptic.
4. Attach a 10 ml syringe to a 23G needle.

5. Insert the needle into the site and pull back on the plunger. Repeat this five times. Do not withdraw the needle from the site.
6. Maintain slight pressure in the syringe by holding the plunger slightly back. Remove the needle from the site.
7. Detach the needle from the syringe. Pull back on the plunger and position the end of the syringe over a microscope slide.

8. Push down on the plunger and express the cells on to the microscope slide.

3. This reduces the risk of infection.

4. These sizes will provide the correct amount of negative pressure to gather the sample.
5. This process draws cells from the biopsy site into the needle.

6. This pressure will prevent cells from being pulled out of the needle when removed from the site.
7. Pulling back on the plunger draws all the cells in the needle into the syringe. The needle can now be removed without wasting any cells.
8. The sample is now ready to be made into a smear and examined.

PROCEDURE: PUNCH BIOPSY

ACTION

1. Place the animal in a comfortable position on a table.
2. Ask an assistant to restrain the animal so that it is relaxed and secure and the site is accessible.
3. Clip the site to be selected for biopsy.
4. Clean the area with surgical scrub and warm water until aseptic.
5. With a 25G needle, inject local anaesthetic around the site. Allow sufficient time for the local anaesthetic to work.
6. Use a sterile punch biopsy to excise the sample. Ensure the full thickness of the skin has been included (Table 8.6).
7. Place the sample in a pot containing 10% formal saline.
8. Close the wound left by the biopsy punch with a simple interrupted suture.

RATIONALE

1. If the animal feels uncomfortable it will try to escape.
2. The assistant will be able to react quickly should the animal try to escape. The animal may resent the site being touched.
3. This will make the site more accessible.
4. This reduces the risk of infection.

5. This will reduce the pain experienced by the animal.

6. Biopsy punches of 4 mm and 6 mm are available. Choice depends on thickness of skin to be sampled.
7. This 'fixes' the sample, preventing cell necrosis and aiding cell examination.
8. As the wound has been incised, it will heal quickly by first-intention healing.

Dentistry

PROCEDURE: SCALING AND POLISHING THE TEETH

ACTION

1. Make sure that the patient is stable under a general anaesthetic and at the correct depth of anaesthesia.
2. Introduce an endotracheal tube of the correct size into the trachea. Tie the tube to the upper jaw using a length of bandage.
3. Position the patient in lateral recumbency, the head slightly lower than the body. This can be achieved by tilting the table or raising the shoulders.
4. Make sure that any fluid is able to drain away from the animal. A tub table is ideal.
5. Put on a facemask, gloves and goggles.

6. Select a gag appropriate to the animal's size. Insert the top and bottom of the gag into the upper and lower canines, respectively.
7. Pack the pharynx with a sterile throat pack appropriate to the animal's size.
8. Examine the teeth for signs of periodontal disease (Table 8.7).
9. Using an ultrasonic scaler, scale the teeth on that side. Refer to manufacturer's instructions. Spend no longer than 10 seconds on one tooth.
10. Check that all calculus (tartar) is removed.

11. Mop up any debris and excess fluid with damp cotton wool swabs.
12. Turn the animal over by swinging the legs under the patient, not over. Ensure that the anaesthetic circuit does not twist and the endotracheal tube is not pulled out.
13. Repeat the scaling process on the other side.

14. Polish the teeth with a polishing handpiece (refer to manufacturer's instructions) using prophylactic paste.
15. When both sides have been completed, clean up any excess paste, check that all teeth have been cleaned and remove the throat pack.

RATIONALE

1. See anaesthetic chapter.

2. It is essential that the animal is intubated to ensure that no fluid from the procedure enters the lungs. The tube must be secure.
3. This will encourage fluid from the procedure to run out of the mouth.

4. This prevents the animal becoming wet and possibly hypothermic.
5. This prevents bacteria in the patient's mouth, disturbed by the procedure, from entering the operator.
6. To keep the mouth open, enabling the operator to work.

7. To prevent fluid entering the lungs.

8. Any problems must be referred to the veterinary surgeon.
9. The vibrating action of the ultrasonic scaler may damage the tooth if used for longer than 10 seconds. You may return to the tooth later if it is still not clean.
10. Calculus is the hard brown deposit on the teeth that forms from plaque as a result of bacterial action.
11. It is important to clean as you work, this prevents the fluid soaking the animal.
12. Dislodging or twisting the anaesthetic tubing are common problems when moving the animal. It may be necessary to disconnect the circuit briefly.
13. It is possible to reach the inside of the far teeth.
14. Polishing the teeth will leave them smooth, which in turn reduces the ability of bacteria to stick to the surface.
15. It is very important always to check that no teeth have been overlooked.

Table 8.7 Periodontal disease

Condition	Description	Treatment
Plaque	A soft layer composed of bacteria in an organic matrix that forms on the surface of a tooth	Brushing pets teeth at home. Change diet if necessary
Calculus	A calcified deposit that forms on the surface of the teeth as a result of bacterial action on plaque	Scaling and polishing
Gingivitis	Inflammation of the gums, which become swollen and bleed easily. Caused by plaque at the base of the teeth	Removal of plaque and calculus by scaling and polishing. Short-term antibiotics to erase the infection
Periodontitis	Resulting from untreated gingivitis, the gum line recedes away from the base of the tooth	Extraction of the tooth. Treatment for gingivitis
Caries	Decay and crumbling of the tooth due to acid produced by bacteria	Extraction or filling
Fracture of the crown	Caused by trauma to the tooth	Extraction or filling
Retained deciduous teeth	Teeth are not shed before permanent ones erupt May cause misplacement of new teeth	Extraction

16. Ensure the animal is clean and dry before finishing.

16. A dental scale and polish is a very wet procedure. If necessary use a hair dryer to dry the animal's fur.

FURTHER READING

Conner J, McKerrel J 1995 A Guide to Animal Bandaging. Millpledge, Retford
Cooper B, Lane DR (eds) 1999 Veterinary Nursing, 2nd edn. Butterworth-Heinemann, Oxford

Hotson-Moore A (ed.) 1999 Manual of Advanced Veterinary Nursing. BSAVA, Gloucester
Tracy DL (ed.) 1994 Small Animal Surgical Nursing, 2nd edn. Mosby, London

9

First aid procedures

T. Samuel

Introduction

Under the Veterinary Surgeons Act 1966 anyone may perform first aid on an animal to save life, to prevent suffering or to prevent the condition from deteriorating but only until such time as a veterinary surgeon is able to attend to the animal. Although by law, lay people and veterinary nurses are able to perform the same procedures, the veterinary nurse will have the greater knowledge and training to be able to assess the situation and deal with the frightened animal and the clinical experience to apply the relevant techniques.

PROCEDURE: EVALUATION OF THE EMERGENCY PATIENT

ACTION

1. Call a veterinary surgeon as soon as possible.

2. Ensure that the environment is safe to treat the animal.

3. Stand back from the animal and evaluate the situation. What are you presented with?

4. Make sure that the patient is restrained appropriately. If the animal is breathing normally, it may be necessary to apply a tape muzzle (see Ch. 1).

5. Check that the animal has a patent airway.

6. Check the animal is breathing. If not, check that the heart is beating, and begin artificial respiration.

7. Check that the animal has a heart beat. If not, start cardiac massage and artificial respiration.

8. Once the patient is stable, check for haemorrhage and control.

9. Examine the patient for fractures and immobilise (see Ch. 8).

10. Check the patient's capillary refill time, mucous membrane colour, pulse and temperature. Record all the information (see Ch. 2).

11. Examine the patient for other wounds.

12. Treat for shock.

RATIONALE

1. This must be done at the first available opportunity. While you are waiting you can assess for 'airway, breathing and circulation'.

2. Do not attempt to treat the animal if there is any risk to you, e.g. fire, electrocution, traffic, radiation or falling masonry.

3. You must remain calm and in control. The owners are likely to be panicking. Avoid rushing in to help before you have assessed the situation.

4. This is made easier if you have an assistant. The animal is likely to be frightened and in pain and its immediate reaction is to escape and/or bite.

5. The animal may be trying to breathe but, if the airway is blocked, respiration will be difficult.

6. Lack of oxygen to the body will kill the animal within a few minutes.

7. If the heart is not beating, blood will not circulate around the body to supply the vital organs.

8. Loss of blood may cause the animal to go into shock.

9. This must be done before attempting to move the patient to reduce pain and prevent the injury deteriorating.

10. These all indicate the condition of the animal.

11. These can be cleaned and dressed as appropriate.

PROCEDURE: CONTROL OF HAEMORRHAGE

ACTION

1. Place the animal in a comfortable position on a table or at a comfortable height for you.

2. Ask an assistant to restrain the animal so that it is relaxed and secure and the wound is accessible for treatment.

3. Clean your hands with a surgical scrub.

4. Assess what type of haemorrhage you are presented with (Table 9.1).

RATIONALE

1. If the animal feels uncomfortable, it will try to escape.

2. The assistant will be able to react quickly if the animal tries to escape. The animal may resent the wound being touched.

3. It is important not to introduce infection into the wound.

4. The extent of the haemorrhage depends on the type of blood vessels that have been

5. Control the haemorrhage using one of the methods described in Table 9.2.

6. Once haemorrhage has been controlled, check for signs of shock and treat if necessary. (Refer to shock.)

7. Monitor the animal closely. If blood soaks through the dressing you have applied, place further dressing material on top of those applied previously.

damaged, e.g. an arterial bleed is much more serious than a capillary bleed.

5. The method used will depend on materials to hand, e.g. you may be in the surgery or at the roadside.

6. Blood loss will reduce the circulating blood volume—hypovolaemic shock. This must be treated or the animal may die.

7. Removing the previous dressing will pull off any clot formed and restart the haemorrhage.

Table 9.1 Types of haemorrhage

Type	Identification	Treatment
Arterial	Bright red and pumps out in spurts. Bleeding point is easy to identify	Very serious. Haemorrhage must be arrested immediately Use directed digital pressure on the ends of the vessels until a more long-term method can be instigated
Venous	Darker red and flows in a steady stream. Bleeding point is easy to identify	Slightly less serious than an arterial bleed; however, haemorrhage must be arrested quickly. Use direct digital pressure or a pressure bandage
Capillary	Multiple, pinpoint haemorrhages. The wound will ooze with little force. Commonly seen in incisional wounds	Less serious than arterial and venous haemorrhage; however, capillary bleeding over a long period of time can be serious. Use of a pressure bandage is recommended
Mixed	Commonly seen. This is a combination of the above	Treatment depends on the extent of the haemorrhage
External	Haemorrhage on the outside of the body Easy to identify	Treatment depends on the extent of the haemorrhage
Internal	Haemorrhage inside the body. Difficult to identify and therefore treat	Treatment depends on the area affected. Possible treatments are a pressure bandage, ice pack, immobilisation of the area and/or treatment for hypovolaemic shock

Table 9.2 First aid treatment of haemorrhage

Type	Method	Comments
Direct digital pressure	With a clean finger and thumb apply pressure to the wound on either side. Care must be taken not to push a foreign body or bone fragments deeper	Quick and easy; however, this is a temporary measure and a pressure bandage must be applied as soon as possible
Pressure bandage	Apply direct pressure by using a sterile dressing and firmly applied bandage. Ensure breathing is not impeded	Deep wounds may need packing with sterile gauze before bandaging. If foreign bodies or bone fragments are suspected, use a ring pad to remove the pressure from the site
Pressure points	An artery is pushed against a bone in order to reduce the flow of blood in that vessel. Can be used in the brachial, femoral and coccygeal arteries	The artery is not always easy to find. Venous bleeding will still continue. This is a temporary measure and a pressure bandage must be applied as soon as possible
Tourniquet	A ready-made or improvised strap is applied above the haemorrhage on a limb. Pressure should be such that it just stops the haemorrhage	This is used as a last resort. The tourniquet should be applied for no longer than 15 minutes, before resting for 1 minute, and then reapplying closer to the wound

PROCEDURE: TREATING BURNS AND SCALDS

ACTION	RATIONALE
1. Ensure the environment is safe to treat the animal.	1. Do not attempt to treat the animal if there is any risk to you, e.g. fire, electrocution, radiation or falling masonry.
2. Place the animal in a comfortable position.	2. The animal may be in extreme pain and may try to escape and/or bite.
3. Ask an assistant to restrain the animal so that it is relaxed and secure and the burn is accessible for treatment.	3. The assistant will be able to react quickly should the animal try to escape. The animal may resent the wound being touched.
4. Clean your hands with a surgical scrub.	4. It is important not to introduce infection into the wound.
5. Cool the area with cold water. A shower hose is ideal as it covers a large area with little pressure. Continue for at least 10 minutes.	5. This will cool the area, limiting the numbers of cells destroyed. The use of an ice pack is not recommended as it puts pressure on to the burnt area.
6. Keep the patient warm by wrapping it in dry blankets. Care must be taken, as the animal will be in severe pain.	6. Although the burns must be cooled, the patient must be warmed to reduce shock. Avoid the use of direct heat, i.e. lamps and pads.
7. Clean the area gently with sterile saline.	7. The area is extremely painful and proper cleaning may only be achieved under a general anaesthetic. General anaesthesia is only recommended if the patient is stable.
8. Dress the wound with wound gel and/or paraffin tulle.	8. The wound must be kept moist at all times.
9. Apply a light, non-adhesive dressing on top.	9. Heat must be able to escape, and moisture loss must be avoided so the dressing must be minimal.
10. Apply a polythene bag or cling film over the dressing.	10. This will prevent moisture evaporating from the area.
11. Gently place a cold wet towel on top. Replace regularly.	11. This will keep the area cool.
12. Observe and treat for shock.	12. Fluid therapy is essential to replace the fluid lost from the wound.
13. Consult the veterinary surgeon on the administration of antibiotics and analgesia.	13. A burn is extremely susceptible to infection so antibiotic cover is essential.

PROCEDURE: TREATING FROSTBITE

ACTION

1. Ensure the environment is safe to treat the animal.
2. Place the animal in a comfortable position.

3. Ask an assistant to restrain the animal so that it is relaxed and secure and the frost burns are accessible for treatment.
4. Clean your hands with a surgical scrub.

5. Apply warm water (body temperature) to the areas. Continue until all areas are warmed to body temperature.
6. **Do not rub the area.**
7. Observe and treat for shock.
8. Consult the veterinary surgeon on the administration of antibiotics and analgesia.

RATIONALE

1. Do not attempt to treat the animal if there is any risk to you.
2. The animal will be in pain and will try to escape and/or bite.
3. Common places for frostbite are anywhere that the blood supply is reduced, e.g. on the ear tip, nose, paws, pads and scrotum.
4. It is important not to introduce infection into the wound.
5. This will gradually warm the area, reducing the number of cells destroyed.

6. This will shatter frozen cells.

8. Frostbite wounds are susceptible to infection so antibiotic cover is essential.

PROCEDURE: TREATMENT OF ASPHYXIA

ACTION

1. Clear any blockages from the mouth and pharynx by opening the mouth and removing any obstruction.

2. Loosen and/or remove the collar.

3. If the animal has water or a foreign body blocking the trachea, the Heimlich manoeuvre can be used.
4. Hold the animal up by its hindlegs, or, for larger animals, hang it upside down over a table or door frame.
5. Administer a sharp punch to the abdominal wall, above the xiphisternum, angled down towards the diaphragm (Fig. 9.1).
6. Repeat up to four times.

7. If attempts to remove the blockage are unsuccessful, provide an emergency airway by pushing a wide-gauge needle through the ventral midline of the neck into the trachea.
8. Prepare the animal for a tracheotomy by clipping and scrubbing the ventral throat area.

RATIONALE

1. The animal may be unconscious but trying to breathe. Examples of obstructions are vomit, balls, toys, blood, water and leaves (if fallen into water).
2. Be aware that the animal may recover quickly and try to escape. A dog running around without its collar is a stray.
3. This technique is designed to force foreign matter from the trachea.

4. The obstructing material may move downwards by gravity.

5. This will force air down the respiratory tract, from the lungs to the trachea, and dislodge the blockage.
6. Repeating the procedure too often can inflict damage.
7. This will act as an air inlet/outlet until a proper tracheotomy can be performed.

8. This is a surgical procedure carried out by the veterinary surgeon.

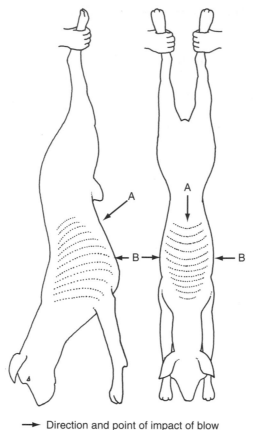

→ Direction and point of impact of blow

Figure 9.1 The Heimlich manoeuvre: A, standard; B, modified version. Reproduced, with permission, from *Veterinary Nursing*, p. 92, 2nd edn, by Lane and Cooper (1994). Butterworth Heinemann, UK.

PROCEDURE: ARTIFICIAL RESPIRATION IN THE INTUBATED PATIENT

ACTION

1. Place an endotracheal tube of an appropriate size in the larynx and trachea of the unconscious animal.
2. Check that the endotracheal tube is free from blockages.
3. Place the animal in the recovery position (Fig. 9.2). Connect the endotracheal tube to an oxygen supply via a closed anaesthetic circuit.
4. Squeeze enough oxygen out of the rebreathing bag to raise the chest slightly. Use gentle pressure at approximately 2 breaths per second.
5. Rest for 5 seconds every 15 seconds.

RATIONALE

1. An endotracheal tube must not be used in a conscious animal as the cough reflex will initiate gagging.
2. The airway must be clear to allow air to pass through.
3. This is the most efficient and hygienic way for the veterinary nurse to perform artificial respiration.
4. This rate mimics the patient's own panting.

5. This time allows you to monitor for the recommencement of the animal's own breathing.

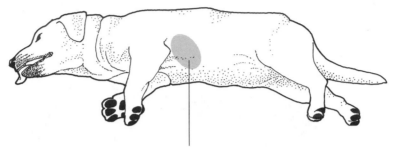

Area to which pressure is applied in artificial respiration

Figure 9.2 The recovery position. Reproduced, with permission, from *Veterinary Nursing*, p. 86, 2nd edn, by Lane and Cooper (1994). Butterworth Heinemann, UK.

6. If there is no oxygen supply to hand, blow down the tube at 1 second intervals.
7. Continue until the animal begins to breathe on its own.

6. The carbon dioxide in your own respiration will act as a respiratory stimulant.
7. This process may be continued for about 30 minutes. If breathing has not restarted by this time, the animal can be pronounced dead.

PROCEDURE: ARTIFICIAL RESPIRATION WITH NO ENDOTRACHEAL TUBE IN PLACE.
ASSUME NO DAMAGE TO CHEST WALL

ACTION

1. Lie the animal on its right side. Extend the head and neck and pull the tongue forwards. Pull the front legs forward so that the upper leg does not lie on the chest.
2. Place the palm of your hand in the middle of the chest wall (Fig. 9.2).
3. Apply firm steady pressure downwards and then release.
4. Apply the pressure at 0.5–1 second intervals, depending on the size of the animal.
5. Continue until the animal begins to breathe on its own.

RATIONALE

1. This is the optimum position for maximum air intake.

2. This hand is used to push the chest wall on to the lungs, forcing air in and out.
3. The elastic rib cage springs back, drawing air into the lungs.
4. The smaller the patient, the faster the respiration rate should be.
5. This process may be continued for about 30 minutes. If breathing has not restarted by this time, the animal can be pronounced dead.

PROCEDURE: MOUTH TO NOSE RESUSCITATION.
ASSUME CHEST WALL IS DAMAGED

ACTION

1. Lie the animal on its right side. Extend the head and neck and pull the tongue forwards.
2. Grasp the nose firmly in the left hand so that the thumb and fingers curl around the nose and mouth and hold the mouth closed.

RATIONALE

1. This is the optimum position for maximum air intake.
2. This creates an air-tight seal.

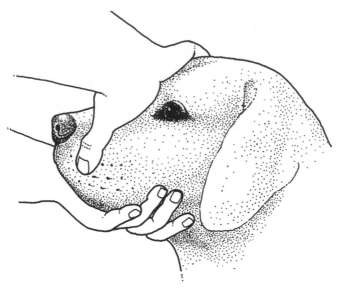

Figure 9.3 Mouth to nose resuscitation: holding the nose. Adapted with permission, from *Veterinary Nursing*, p. 87, 2nd edn, by Lane and Cooper (1994). Butterworth Heinemann, UK.

3. Place the right hand under the lower jaw (Fig. 9.3).
4. If possible, wear a facemask or use a cloth or handkerchief to blow through.
5. Blow down the nose at 1 second intervals. Turn your head away after each blow to avoid inhaling the expired air and saliva.
6. Do not overinflate the lungs. Use just enough air to raise the chest slightly.

3. The weight of the head is now supported.

4. This method is more hygienic for the veterinary nurse.
5. This procedure provides the animal with your expired breath. This is rich in carbon dioxide, which acts as a respiratory stimulant.
6. Some animals, especially the small and/or young, have very delicate lung tissue that can easily be damaged.

PROCEDURE: CARDIAC MASSAGE

ACTION

1. This procedure should be started as soon after lack of a pulse or heartbeat has been detected.
2. Lie the patient in right lateral recumbency.

3. Locate the position of the heart.

4. Place the fingertips of both hands on either side of the chest, over ribs 3–6. Use rhythmical but gentle compression to push the rib cage down. Use a method appropriate to the animal's size.

RATIONALE

1. Lack of blood to the cells, pumped around by the heart, very quickly results in cell death and eventually death of the patient.
2. In this position the heart is situated slightly uppermost and so is easier to palpate.
3. This is within the rib cage, between ribs 3 and 6.
4. For cats and small dogs use pressure with the fingertips of both hands on either side of the thorax. For medium-sized dogs use the lower palm of the hand, and large dogs will require the operator to punch with a closed fist.

5. Apply compression at 0.5–1 second intervals, depending on the animal's size.

6. Carry out artificial respiration at the same time as cardiac massage.

7. If only one person is available, apply cardiac massage for five compressions and inflate the chest three times. Repeat the procedure continuously.

8. If the heart does not restart within 3 minutes, the animal may be declared dead.

5. Small dogs and cats have a faster heart rate than larger dogs so need a faster compression rate.

6. This is easier with two people.

7. This method requires one operator to do both cardiac massage and artificial respiration and can be exhausting after a time.

8. Beyond this time there will be extensive brain damage due to lack of oxygen.

PROCEDURE: TREATMENT OF POISONING

ACTION

1. Take a comprehensive history from the owner of the animal (Table 9.3).

2. Inform the veterinary surgeon.

3. If the animal is still in contact with the poison, then remove it from the source. In the first instance, this is likely to be done by the owner: explain clearly what you expect owners to do—they may be panicking.

RATIONALE

1. The history may be taken over the telephone or when the patient is brought into the surgery. It will provide information to help identify the poison and the time at which it was taken.

2. This must be done at the first available opportunity.

3. For example, if the animal has the poison on its coat or is close to the source, e.g. gas. If the coat is contaminated, wipe the poison away with paper towelling until professional advice can be sought. The use of an Elizabethan collar or towel wrapped around the patient will prevent further ingestion.

Table 9.3 Questions to ask the owner

Question	Rationale
Do you know the cause of the poisoning?	Time is saved if the owner can give you the details of the poison or bring the packet or container to the surgery*
Do you know at what time the patient ate, or came into contact with, the poison?	This will determine whether inducing emesis will be effective
Did the patient eat anything unusual prior to the onset of symptoms?	If a sample is available then advise the owner to bring it to the surgery
Was the patient missing prior to the onset of symptoms? If so, then where?	If the owner knows that the patient has been in a certain place, e.g. shut in a garden shed or garage, then this should be searched for a possible source
Is there any substance on the patient's coat or around or in its mouth?	Advice can be given about obtaining a sample and preventing further absorption
Is there any medication, human or animal, that is damaged or missing?	This may help identify the poison. If a sample is available then advise the owner to bring it to the surgery
Did the owner use any product in the house or garden prior to the onset of symptoms	This may help identify the poison. If a sample is available, advise the owner to bring it to the surgery

* If the poison is known the Veterinary Poisons Information Service can be contacted with the consent of the veterinary surgeon. The telephone number is 0171 6359195 or 0113 2430715. A charge will be made for the use of this service; however, many veterinary practices subscribe yearly.

Table 9.4 Toxic agents

Type	Causes	Effects	Treatment
Medicines ACP misuse	Accidental overdosing with tablets in the house Idiosyncratic reaction to the drug	Depression or collapse. (Cats may become hyperaesthetic) Vasodilatation leads to decreased blood pressure and increased susceptibility to heatstroke on warm days Brachiocephalic dogs are especially likely to suffer Increased likelihood of fits in epileptic animals	Induce vomiting if many tablets have been eaten (unlikely, since few surgeries prescribe more than a few tablets for specific occasions) Treat symptoms of collapse/shock, heatstroke and epilepsy
Abnormal response (anaphylactic reaction)	Allergic-type response to medication, e.g. vaccination, antibiotics	Depression, occasionally vomiting and diarrhoea, swelling of injection sites Severe reactions result in collapse, with signs of shock	Swellings may have cold compresses applied Treat for shock if collapsed and maintain if unconscious Prepare corticosteroid injection
Non-steroidal anti-inflammatory drugs (NSAIDs)	Owners using human preparations on their animals (dosing their pets with so-called pain killers). Dogs 'stealing' owners' medications *Aspirin*—particularly toxic in cats. *Ibuprofen, flurbiprofen* and *naproxen*—may be rapidly fatal in some dogs. *Phenylbutazone*—more toxic to cats than dogs	*Aspirin*—Depression. Gastric irritation, leading to vomiting and anorexia. Cats may show some incoordination *Ibuprofen* and *flurbiprofen*—Gastric ulceration and perforation in dogs leads to vomiting and haematemesis, followed by diarrhoea with melaena. Kidney damage may cause acute and fatal renal failure. Dehydration due to fluid losses *Naproxen*—Gastric inflammation and ulceration leading to vomiting and melaena Anaemia due to low-grade blood loss Dehydration	Stop medication with the drugs *Before symptoms show*, induce vomiting as soon as possible *If showing symptoms*, give absorptive preparations and/or demulcents. Dosing with activated charcoal is vital in cases of aspirin poisoning and should be given immediately after vomiting ceases Prepare intravenous fluids Prepare **cimetidine** for intravenous injection in cases of naproxen poisoning
Paracetamol	Owner administered dose or tablet packet chewed	Dogs tolerate paracetamol well but cats are easily poisoned by as little as half a 500 mg tablet. Poisoning with paracetamol results in haemoglobin being changed to methaemoglobin, which is incapable of transporting oxygen *Signs* Cyanosis Depression or excitement Incoordination due to hypoxia Facial swelling	Induce vomiting if no symptoms shown Give absorptive material by mouth but NOT before consulting veterinary surgeon—if **N-acetyl cysteine** is to be used, the absorptive material may also prevent the absorption of this antidote Provide oxygen if any sign of cyanosis; ensure that the animal rests as much as possible. Prepare **methionine** or *N*-acetyl cysteine (human preparation 'Parvolex') for oral administration

Poison	Cause	Signs	Treatment
Salbutamol	Human preparations that are used to treat asthma and for premature labour	Stimulation of the sympathetic nervous system, causing peripheral vasodilatation and rapid heart rate (tachycardia). Panting respiration. Muscle weakness	General first aid treatment but beta blockers may be needed if the heart rate becomes excessively high
Calcipotriol	Vitamin D derivative contained in psoriasis creams and ointments, chewed by pups	Similar to vitamin D overdose. Poisoning leads to hypercalcaemia and hyperphosphataemia, causing acute nephritis and damage to gastrointestinal tract. *Signs* Haemorrhagic diarrhoea. Polyuria and polydipsia. Collapse with or without convulsions. Death may occur within 24 hours	Induce vomiting if ingested within 2–4 hours. Prepare activated charcoal solution. Prepare Hartmann's solution for i.v. administration—it is important to flush the calcium and phosphates through the kidneys to minimise renal damage. Prepare furosemide (frusemide) diuretic injection
Herbicides			
Chlorates	Ingestion of weedkillers or drinking from contaminated puddles—this substance does not degrade readily after use	Vomiting and diarrhoea with abdominal pain. Cyanosis of mucosa, turning to a muddy brown colour (blood becomes chocolate in colour because poison causes the formation of methaemoglobin—see Paracetamol)	General first aid treatment. Prepare **methylene blue** injection
Dinitro compounds	Ingestion of 2,4-dinitrophenol (2,4-D) or dinitro-orthocresol (2,4,5-T)	Depression, listlessness, muscle weakness. Rapid respiration and dyspnoea. Hyperthermia with sweating. Urine is almost fluorescent yellow/green	General first aid treatment. Monitor rectal temperature to detect hyperthermia
Paraquat	Ingesting weedkiller (although this product is rapidly absorbed on to the soil after application, which renders it harmless). Paraquat has been used in malicious poisonings, but most cases are due to accidents	Inflammation of the mouth and tongue. Vomiting and diarrhoea, with abdominal pain. Depression and progressive respiratory distress and cyanosis over a period of days, resulting in death	**Induce vomiting** as soon as ingestion of this chemical is suspected. Even though this is an irritant poison, the effects of the absorbed poison are so severe that treatment is usually hopeless and the only hope is to remove the poison from the alimentary tract as soon as possible. Administering fuller's earth is also helpful because the poison will bind to the fuller's earth and be rendered inactive
Insecticides			
Borax	Ant killers (e.g. Nippon) which are based on honey and therefore very attractive to dogs	Vomiting and diarrhoea. Collapse, convulsions and possible paralysis. Poisoning may be fatal	General first aid treatment
Organophosphates	Overdosing with insecticidal sprays, chewing insecticidal collars, etc.	Vomiting and diarrhoea. Salivation. Constricted pupils. Muscular twitching, excitement, followed by weakness, incoordination. Depression or convulsions	General first aid treatment. Prepare **atropine sulphate** for injection

Continued

Table 9.4 Toxic agents (*Cont'd*)

Type	Causes	Effects	Treatment
Organochlorines	Woodworm treatments and other insecticides (aldrin, dieldrin, gamma BHC, etc.). Many products are now withdrawn from sale but old stocks still exist	Involuntary twitching of muscles, especially facial, fore- and hindlimbs and convulsions Behavioural changes, e.g. aggression, pacing, apprehension, frenzy	Wash off contamination Administer absorptive material and/or liquid paraffin to decrease absorption **Fatty foods and drinks** (including milk) **must not be given** as they may increase absorption of the poison Prepare **barbiturate** injection to control convulsions
Molluscicides Carbamate Metaldehyde	See Organophosphates Ingestion of slug bait, which some dogs and cats seem to find very palatable	Incoordination leading to hyperaesthesia and convulsions Rapid pulse and respiration and possibly cyanosis	General first aid treatment Dosing with liquid paraffin may delay absorption of poison as long as it is given before the patient shows any symptoms (do not dose the unconscious patient) Prepare **barbiturate** injection to control convulsions
Rodenticides Alphachloralose	Rat baits and preparations to control pigeon and seabird populations	Poison acts by lowering the body temperature Progressive depression, incoordination and coma with hypothermia	General first aid treatment but warmth is essential
Calciferol Anticoagulant preparations	Ingestion of rat bait Rat baits. Several different compounds come under this heading: warfarin, coumatetralyl, chlorophacinone, difenacoum, brodifacoum, bromadiolone	See Calcipotriol (Medicines) Interference with clotting mechanism results in haemorrhages in the mucosae, bruising and haematomata, swollen joints, etc.	General first aid treatment Prepare injections of vitamin K. Large and repeated dosing may be necessary
Household chemicals Alcohol	Ingestion of alcoholic drink or fermenting grain (especially likely with pups)	Hyperaesthesia, incoordination, collapse and even death	Induce vomiting and provide general first aid treatment
Chocolate	Ingestion of large amounts of high cocoa content chocolate or cocoa powder. (Not a common poisoning, but causes much public concern)	Nervous excitement progressing to fits and coma Tachycardia Panting	Induce vomiting (may not be effective if chocolate ingested because of its sticky consistency). Gastric lavage may be required Prepare activated charcoal solution. Prepare diazepam/phenobarbitone to control fits

Disinfectants	Household disinfectants, when diluted to correct strength, do not cause a problem but are often used undiluted or incorrectly diluted by overzealous owners Phenols—**Cats are particularly susceptible to poisoning by phenols.** Licking paws after walking on wet surfaces recently cleaned with undiluted or incorrectly diluted solutions of disinfectant. Grooming coat after accidental spraying or splashing with strong disinfectant solutions	**These are corrosive poisons with a strong, distinctive odour**, e.g. pine disinfectants Convulsions, coma and death in acute poisoning cases Less acute cases may have inflamed mouths (stomatitis) and occasionally ulcers in the mouth. Animals may also vomit and have diarrhoea and abdominal pain	**Do not induce vomiting** General first aid treatment, including thorough washing of contaminated fur
	Quarternary ammonium compounds—as for phenols	These are also corrosive poisons but are odourless Depression and anorexia. Occasionally vomiting Salivation, stomatitis and mouth ulcers, especially on the tongue tip Skin ulcerations if compound not washed off quickly	As for phenols
Ethylene glycol (antifreeze)	Ingestion of water drained from car radiators (dogs seem particularly prone to drink this)	Incoordination, depression and rapid breathing. Later animal may become uraemic	General first aid treatment. **Ethanol** is the specific antidote and intravenous injections may be prepared if available at the surgery
Petroleum products	Usually a problem in cats which have fallen into containers of sump oil, drained from cars Accidental spillages of petrol, paraffin, etc. Caking of tar in the paws	These are very corrosive poisons with a distinctive odour Depression, vomiting, collapse and death if enough ingested. If submersed in the liquid, may also suffer an aspiration pneumonia, which is very severe because of the extremely irritant nature of the inhaled liquid Inflammation of the in-contact skin and mouth, especially the tongue if the animal has been allowed to groom	**Do not induce vomiting** General first aid treatment, including giving olive oil by mouth to decrease the absorption of the toxins

Table 9.5 Emetic agents

Agent	Method
Washing soda crystals	Two crystals on the back of the tongue
Apomorphine	Only given under the direction of the veterinary surgeon; 0.1 mg/kg subcutaneously
Xylazine	Only given under the direction of the veterinary surgeon; 3.0 mg/kg intramuscularly
Mustard	Not as effective as above; two teaspoonfuls in a cup of warm water

Table 9.6 Demulcent agents—used to bind poison in the gut

Agent	Method
BCK granules	1–3 heaped teaspoons orally. May need to mix with food or water and syringe in
Charcoal	1 g/kg orally. May need to mix with food or water and syringe in
Kaolin	1–2 ml/kg orally

4. Identify the poison (Table 9.4). Ask the owner to bring in the packet or label if applicable.

5. Prevent further absorption of the poison. The use of an emetic (Table 9.5) and/or a demulcent (Table 9.6) may be used. **Never** induce vomiting if the poison is corrosive or the patient is unconscious or fitting.

6. Collect a clearly labelled sample of any poison, vomit and/or urine/faeces. This may be used for analysis at a later date.

7. Treat the symptoms shown by the patient. Administer drugs as directed by the veterinary surgeon.

8. Administer an antidote if it is available.

9. Administer fluids orally if the patient is conscious, or set up an intravenous drip.

10. Make the patient warm and comfortable. Monitor its rectal temperature. Ensure that the body temperature is maintained.

11. Monitor the patient continually.

12. If the owner implies that this poisoning is malicious, maintain a diplomatic silence and do not express opinions that may be used in a subsequent legal case.

4. The type of poison will determine your actions. The information may be obtained from your questions to the owner.

5. If the identity of the poison is known and it is non-corrosive, advise the owners to induce emesis at home. Emesis is ineffective if the substance has been ingested over 4 hours previously.

6. Analysis may aid identification of the substance.

7. If the patient is collapsed or unconscious, administer oxygen. If advised, administer demulcents (Table 9.6) to bind the poison.

8. Very few poisons have an antidote. If there is one, it is given under the direction of a veterinary surgeon.

9. Oral fluids will dilute any poison that has been absorbed. In some cases fluids will reduce the damage to the kidneys caused by excretion of the poison in the urine.

10. Some poisons will depress or raise the body temperature.

11. Any changes in the patient's condition must be acted upon quickly.

12. The case history and the laboratory results may be used as evidence in a legal case, should the poisoning be malicious. Make sure that all records are accurate and kept safely.

PROCEDURE: TREATMENT OF BITES AND STINGS

ACTION

1. Place the animal in a comfortable position on a table.
2. Ask an assistant to restrain the animal so that it is relaxed and secure and the area is accessible for treatment.
3. Clean your hands with a surgical scrub.

4. Assess the type of wound (Table 9.7).

5. Treat the area with the appropriate action.
6. Monitor the patient continually.

RATIONALE

1. If the animal feels uncomfortable it will try to escape.
2. The assistant will be able to react quickly should the animal try to escape. The animal may resent the area being touched.
3. It is important not to introduce infection into the wound.
4. Treatment depends on the cause of the injury. There may be multiple bites or stings.
5. Refer to Table 9.7.
6. Any changes in the patient's condition can be acted upon quickly.

Table 9.7 Treatment of stings and bites

Type	Symptoms	Complications	Treatment
Wasp sting	Commonly seen in dogs. Stings are usually around the mouth and nose, and also the feet. The result is a painful swelling and, if in the mouth area, excessive salivation Stings to the pharynx can inhibit respiration. The sting is **not** left in the animal	Some animals may be allergic to the sting and may show an excessive reaction, anaphylaxis Collapse, dyspnoea and symptoms of shock may be seen	Wash the area with warm water and apply a dilute solution of water and acetic acid (vinegar). If the patient is collapsed, treat as for shock. If the patient is dyspnoeic, treat for asphyxia
Bee sting	Commonly seen in dogs. Stings are usually around the mouth and nose, and also the feet. The result is a painful swelling and, if in the mouth area, excessive salivation Stings to the pharynx can inhibit respiration. The sting **is** left in the animal	Some animals may be allergic to the sting and may show an excessive reaction, anaphylaxis Collapse, dyspnoea and symptoms of shock may be seen	The sting has a pumping sac attached. This must be removed carefully to avoid further liquid entering the site. Hold the sting at the point of entry with a pair of tweezers and remove. Wash the area with warm water and apply a solution of water and bicarbonate of soda (1 teaspoon in 1 pint of water)
Snake bite	Commonly seen in dogs. Bites are usually around the head and neck. The area is painful and oedamatous. Two fang marks may be visible The patient may be dull and depressed; condition may lead to collapse	The severity of the reaction depends on the type of snake, the amount of venom injected and the patient's reaction to the venom	Call a veterinary surgeon. Keep the patient as still as possible Thoroughly wash with warm water, but **do not rub**. This will push the venom deeper into the tissue. Apply a cold compress to reduce tissue perforation Administer antivenom and medication under the directions of the veterinary surgeon
Toad skin venom	Commonly seen in dogs that have picked up a toad in their mouths Excessive salivation may be seen	Occasionally the animal may swallow the toad	Constant observation of the patient. Occasionally nervous symptoms may develop Administer medication as directed by the veterinary surgeon

PROCEDURE: TREATMENT OF ELECTROCUTION

ACTION

1. Assess the environment that you are in: is there any risk to you or to others?

2. If the power cannot be disconnected, push the animal from the source with a **dry, wooden** pole.

3. Check the patient's airway, breathing and circulation. Resuscitate as appropriate.

4. When stable, examine the patient for burns and other injuries. Treat as appropriate.

RATIONALE

1. **Never** touch an electrocuted animal until the power supply is disconnected, as you may get an electric shock via the animal.

2. Such a pole will not conduct the electricity.

3. The animal may be found collapsed or even dead. Electric shocks may induce a cardiac arrest.

4. Burns may appear on the entry and exit points of the electric current. Pieces of skin that touch other skin, e.g. toes or scrotum, may also be affected.

PROCEDURE: TREATMENT OF SHOCK

ACTION

1. Assess the animal for clinical signs of shock (Tables 9.8, 9.9).

2. Restore the circulating blood volume to its original level by using intravenous fluid therapy.

3. The fluid used should resemble that which is lost. In cases of severe shock the use of a plasma expander is recommended.

4. Provide oxygen to the patient via a closed anaesthetic circuit.

5. Provide warmth. This should be by indirect heat, i.e. a warm environment, and/or conserving body heat with bubble wrap and blankets.

6. Monitor the patient closely.

7. Administer medication under the direction of a veterinary surgeon.

RATIONALE

1. From this examination you can assess the severity of the problem.

2. This will increase blood pressure and therefore improve the circulation to the body tissues.

3. Replace blood with blood or a plasma expander, and replace electrolytes with a crystalloid solution such as Hartmann's solution. Plasma expanders increase the osmotic pressure of blood, which draws fluid into the blood vessels, increasing circulating blood volume.

4. This will correct hypoxia caused by low haemoglobin levels due to blood loss.

5. Direct heat will increase surface dilatation of the capillaries and take blood away from the vital organs to the skin surface.

6. Any changes in the patient's condition can be noted and treated.

7. Drugs used may include sodium bicarbonate to correct metabolic acidosis, corticosteroids, anticoagulants, adrenaline (epinephrine) and antibiotics.

For treatment of injuries to the different body systems refer to Table 9.10.

Table 9.8 Clinical signs of shock

Symptom	Reason
Rapid, weak pulse	The heart is working harder because of low blood volume/pressure
Quiet heart sounds	Poor cardiac filling
Pale mucous membranes	Vasoconstriction due to the blood going to the vital organs, e.g. heart, brain and lungs
Increased capillary refill time	Vasoconstriction due to the blood going to the vital organs, e.g. heart, brain and lungs
Cold extremities	Due to vasoconstriction and low metabolic rate
Depressed level of consciousness	Reduced blood flow to the brain
Reduce urine output	Reduced blood flow to the kidneys

Table 9.9 Types of shock

Type	Cause
Cardiogenic	Cardiac output is reduced, e.g. reduced cardiac filling, pericardititis, or reduced cardiac emptying, cardiomyopathy
Hypovolaemic	Low circulating blood volume, e.g. haemorrhage, excessive vomiting or diarrhoea

Vasculogenic
  Neurogenic—trauma to the CNS
  Anaphylactic—an abnormal reaction to an antigen. Causes widespread histamine release, which in turn causes vasodilation
  Endotoxic—endotoxins from bacteria release chemicals, which cause vasodilation
	The capacity of the blood vessels increases due to vasodilation

Table 9.10 Injuries to the body systems

Area/disorder	Possible causes	Symptoms	Treatment
Respiratory system			
Nose	Trauma	Head shaking, epistaxis, mouth breathing crepitus, deformity and/or dyspnoea	Cold compress to control swelling/haemorrhage Oxygenation if dyspnoeic. Rest to lower blood pressure. Constant monitoring in case of concussion
	Foreign body, e.g. grass/grass seed	Sneezing, head shaking, epistaxis, discharge and/or mouth breathing	Remove if visible. Prepare for GA/sedation
	Tumour	Head shaking, epistaxis, mouth breathing crepitus, deformity and/or dyspnoea	Cold compress to control haemorrhage. Oxygenation if dyspnoeic. Rest to lower blood pressure
Pharynx and oesophagus	Foreign body, e.g. grass, fish hook, string, balls and sticks	Gagging, retching, salivation, dysphagia, dyspnoea and/or asphyxia	Remove if visible. Prepare for GA/sedation. Fish hooks must be cut out (not pulled). Treat asphyxia. The Heimlich manoeuvre may be required
Larynx and trachea	Foreign body, e.g. grass, balls and sticks	Gagging, retching, salivation, dyspnoea and/or asphyxia	Remove if visible. Treat asphyxia. The Heimlich manoeuvre may be required
	Trauma, e.g. dog bites, strangulation from a caught collar	Open and closed wounds, pain, swelling, emphysema (air in tissues), dyspnoea, air hissing and/or asphyxia	Clean and dress wounds. Ensure that no fluid enters the trachea. Cover holes into the trachea with clean cling film before dressing. Treat dyspnoea with oxygen. Treat asphyxia. Treat for shock

Continued

Table 9.10 Injuries to the body systems (*Cont'd*)

Area/Disorder	Possible causes	Symptoms	Treatment
Lungs and chest wall	Trauma, e.g. bites, gunshot wounds	Open and closed wounds, pain, swelling, emphysema (air in tissues), dyspnoea, air hissing and/or asphyxia	Clean and dress wounds. Ensure that no fluid enters the trachea. Cover holes into the trachea with clean cling film before dressing. Treat dyspnoea with oxygen. Treat asphyxia. Treat for shock
	Fluid in the alveolar spaces	Dyspnoea and asphyxia	Treat dyspnoea with oxygen. Treat asphyxia. Treat for shock
	Paraquat poisoning	Dyspnoea and cyanosis	Refer to poisoning
	Trauma resulting in a pneumothorax and/or haemothorax	Open and closed wounds, pain, swelling, emphysema (air in tissues), dyspnoea, air hissing and/or asphyxia	Clean and dress wounds. Ensure that no fluid enters the thorax. **Do not** remove any penetrating foreign bodies. The use of a ring pad will prevent displacement of the foreign body and/or fractures. Cover holes with clean cling film before dressing. Treat dyspnoea with oxygen. Treat asphyxia. Treat for shock
Diaphragm	Trauma, e.g. traffic accident	Commonly seen in cats. Dyspnoea, abdominal respiration and lung collapse	Treat dyspnoea with oxygen. Encourage abdominal organs back into place by lifting the patient up under the shoulders. Rest with the head and shoulders higher than the body
Digestive system			
Mouth	Stings	Swelling and salivation	Refer to stings
	Foreign body, e.g. bones, sticks, string and fish hooks	Gagging, retching, salivation, dysphagia, dyspnoea and/or asphyxia	Remove if visible. Prepare for GA/sedation. Fish hooks must be cut out (not pulled). Treat asphyxia. The Heimlich manoeuvre may be required
	Trauma	Fractures, crepitus and/or wounds	Compress wounds if possible. Fractures will need immobilising under GA
Stomach and intestines	Infection	Vomiting and/or diarrhoea. Pain and dehydration	Supportive therapy such as intravenous fluids. Nil by mouth. Treat shock
	Gastric dilatation volvulus. The stomach distends with gas and then twists (volvulus) at the cardia and pylorus	Restlessness, vomiting and belching. Swelling of the abdomen, laboured breathing, progressing to collapse and death	Call a veterinary surgeon as soon as possible. Relieve pressure in the stomach by passing a stomach tube. Use a roll of bandage as a mouth guard to prevent chewing. If that is unsuccessful then insert a wide-bore needle into the left abdominal wall at the point of maximum distension
	Intussusception or foreign body, e.g. toys, bones and balls	Vomiting, pain and dehydration	Supportive therapy such as intravenous fluids. Nil by mouth. Treat shock. Prepare for X-rays and surgery
Rectum	Prolapse caused by tenesmus or diarrhoea	Protrusion of the rectum through the anal sphincter. Common in hamsters. Can be partial or total. Swelling can occur if left for too long	Moisten the area with warm saline and lubricate with liquid paraffin. Attempt to replace by turning the prolapse back on itself. Ensure that hands are scrubbed. Prevent further straining with an analgesic suppository or local anaesthetic. Prevent self-trauma with the use of an Elizabethan collar

Anus	Impacted faeces or foreign body, e.g. bones	Tenesmus, discomfort, haemorrhage and licking the area	Lubricate the area with liquid paraffin. Remove obstruction with fingers or forceps. Wear gloves
Perineum	Fly strike	Smelly, inflamed and burnt area. Eggs and maggots visible	Remove **all** maggots. Clip and clean the area. An application of an insecticide can be used. Treat for shock if extensive
Urogenital system			
Prolapsed uterus and polyps	Sometimes seen at time of oestrus	Red mass protruding from the vulva	Ensure hands are scrubbed. Lubricate with liquid paraffin and apply gentle pressure to replace. Prevent self-trauma with the use of an Elizabethan collar
Penis	Paraphimosis: penis is engorged with blood and too big to slide back into the prepuce	Swelling and redness	Apply a cold compress on to the area. This will reduce the blood supply and the size of the penis. Lubricate and replace
	Trauma, e.g. cuts or haemorrhage from an over-amorous dog	Open wounds and haemorrhage	Apply a cold compress on to the area. Pinching the skin in front of the scrotum will reduce the haemorrhage
	Foreign body, e.g. grass/grass seed	Swelling, pain and anuria	Remove if visible. GA/sedation may be required. Prepare theatre
Special senses			
Eye	Foreign body, e.g. grass seed	Blepharospasm (eye screwed up), photophobia (fear of light), tears, redness and rubbing	Remove by flushing with sterile saline and/or use a damp cotton bud. GA/sedation or local anaesthetic may be necessary. **Do not** remove a penetrating foreign body
	Prolapse	The eyeball is outside the patient's head. It will become more inflamed the longer it is out	Replace the eyeball as soon as possible. With scrubbed hands, lubricate the eyeball and lids with 'false tears'. Pull back the eyelids and attempt to replace. Never put any pressure on the eyeball Advise the owner to keep the eyeball damp with dilute salt water (1 teaspoon to 1 litre of water) before bringing to the surgery
	Chemical splashes	Blepharospasm (eye screwed up), photophobia (fear of light), tears, redness and rubbing	Flush with copious amounts of sterile saline. Dilute vinegar may be used to 'neutralise' alkali splashes, and sodium bicarbonate will neutralise acid splashes Follow with sterile saline
Ear	Trauma	Open wounds or haematoma	Control haemorrhage with a cold compress or pressure bandage. Clean and dress wounds. Apply an ear bandage. The haematoma may need draining under a GA
Metabolic disorders			
Hypocalcaemia	Low blood calcium. Commonly seen in bitches at the peak of lactation (usually 2–3 weeks). Calcium is transferred from the bloodstream to the milk. This leaves little calcium in the rest of the body	Restlessness, panting and shivering, progressing into collapse, hyperaesthesia and eventually death	Extra calcium must be provided in the diet. If the patient is already hypocalcaemic, an injection of intravenous calcium 10% must be given under the direction of the veterinary surgeon. Wean the offspring immediately

Continued

Table 9.10 Injuries to the body systems (*Cont'd*)

Area/Disorder	Possible causes	Symptoms	Treatment
Hypoglycaemia	Occurs in diagnosed diabetics where there is an imbalance between the insulin given and glucose available. This can be due to an overdose of insulin, anorexia, strenuous exercise and/or extreme temperatures	Slowed metabolic rate, lethargy, incoordination and dry mucous membranes, leading to collapse, hyperaesthesia, convulsions and eventually death	If the animal is conscious, administer oral glucose solution. Honey or sugar is the best alternative. If the animal is unconscious then an intravenous injection of glucose must be given under the direction of a veterinary surgeon. Glucose can also be given via a stomach tube. This is metabolised at a slower rate
Uraemia	Usually occurs in old dogs and cats with chronic renal failure. The kidneys, which normally excrete toxins, are not working, so the toxins remain in the blood	Polydipsia and polyuria, loss of weight, vomiting, halitosis and mouth ulcers, progressing into epileptiform fits and death	Make the patient comfortable. The use of intravenous fluids can help to alleviate the symptoms; however, there is no cure and euthanasia is often performed
Hyperthermia	Often caused by heat stroke, e.g. dogs left in hot cars. The temperature-regulating centre in the brain is unable to control the body temperature	Restlessness, panting, salivation and distress, progressing into collapse, coma and death. High rectal temperature	Cool the patient as soon as possible. Use a cold shower or hosepipe. Ice packs and wet towels are useful. Monitor rectal temperature every 15 minutes Cool until normal temperature is reached. Continue to monitor every 30 minutes in case it rises again
Hypothermia	Often seen in young or small animals under anaesthetic. Heat loss is great because they have a large surface area compared to body mass	Lethargy, reluctance to move or feed, cold to touch, progressing to collapse and death	Warm the animal as soon as possible. Use a warm environment, blankets, heat pad and/or hot water bottle. Monitor rectal temperature every 15 minutes until normal temperature is reached. Continue to monitor every 30 minutes in case it should fall again

FURTHER READING

British Veterinary Nursing Association—Bandaging Fact Sheets. BVNA, Harlow

Conner J, McKerrel J 1995 A Guide to Animal Bandaging. Millpledge, Retford

Cooper B, Lane DR (eds) 1999 Veterinary Nursing, 2nd edn. Butterworth-Heinemann, Oxford

Hotson-Moore A (ed.) 1999 Manual of Advanced Veterinary Nursing. BSAVA, Gloucester.

- Setting up the X-ray machine
- Preparing the X-ray room for a radiographic examination
- Preparing the patient for a radiographic examination

Positioning the patient
- Lateral thorax
- Dorsoventral thorax
- Lateral abdomen
- Ventrodorsal abdomen
- Lateral pelvis
- Ventrodorsal pelvis (extended hip position)
- Ventrodorsal skull
- Dorsoventral skull
- Open mouth rostrocaudal view of the tympanic bullae
- Dorsoventral intra-oral view of the nasal chambers
- Nasopharynx
- Mediolateral view of a distal limb extremity—general rules
- Dorsopalmar, dorsoplantar or craniocaudal view of a limb—general rules
- Lateral shoulder
- Craniocaudal shoulder
- Lateral spine
- Ventrodorsal spine

Use of contrast media
- Use of barium in the evaluation of the gastrointestinal tract
- Barium swallow
- Barium meal or 'follow through'
- Barium enema
- Intravenous urography
- Urethrogram (retrograde urethography)—male
- Urethrogram (retrograde vagino-urethography)—female
- Cystography
- Myelography—cisternal and lumbar puncture

Techniques for processing radiographs
- Manual processing
- Starting up an automatic processor
- Automatic processing
- Shutting down the automatic processor
- Cleaning an automatic processor

Maintenance of radiography equipment
- Care of intensifying screens
- Checking safelight function
- Checking for light leakage in a cassette
- Checking the X-ray tube for leakage of X-rays
- Checking for the accuracy of the light beam diaphragm
- Checking a cassette for poor film–screen contact

Diagnostic ultrasound
- Preparing the patient for an ultrasound examination
- Care of the ultrasound machine

10

Diagnostic imaging

S. Easton

Introduction

The term radiography covers all the procedures involved in the production and processing of a radiograph. The veterinary nurse is often given the responsibility for positioning the patient, setting up the X-ray machine ready for the exposure, and then processing the radiograph either in an automatic or a manual processor. It is important that the quality of the resulting radiograph is such that it aids the diagnosis of the veterinary surgeon: if it does not, there is little point in the technique. To achieve a high standard of radiography the nurse must have a clear understanding of the steps involved in each procedure and how each step contributes to the final product. In addition, health and safety considerations are of particular importance when dealing with ionising radiation and the veterinary nurse must always be aware of the danger to herself or himself and to others in the vicinity of the machine.

Nowadays, radiography is not the only diagnostic imaging technique available in a veterinary practice. Ultrasonography (the use of high-frequency sound waves to create a moving image) is becoming commonplace and the veterinary nurse is likely to be responsible for the preparation of the patient and setting up and maintaining the machine. The advantage of diagnostic ultrasound is that there is little danger to the patient or to the personnel involved in its use.

This chapter describes the procedures involved in the use of both X-rays and ultrasound and in the care of the equipment associated with both diagnostic techniques.

PROCEDURE: SETTING UP THE X-RAY MACHINE

ACTION

1. Place the X-ray machine in the designated room or controlled area.

2. Make sure that the radiation warning signs are displayed and visible.

3. Plug the machine into the mains.

4. Switch the X-ray machine on at the console or the main body of the machine.

5. Check that the mains voltage compensation is accurate.

6. Adjust the mains voltage compensation if needed.

7. Set the X-ray tube to the correct height above the film.

8. Set the exposure factors suitable for the examination, patient type and the equipment being used.

RATIONALE

1. To ensure that the local rules are followed, the X-ray machine must be used in a specifically designated area, as outlined in the rules.

2. Warning signs must be displayed when X-rays are being used. The position of these warning signs will be specified in the local rules.

3. Most machines rely on mains electricity to work.

4. The machine must be plugged in prior to switching on the machine.

5. Mains voltage compensation ensures that the voltage received by the machine remains constant despite fluctuations within the mains voltage.

6. Without adjustment of the mains voltage, radiographic exposure factors will not be accurate.

7. The X-ray tube should always be at a standard distance from the film: the film–focus distance.

8. Exposure factors depend on the type of machine, the film–screen combination, the size of the patient and the region being examined.

PROCEDURE: PREPARING THE X-RAY ROOM FOR A RADIOGRAPHIC EXAMINATION

ACTION

1. Place the X-ray machine in the room and ensure that the correct exposure factors are set.

2. Place the cassette on the table and centre it under the X-ray tube.

3. If a stationary grid is being used, place this in the correct position over the cassette.

4. Place sandbags, ties and foam pads so that they can be easily reached if needed to position the patient.

RATIONALE

1. Setting the exposure factors before positioning the patient ensures that, once the animal is positioned, an exposure can be made immediately.

2. The cassette should be placed securely on the table to prevent it falling on to the floor and breaking.

3. Incorrect use of the grid will result in poor quality/non-diagnostic images.

4. Sandbags, ties and foam pads are used to hold the patient in the required position.

5. Remove unnecessary equipment from the room.
6. Remove any distractions from the room.

5. This includes any objects that may cause an accident if left around on the floor.
6. Anything that may prevent the animal cooperating or cause unnecessary distress.

PROCEDURE: PREPARING THE PATIENT FOR A RADIOGRAPHIC EXAMINATION

ACTION

1. Ensure that there is a valid clinical indication for the examination.

2. Use some form of chemical restraint, either sedation or general anaesthesia, as appropriate to the patient.

3. Remove any artefacts from the patient, e.g. leads, collars, clips, matted or wet hair.
4. If required for the procedure, ensure that any preparation of the patient, e.g. fasting, use of an enema or emptying the bladder, has taken place.
5. Position the animal correctly for the radiograph.

RATIONALE

1. Under the Ionising Radiation Regulations 2000, all examinations must be clinically justified and all exposures must be kept to a minimum.
2. Suitable chemical restraint should be used unless the patient is considered to be an anaesthetic risk. Manual restraint should be used only in extreme circumstances as it poses a risk to the health and safety of personnel.
3. Artefacts may distract the attention from, and may overlie, the main point of interest.
4. In some examinations the presence of faeces or urine or food in the stomach may restrict the view of the diagnostic points.

5. If the animal is conscious and/or sedated, it may be necessary to calm the animal while it is positioned.

POSITIONING THE PATIENT (TABLES 10.1, 10.2, FIG. 10.1)

Thorax

PROCEDURE: LATERAL THORAX (FIG. 10.2)

ACTION

1. Place the patient in right lateral recumbency.

2. Extend the forelegs and secure them using sandbags or ties.

3. Place a pad under the sternum.

RATIONALE

1. This is the conventional position for a thoracic radiograph.
2. Extending the forelegs prevents the soft-tissue mass of the shoulder girdle impeding the view of the thoracic contents.
3. This prevents rotation of the chest and ensures that it is in the same horizontal plane as the spine. This prevents distortion of structures in the thorax.

Table 10.1 Positioning aids

Type	Use	Radiographic density
Troughs—range of sizes	To restrain animal on its back. Prevents rotation of the trunk	Radiolucent
Foam wedges—range of shapes and sizes. Covered in plastic for ease of cleaning	For lateral views to provide support and prevent rotation of the trunk and for accurate limb positioning. May be useful for supporting the spine and trunk to achieve a horizontal plane	Radiolucent
Sandbags—loose filling allows bending and twisting. Covered in plastic for ease of cleaning	Can be wrapped around to hold limbs in position or placed over the neck	Radio-opaque—do not place in the primary beam
Tapes or ties—range of lengths	Looped around limbs to pull them into position and tie them to cleats on the table	Radiolucent
Wooden blocks	For raising the cassette up to the area of interest	Radio-opaque—do not place in the primary beam

Table 10.2 General principles of positioning

Action	Rationale
Centre the primary beam over the main point of interest	To prevent distortion of the area by an oblique view
Place the area of interest as close as possible to the film	To prevent gross magnification of the part due to an excessive object–film distance. The image may also be blurred
Ensure that the centre of the primary beam is at right angles to the film	To avoid distortion of the image. This is important when examining joint or intervertebral disc spaces
Collimate the beam to as small an area as is realistically possible	To reduce the amount of scattered radiation
Take two views at right angles to each other	To assist in accurate location of a lesion and to visualise the area completely
Try to contain the whole area of interest on a single film	To reduce the number of exposures. If this means that important parts are viewed obliquely, e.g. whole spine, it is better to take views of several smaller areas
When imaging the spine, the body must be supported so that the vertebrae are in the same horizontal plane	To prevent distortion and magnification of individual vertebrae and of the intervertebral disc spaces

4. Place sandbags over the neck and hindlegs to hold them in place.
5. Centre the beam (indicated by the cross of the light beam diaphragm) midway between the sternum and spine, level with the border of the caudal border of the scapula.
6. Collimate the beam to include the front of the shoulder and the edge of the sternum.
7. Expose on inspiration.

4. The hindlegs should be secure but should not be extended as this rotates the chest.
5. This ensures that the centre of the primary beam coincides with the base of the heart.

6. All regions of the lung field will be included.
7. The lungs are fully inflated during inspiration, which provides better contrast between the air and the soft tissues.

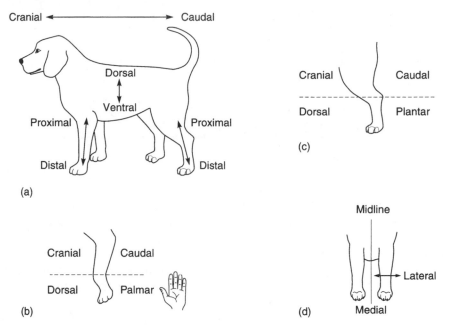

Figure 10.1 Standard nomenclature for body regions. Reproduced, with permission, from *Preveterinary Nursing Textbook*, by Masters and Bowden (2001). Butterworth Heinemann, UK.

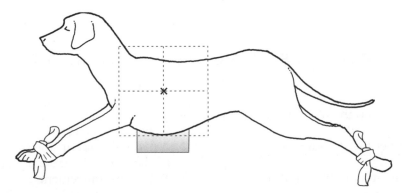

Figure 10.2 Positioning for lateral thorax.

PROCEDURE: DORSOVENTRAL THORAX (FIG. 10.3)

ACTION

1. Place the patient in sternal recumbency.

2. Place a sandbag over the neck.
3. Extend the forelegs and adduct them with the elbows out to the sides.
4. Centre the beam (indicated by the cross of the light beam diaphragm) in the midline on the caudal border of the scapula.

RATIONALE

1. This is particularly used for examination of the heart.
2. To prevent movement.
3. This prevents the muscle mass of the shoulder girdle overlying the thoracic cavity.
4. This ensures that the heart base is in the centre of the image.

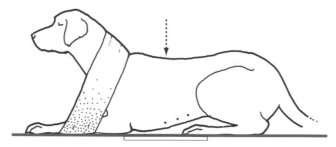

Figure 10.3 Positioning for dorsoventral thorax.

5. Collimate the beam to include the skin surfaces laterally, the thoracic inlet and the diaphragm.
6. Expose on inspiration.

5. The image will include the cranial and caudal extent of the lung field.

6. The lungs are fully inflated during inspiration, which provides better contrast between the air and the soft tissues.

Abdomen

Note. A ventrodorsal view of the thorax may be used to examine the lungs; however, if the animal is in respiratory distress, this position should be avoided, as it may make respiration even more difficult.

PROCEDURE: LATERAL ABDOMEN (FIG. 10.4)

ACTION

1. Place the patient in right lateral recumbency.

2. Place a pad under the sternum.

3. Extend the fore- and hindlegs and secure them with sandbags or ties.

RATIONALE

1. This is the conventional position for viewing the abdomen.
2. A pad will support the sternum, keeping the body in a horizontal plane.
3. To prevent movement.

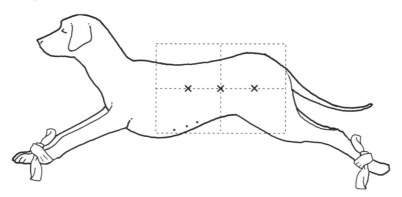

Figure 10.4 Positioning for lateral abdomen.

4. Centre the beam (indicated by the cross of the light beam diaphragm) at the 11–12th intercostal space, just cranial to the last rib.

4. This ensures that the entire abdomen is included.

5. Collimate the beam to include the dorsal and lateral skin edges, the diaphragm and pubic symphysis. If the patient is large, move the beam towards the diaphragm or pubic symphysis, depending on the area of interest.

5. The top of the liver should be included in all radiographs of the complete abdomen.

6. Expose on expiration.

6. During expiration the diaphragm relaxes into its characteristic dome shape and the lungs contract, providing the maximum amount of space for the abdominal contents.

PROCEDURE: VENTRODORSAL ABDOMEN (FIG. 10.5)

ACTION

1. Place the patient in dorsal recumbency.

2. Extend each foreleg cranially and secure with a tie or sandbag placed over the carpus.

3. Make sure that the body does not rotate, so that the sternum and spine are kept in vertical alignment.

RATIONALE

1. Care must be taken if the animal is only lightly anaesthetised.

2. This prevents rotation of the body. Do not place sandbags over the axillae as this can be uncomfortable.

3. The use of a trough or sandbags placed on either side may help to support this position.

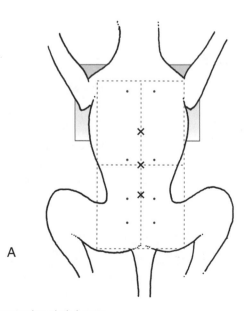

Figure 10.5A, B Positioning for ventrodorsal abdomen.

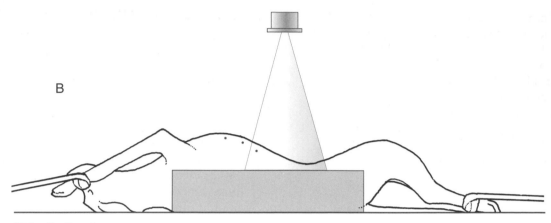

Figure 10.5 *Continued.*

4. Centre the beam (indicated by the beam of the light beam diaphragm) on the midline at the level of the umbilicus. This point may be adjusted towards the diaphragm or the pubic symphysis in larger breeds of dog.
5. Collimate the beam to include the lateral skin surfaces, the diaphragm and the pubic symphysis.
6. Expose on expiration.

4. This ensures that the whole abdominal area is included.

5. The cranial border of the liver must be shown in an abdominal radiograph.

6. During expiration the diaphragm relaxes into its characteristic dome shape and the lungs contract, providing the maximum amount of space for the abdominal contents.

Pelvis

PROCEDURE: LATERAL PELVIS (FIG. 10.6)

ACTION

1. Place the patient in right lateral recumbency.

2. Place pads between the hindlegs.
3. Centre the beam (indicated by the cross of the light beam diaphragm) over the greater trochanter of the left femur.
4. Collimate the beam to include the entire pelvic area.

RATIONALE

1. This is the only way of providing a true lateral projection of the pelvis.
2. This ensures that the pelvis does not rotate.
3. This ensures that the wings of the ilium and the acetabulum are visible.

PROCEDURE: VENTRODORSAL PELVIS (EXTENDED HIP POSITION) (FIG. 10.7)

This is the position required by the British Veterinary Association/Kennel Club hip dysplasia scheme. It is important to make sure that the radiograph is correctly positioned, as those that are not will be returned to the veterinary surgeon. The radiograph must also be labelled with the dog's Kennel Club registration number, the date of radiography and left and/or right markers.

ACTION	RATIONALE
1. Place the patient in dorsal recumbency, ensuring that the body is straight.	1. This may be helped by the use of a trough or sandbags placed on either side of the upper abdomen. If the upper body is straight, the pelvis should also be straight. If the pelvis rotates, a foam pad may be placed under the lower hip.

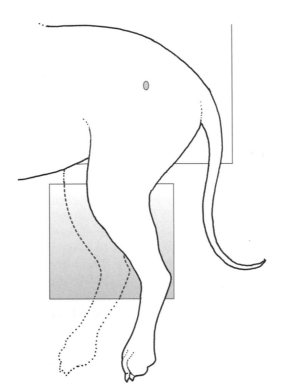

Figure 10.6 Positioning for lateral pelvis.

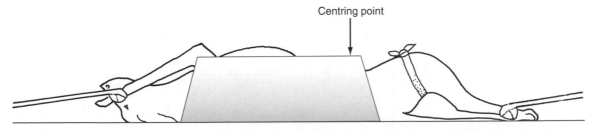

Figure 10.7 Positioning (ventrodorsal pelvis) and centring point (arrowed) for assessment of hip dysplasia. Adapted with permission, from *Veterinary Nursing*, p. 676, 2nd edn, by Lane and Cooper (1994). Butterworth Heinemann, UK.

2. Extend the hindlegs caudally so that the hips and stifles are fully extended. Secure with ties at the hocks.
3. Rotate the hindlegs medially so that the femurs lie parallel to each other and the patellae are centred over the distal femurs.
4. Hold the femurs together by placing a tie around the level of the mid-femurs. Adhesive tape may be a convenient way of doing this.
5. Added security may be achieved by placing another tie around the legs at the level of the mid-tibia. Again adhesive tape may be of use.
6. Centre the beam (indicated by the cross on the light beam diaphragm) in the midline over the pubic symphysis.
7. Collimate the beam to include the wings of the ilium and the proximal half of the femurs.

2. This will further ensure that the pelvis is straight.
3. Rotation of the femur places the femoral head into the acetabulum, which gives an indication of the degree of hip dysplasia.
4. The use of ties will ensure that the patient remains in this position.

6. This should provide equal detail on either side of the pelvic girdle.

7. This should demonstrate the entire pelvic girdle and the hip joints. The obturator foramina should be of equal size. Any inequality may be due to tilting of the pelvis and poor positioning.

Skull

PROCEDURE: VENTRODORSAL SKULL (FIG. 10.8)

ACTION

1. Place the patient in dorsal recumbency.

2. Extend the neck.

3. Place a foam pad under the neck.

4. Centre the beam (indicated by the cross on the light beam diaphragm) in the midline at a point halfway along the interpupillary line.
5. Collimate the beam to include the entire skull.

RATIONALE

1. This ensures that the skull is as close as possible to the film.
2. Extension makes sure that the head is horizontal.
3. This forces the head back, so that the hard palate is parallel to the table top.
4. This point may vary with the area to be examined.

5. If necessary, collimate more tightly over the area of interest, e.g. tympanic bulla.

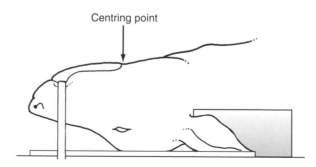

Centring point

Figure 10.8 Positioning for ventrodorsal skull to show the position of the hard palate.

PROCEDURE: DORSOVENTRAL SKULL (FIG. 10.9)

ACTION

1. Place the patient in sternal recumbency.

2. Support the head on a pile of pads or wooden blocks.

3. Place the cassette on top of the pile.

4. Centre the beam (indicated by the cross on the light beam diaphragm) in the midline at a point midway along the interpupillary line.

5. Collimate the beam to include the entire skull.

RATIONALE

1. This ensures that the dorsal surface of the skull is closest to the X-ray tube head.

2. This ensures that the median sagittal plane is perpendicular to the cassette. Make sure that the line between the pupils is parallel to the cassette.

3. The head is as close as possible to the cassette. If you place the cassette under the supporting pile you may distort the image by magnification.

4. This point may vary with the area to be examined.

5. If necessary, collimate more tightly over the area of interest, e.g. tympanic bulla.

PROCEDURE: OPEN MOUTH ROSTROCAUDAL VIEW OF THE TYMPANIC BULLAE (FIG. 10.10)

ACTION

1. Place the animal in dorsal recumbency, with the hard palate perpendicular to the cassette. Tip the nose slightly past the vertical.

RATIONALE

1. This position ensures that the bullae are as close as possible to the cassette. By tilting the head, the skull bones do not obstruct the view of the tympanic bullae.

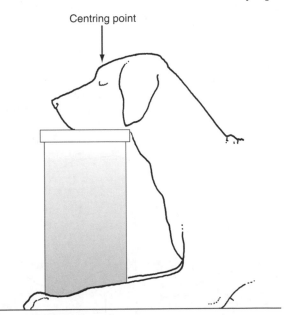

Centring point

Figure 10.9 Positioning for dorsoventral skull.

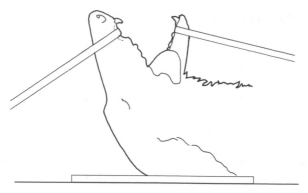

Figure 10.10 Positioning for open mouth rostrocaudal view.

2. Hold the mouth open to form a V-shape, using tapes around each jaw, or place an old needle case (with one end cut off to create a hole) between the teeth of the upper and lower jaws.

2. In this position, the mandible and the maxilla are removed from the area of interest.

3. Aim the primary beam parallel to the hard palate and centre it (indicated by the cross of the light beam diaphragm) on the base of the tongue.

3. The tympanic bullae are located directly behind the base of the tongue in this position.

4. Remove the endotracheal tube before exposure.

4. The endotracheal tube will be superimposed on the tympanic bullae if not removed.

PROCEDURE: DORSOVENTRAL INTRA-ORAL VIEW OF THE NASAL CHAMBERS (FIG. 10.11)

ACTION

1. The patient must be fully anaesthetised.

RATIONALE

1. The cassette must be placed in the patient's mouth: without anaesthesia the animal will chew on the film.

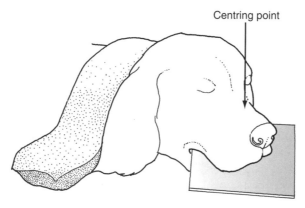

Centring point

Figure 10.11 Positioning for dorsoventral intra-oral view of the nasal chambers.

2. Place the animal in sternal recumbency

3. Extend the neck.

4. Place a sandbag over the neck.
5. Place a non-screen film into the mouth, corner first, as far into the mouth as possible.
6. Centre the beam (indicated by the cross on the light beam diaphragm) on a line midway between the external nares and the interpupillary line.
7. Place a left/right marker on the relevant side.

2. This position ensures that the maxilla does not overlie the nasal chambers and provides a comfortable supported position for the animal.
3. The position of the head is straighter if the neck is extended.
4. This prevents the head from rotating.
5. Non-screen film is used as it provides excellent definition.
6. This allows visualisation of the entire area of the nasal chambers.

7. This ensures that any lesion can be related to the relevant nasal chamber. Most non-screen film cannot be labelled after processing so this must be done prior to exposure.

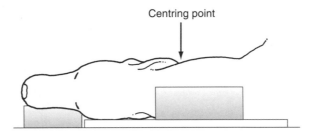

Centring point

Figure 10.12 Positioning for nasopharynx.

PROCEDURE: NASOPHARYNX (FIG. 10.12)

ACTION

1. Place the patient in lateral recumbency.

2. Place pads under the nose and under the neck.

3. Pull the forelegs caudally to lie against the wall of the thorax using ties.

4. Centre the beam (indicated by the cross on the light beam diaphragm) on the mid-cervical area to include the pharynx and thoracic inlet.
5. Remove the endotracheal tube before exposure.

RATIONALE

1. This will provide radiographic access to the nasopharynx.
2. These maintain the skull in a horizontal line and prevent rotation.
3. This pulls the shoulders and associated soft-tissue structures away from the area of interest.
4. The areas cranial and caudal to the pharynx must be included.

5. The endotracheal tube may mask a stricture or a mass.

Limbs

PROCEDURE: MEDIOLATERAL VIEW OF A DISTAL LIMB EXTREMITY (FIG. 10.13)—GENERAL RULES

ACTION

1. Place the patient in lateral recumbency, with the limb to be X-rayed closest to the cassette, e.g. right forelimb—place body in right lateral recumbency.
2. Extend the uppermost limb caudally (forelimb) or cranially (hindlimb) and support it on the flank using a tie.
3. The limb to be X-rayed should lie parallel to the cassette. It may be necessary to use a pad to prevent rotation of the limb.
4. Stifles and elbow joints should be flexed.
5. Centre the beam (indicated by the cross on the light beam diaphragm) at the level of the joint or mid-shaft.
6. Collimate the beam to include the joint above and below the long bone, or a small area above and below the joint in question.

RATIONALE

1. This ensures that the area is in close contact with the film, minimising distortion of the image.

2. The limb and any associated tissue that is not required are pulled out of the area of interest.
3. Rotation of the limb should be avoided as the image should show a true mediolateral view.
4. Flexion enables a full examination of the joint.
5. Accurate centring will avoid distortion.

6. Viewing adjacent structures may aid diagnosis.

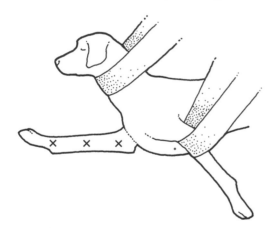 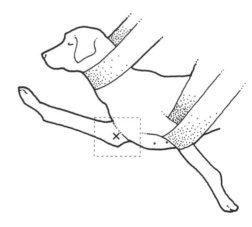

Figure 10.13 Positioning for mediolateral view of a distal extremity.

PROCEDURE: DORSOPALMAR, DORSOPLANTAR OR CRANIOCAUDAL VIEW OF A LIMB (FIG. 10.14)—GENERAL RULES

ACTION

1. Place the patient in sternal (forelimb) or dorsal (hindlimb) recumbency so that the limb under investigation is parallel to the cassette.

RATIONALE

1. Joints of the hindlimb are better imaged with the patient in dorsal recumbency. This allows the limb to be extended more easily, while still keeping the limb in good contact with the film.

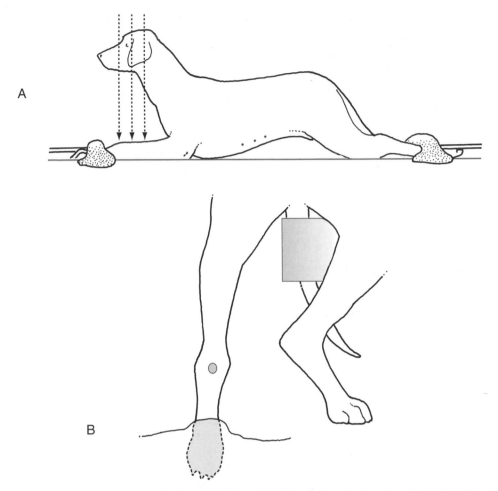

Figure 10.14 Positioning for craniocaudal view of distal forelimb (A) and dorsoplantar view of distal hindlimb (B).

2. Keep the limb under investigation straight.

3. Centre the beam (indicated by the cross on the light beam diaphragm) at the level of the joint or the midshaft.

4. Collimate the beam to include the joint above and below the long bone, or a small area above and below the joint under investigation.

2. On extension, the limb may rotate inwards. To prevent this it may be necessary to lift and rotate the opposing limb.

3. This must be accurate to avoid distortion.

4. Viewing adjacent structures may aid diagnosis.

PROCEDURE: LATERAL SHOULDER (FIG. 10.15)

ACTION

1. Place the patient in lateral recumbency, making sure that the limb to be examined is closest to the cassette.
2. Extend the head and neck and secure by placing a sandbag over the neck; be careful to avoid interfering with normal respiration.
3. Pull the affected leg cranially and secure with a tie.

4. Pull the opposing limb caudally and secure with a tie.

5. Centre the beam (indicated by the cross on the light beam diaphragm) through the joint space of the shoulder.
6. Collimate the beam to include the proximal third of the humerus and the distal part of the scapula.

RATIONALE

1. Lateral recumbency gives adequate access to the shoulder joint.

2. This ensures that an endotracheal tube lying in the trachea and larynx is pulled away from the area of the shoulder.
3. This ensures that the area of the shoulder joint is not overlain by the soft tissues of the other shoulder.
4. This draws the soft tissues of the opposing limb away from the shoulder joint to be examined.
5. Palpating the greater tuberosity of the humerus on the lateral aspect of the bone will provide the correct location.
6. This will cover the complete shoulder joint.

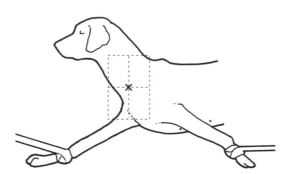

Figure 10.15   Positioning for lateral shoulder.

PROCEDURE: CRANIOCAUDAL SHOULDER (FIG. 10.16)

ACTION

1. Place the patient in dorsal recumbency and support in a cradle or with sandbags.
2. Fully extend the limb to be examined cranially and secure with a tie.
3. Rotate the thorax until the limb is in the craniocaudal position.
4. Centre the beam (indicated by the cross on the light beam diaphragm) over the acromion of the scapula.

RATIONALE

1. This allows extension of the limb while preventing obstruction by the chest wall.
2. Full extension of the limb will demonstrate the joint, without the elbow overlying the area.
3. Rotation of the thorax enables the limb to be placed in a true craniocaudal position.
4. The acromion can be palpated on the lateral aspect of the joint, at the distal end of the spine of the scapula. The joint will be in the centre of the radiograph and demonstrated without distortion.

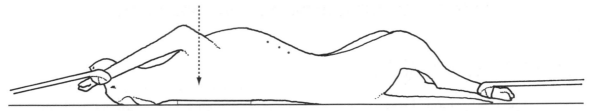

Figure 10.16 Positioning for craniocaudal shoulder.

5. Collimate the beam to include the proximal third of the humerus and the distal part of the scapula.	5. This will cover the complete shoulder joint.

Spine

PROCEDURE: LATERAL SPINE (FIG. 10.17)

ACTION

1. Place the patient in right lateral recumbency.

2. Place supporting pads under the natural curves of the spine, i.e. the neck and the lumbar region, and a pad under the nose.

3. Place pads under the sternum and between the limbs.

4. If the cervical spine is to be examined, pull the forelimbs caudally.

5. Centre the beam (indicated by the cross of the light beam diaphragm) over the area of interest.

6. Collimate the beam to cover about three vertebrae either side of the centre. Include muscle mass but not fat and skin. If the entire spine is to be examined, each image should overlap with the ones on either side.

RATIONALE

1. This will provide an image on which to base a diagnosis.

2. These supports keep the spine horizontal and parallel with the table top. Placing a pad under the nose keeps the head in line.

3. These prevent rotation, which will pull the spine out of its horizontal position.

4. This ensures that the soft tissues of the shoulder do not overlie the spine.

5. Centring must be accurate and care must be taken to avoid trying to cover too large an area at one time: divergence of the beam at the edges of the field will cause artificial narrowing of the joint spaces.

6. By ensuring overlap, a complete study of each vertebra can be achieved with a minimum of distortion.

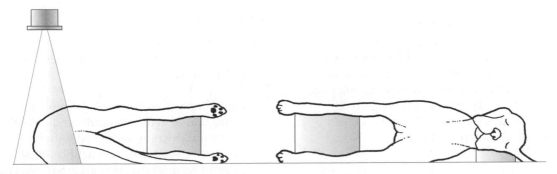

Figure 10.17 Positioning for lateral spine.

PROCEDURE: VENTRODORSAL SPINE (FIG. 10.18)

ACTION

1. Place the patient in dorsal recumbency supported in a trough or with sandbags.

2. The spine must be positioned so that the sternum and the spine are in the same vertical plane.
3. Extend the fore- and hindlegs and secure with ties.
4. Centre the beam (indicated by the cross of the light beam diaphragm) over the area of interest.

5. Collimate the beam to cover about three vertebrae either side of the centre. Include the transverse processes and include muscle mass but not fat and skin. If the entire spine is to be examined, each image should overlap with the ones on either side.

RATIONALE

1. Support must be provided to prevent rotation. This is even more important if a spinal injury is suspected.
2. Lack of alignment and rotation will affect the image and may provide an incorrect diagnosis.
3. This provides additional support and prevents rotation of the spine.
4. Try to select the areas that correspond to those radiographed in the lateral view. In this way you have two planes for each area of the spine.
5. By ensuring overlap, a complete study of each vertebra can be achieved with a minimum of distortion.

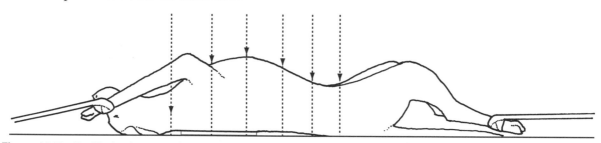

Figure 10.18 Positioning for ventrodorsal spine.

USE OF CONTRAST MEDIA

PROCEDURE: USE OF BARIUM IN THE EVALUATION OF THE GASTROINTESTINAL TRACT

ACTION

1. Prepare the barium sulphate. It may require mixing with a prescribed amount of water or may be ready-made. This must be done in the preparation room, away from the patient.
2. Ensure that the patient is prepared as appropriate, e.g. fasted, given an enema. Do not sedate the animal.

RATIONALE

1. Barium should not be prepared near to the X-ray table as it may contaminate the table or the patient.

2. Good patient preparation prevents the formation of artefacts on the radiograph, e.g. stomach contents mixed with barium. The use of sedatives will artificially slow gastrointestinal function and may affect the final diagnosis.

3. Take plain radiographs before the introduction of contrast material.

4. If the patient is to be given a barium swallow, mix the barium with a small amount of normal food. Place a small amount of normal food on the top to entice the animal to eat.

5. If the patient is to be given a barium 'follow through' or meal, draw up approximately 5 ml/kg of liquid barium into a syringe. The patient may lap up the liquid or be force-fed with it.

6. If the patient is to be given a barium enema, the barium must be as liquid as possible. Introduce the barium into the rectum using a catheter (retrograde filling). Air may be introduced to provide a double-contrast examination (Fig. 10.19).

7. Always use the correct volume and consistency of contrast material.

8. Select the correct patient position and collimate accurately.

3. These can be used for comparison with the contrast radiographs. Contrast media may mask some diagnostic features.

4. The use of food allows the processes of eating and swallowing to be seen more clearly.

5. A larger volume of barium is needed to prevent dilution as it passes down the gastrointestinal tract.

6. Barium is used to outline the colon and must be as liquid as possible. Air can be used to enhance the image.

7. If the wrong type and volume of contrast material is used, the radiographs may not be diagnostic.

8. Incorrect positioning may miss the area of interest and alter the appearance of the pathology present. Collimation will enhance the image.

PROCEDURE: BARIUM SWALLOW

ACTION

1. The patient remains conscious, but mild sedation may be needed.

2. Place the patient in right lateral recumbency and take a plain radiograph.

3. Offer the patient food mixed with barium or restrain the patient, as described in Chapter 1, and place a syringe-full of liquid barium into the corner of the mouth, avoiding spillage. Administer in one bolus.

4. Place the patient in right lateral recumbency and take the X-ray of the oesophageal/thoracic area.

RATIONALE

1. The use of general anaesthesia is not recommended, as the animal will be unable to swallow. Sedation should be avoided as this may slow the passage of ingesta down the gastrointestinal tract. If the animal seems likely to object to the taking of serial radiographs, sedation may be necessary.

2. Plain radiographs can be used to compare with the contrast radiographs.

3. The barium must be given as a bolus to aid visualisation on the radiograph. Any spillage of barium may appear as an artefact on the radiograph.

4. Food takes 15–30 seconds to pass down the oesophagus, so the radiograph must be taken quickly. Any barium remaining in the oesophagus will line the mucosa and outline any lesions.

PROCEDURE: BARIUM MEAL OR 'FOLLOW THROUGH'

ACTION

1. The patient should be fasted for 12 hours. Water should be withheld for 2 hours

2. Moderate sedation may be needed.

3. Take plain radiographs: lateral and ventrodorsal views.

4. Restrain the patient and place a syringe containing barium into the corner of the mouth, avoiding spillage. Administer slowly. It may be necessary to use a stomach tube.

5. If fluoroscopy is available, it may be used to observe the movements of the stomach.

6. Take a series of radiographs, right lateral, left lateral, ventrodorsal and dorsoventral centred over the mid-abdomen, immediately after administration of the barium.

7. Repeat these views 10 minutes later and then at intervals of 30 minutes until the stomach is empty.

8. To demonstrate the small intestine, radiographs should be taken every hour until the stomach is empty.

RATIONALE

1. The presence of food and water will effect stomach function and the appearance and movement of the barium.

2. The patient may object to serial radiographs being taken. Acepromazine has the least effect on gut motility.

3. These provide a comparison with contrast radiographs. Taking two views allows accurate localisation of any lesions.

4. The barium must be administered over a short period, so the procedure must be carried out quickly and cleanly. Any spillage of barium may appear as an artefact on the radiograph.

5. Fluoroscopy produces 'live' X-ray pictures and can be used for real-time investigations.

6. These four views ensure that all parts of the stomach are examined.

7. These time intervals allow the movement of barium to be monitored without missing too much detail.

8. This ensures that the complete intestinal tract is demonstrated.

PROCEDURE: BARIUM ENEMA (FIG. 10.19)

ACTION

1. The patient should be fed on a low residue diet for 3 days.

2. Prepare the patient by giving a non-irritant enema 2–3 hours before the examination.

3. The patient should be given a general anaesthetic or heavy sedation.

4. Place the patient in ventrodorsal and right lateral recumbency and take plain radiographs of the abdomen.

5. Hang an old drip bag, containing a 50:50 mixture of barium and water, from a drip stand.

RATIONALE

1. This will ensure that a minimum amount of faeces is present in the colon.

2. This removes the faeces and ensures that barium does not adhere to anything other than the wall of the colon. The presence of faeces may obscure much of the abdominal detail.

3. This is essential to allow catheterisation of the rectum and the introduction of barium, which can be uncomfortable.

4. These will demonstrate any pathology present and may be used for comparison with the contrast radiographs.

5. This mixture allows the barium to flow into the colon.

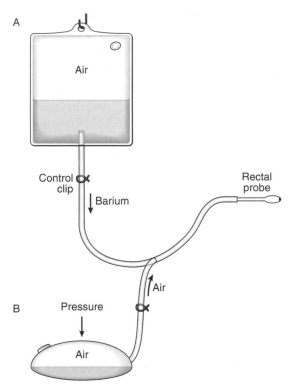

Figure 10.19 Barium enema bag. In position A, the barium flows under gravity into the colon. In position B, barium empties from the colon into the bag and then pressure on the bag will distend the colon with air for the double contrast effect. Adapted with permission, from *Veterinary Nursing*, p. 669, 2nd edn, by Ouster (2000). Butterworth Heinemann, UK.

6. Insert a Foley catheter into the rectum. This is attached by means of a length of rubber tubing to the drip bag. Attach a clamp to control the flow from the bag.

7. Adjust the clamp to allow barium to flow slowly into the rectum and colon. Continue until the barium just begins to leak out around the catheter.

8. Place the patient in right lateral, left lateral and ventrodorsal recumbency; take radiographs.

9. kV should be increased above that used for the plain radiographs.

10. If a double-contrast technique is used, lower the drip bag and allow barium to flow back into the bag by gravity.

11. Gently squeeze the bag, forcing air into the rectum and colon.

12. Repeat the radiographs as in step 8.

6. Control of the barium flow is essential to prevent backflow and overfilling of the colon.

7. Hanging the bag from a drip stand allows the barium to flow into the rectum by gravity.

8. These views allow the entire colon to be demonstrated.

9. This ensures that the edges of the barium are clearly delineated, which aids interpretation of the radiograph.

10. If the radiograph is taken with both barium and air in the colon, it will not be diagnostic.

11. Air distends the colon, while the remains of the barium sticks to the colonic mucosa.

12. Reduce the kV, as air is of a lower density than barium.

PROCEDURE: INTRAVENOUS UROGRAPHY (IVU) (FIG. 10.20)

ACTION

1. The patient should be starved for 12 hours. Water should be withheld for 2 hours prior to the procedure.
2. Administer an enema.

3. Administer a general anaesthetic to the patient.

4. Take plain radiographs in right lateral and ventrodorsal recumbency, centred on the umbilicus.

RATIONALE

1. This procedure is performed under a general anaesthetic; starvation ensures that the patient does not vomit and choke.
2. The presence of faeces in the colon may mask the view of the kidney and ureters.
3. Intravenous iodine may cause an unpleasant feeling of nausea and may be irritant if perivascular leakage occurs. A large number of radiographs may be needed. If the patient is anaesthetised, these are all made easier.
4. These views will demonstrate all the areas of the urinary tract and can be used for comparison with the later contrast radiographs.

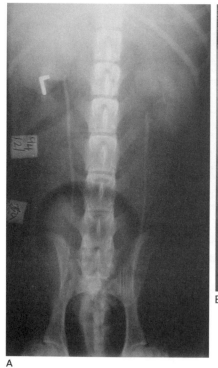

A

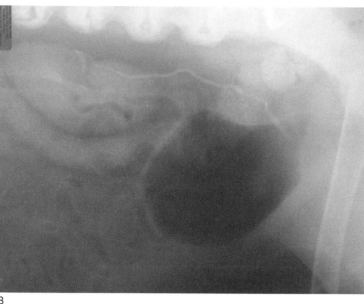

B

Figure 10.20 Ventrodorsal (A) and lateral (B) radiographs of the abdomen to show the effects of intravenous urography.

5. Introduce a urinary catheter into the bladder and empty it by gentle compression on the bladder or by drawing urine out by syringe. Introduce a small amount of air.

6. Administer the contrast medium intravenously.

7. Inject either:

   - A bolus of warmed contrast medium (iodine 300–400 mg/ml conc.) at a dose of 850 mg iodine/kg.
   - An infusion of warmed contrast medium (iodine 150–200 mg/ml conc.) at a dose of 1200 mg iodine/kg. May be administered using a giving set over a period of 10–15 minutes.

8. As soon as the intravenous injection has been completed, take a ventrodorsal radiograph of the abdomen, centring on the area of the umbilicus.

9. Take another radiograph after 5 minutes.

10. Place the patient in right lateral recumbency and take another radiograph after 10 minutes.

11. Place the patient in right lateral recumbency and take another radiograph after 15 minutes. Centre at the level of the neck of the bladder.

12. Further radiographs can be taken if abnormalities are detected or if excretion rates are slowed.

5. The presence of urine in the bladder will dilute the contrast medium. Air in the bladder enables the ureters passing over the bladder and the position of the neck of the bladder to be seen.

6. The cephalic vein is the easiest intravenous route to use in the dog and the cat.

7. Bolus IVU is recommended for kidney examination. Infusion IVU is used for patients with urinary incontinence and ureteric problems. Warming the iodine solution reduces its viscosity and makes intravenous injection easier.

8. Clear colourless iodine appears as a radio-opaque material within the urinary system. The kidneys will fill with iodine, demonstrating the size and shape of the kidneys. A ventrodorsal view enables a comparison of both kidneys to be made.

9. The pelvis of each kidney will be outlined by contrast medium.

10. The ureters will be filled and their size and position can be evaluated.

11. The bladder will be filling and the trigone area should be visible.

12. Taking additional views can be decided on the basis of individual findings.

PROCEDURE: URETHROGRAM (RETROGRADE URETHROGRAPHY)—MALE

ACTION

1. Administer an enema to the patient, but this is not essential.
2. Administer a sedative to the patient. In some cases a general anaesthetic may be given.

3. Place the patient in right lateral recumbency and take a plain radiograph centred to the neck of the bladder and collimated to include the entire urethra.
4. Introduce a urinary catheter into the bladder and drain the urine. Remove the catheter.
5. Select a Foley catheter and flush with contrast material before it is inserted.

6. Place the patient in right lateral recumbency.

7. Gently introduce the Foley catheter into the penile urethra and inflate the cuff.
8. Inject 5–15 ml of iodine (150 mg/ml) slowly up the catheter.

9. Stand back from the patient and take a lateral radiograph. Pull the hindlegs cranially to show the ischial arch and pull them caudally to show the penile urethra.

RATIONALE

1. The presence of faeces may alter the position of the bladder or urethra.
2. This procedure can be performed with care in a conscious animal but it may cause the urethra to constrict: the interpretation of the radiograph should take this into account.
3. This may indicate any lesions that may later be masked by the contrast material.

4. The presence of urine in the bladder will dilute the contrast medium.
5. This flushes air out of the catheter. The presence of air in the catheter when it is inserted into the urethra may appear to be in the urethra itself and thus affect the diagnosis.
6. This is the most comfortable position for the patient and provides easy access to the penis and urethra.
7. Inflating the cuff prevents backflow of contrast material out of the urethra.
8. The addition of KY jelly to the contrast medium will increase the degree of urethral distension and may produce a better image.
9. Hands and forearms must be protected from scattered radiation by a lead sheet or gloves during the exposure.

PROCEDURE: URETHROGRAM (RETROGRADE VAGINO-URETHROGRAPHY)— FEMALE

ACTION	RATIONALE
1. Administer an enema to the patient, but this is not essential.	1. The presence of faeces may alter the position of the bladder or urethra.
2. Administer a general anaesthetic to the patient.	2. The use of Allis tissue forceps later in the procedure is painful so a general anaesthetic is recommended.
3. Place the patient in right lateral recumbency and take a plain radiograph, centred to the neck of the bladder and collimated to include the entire urethra.	3. This will demonstrate any lesions and provide a comparison with later contrast radiographs.
4. Introduce a urinary catheter into the bladder and drain the urine. Remove the catheter.	4. The presence of urine in the bladder will dilute the contrast medium.
5. Select a Foley catheter and flush with contrast material.	5. This flushes air out of the catheter. The presence of air in the catheter when it is inserted into the vestibule may appear to be in the vestibule itself and thus affect the diagnosis.
6. Place the animal in right lateral recumbency.	6. This is the most comfortable position for the patient and provides easy access to the vagina and vestibule.
7. Insert the Foley catheter through the vulval lips and into the vestibule, and inflate the cuff.	7. Inflating the cuff prevents backflow and leakage of contrast material out of the vagina and vestibule.
8. Hold the catheter in place and attach a pair of Allis tissue forceps across the vulva.	8. This procedure prevents further loss of the contrast medium, but can be painful in a conscious bitch.
9. Inject up to 1 ml/kg of iodine (150 mg/ml) slowly up the catheter.	9. The contrast medium enters the vagina under pressure and care must be taken not to overfill the vagina and urethra as rupture can occur.
10. Stand back from the patient and take a lateral radiograph.	10. Hands and forearms must be protected from scattered radiation by a lead sheet or gloves during the exposure.

PROCEDURE: CYSTOGRAPHY

Pneumocystogram, positive contrast cystogram, double-contrast cystogram.

ACTION

1. Administer an enema to the patient.

2. Administer a general anaesthetic, although the procedure can be performed under sedation.

3. Place the patient in right lateral recumbency and take a plain radiograph centred on the neck of the bladder.

4. Introduce a urinary catheter into the bladder and drain the urine.

5. With the patient in right lateral recumbency, gently introduce room air into the bladder using a syringe and a three-way tap at a rate of approximately 10 ml/kg.

6. Take a lateral radiograph.

7. For a positive contrast cystogram, introduce diluted iodine contrast material at a rate of 10 ml/kg after draining the urine from the bladder. Take a lateral radiograph. kV must be increased.

8. For a double-contrast cystogram, inject 2–15 ml of iodine (150 mg/ml) into the empty bladder via the catheter and gently roll the patient from side to side.

9. Inflate the bladder with air until it feels taut. Take a lateral radiograph.

10. In all cases exposure should be carried out immediately after the contrast material has been injected.

RATIONALE

1. The presence of faeces may alter the position of the bladder.

2. This is not necessarily a painful procedure but it may be easier to position the animal if it is sedated or anaesthetised. The urethra may constrict when a fully conscious animal is catheterised and interpretation of the radiograph should take this into account.

3. This can be used as a comparison with later contrast radiographs.

4. The presence of urine in the bladder will dilute the contrast material.

5. The bladder should feel moderately distended when the abdomen is palpated. Care must be taken to avoid rupturing the bladder.

6. This is known as a pneumocystogram; the bladder will appear as a dark mass in the caudal abdomen. The examination is used to detect the presence of calculi in the bladder.

7. The bladder appears as a radio-opaque mass in the caudal abdomen. kV must be increased as positive contrast is denser than the air in the pneumocystogram.

8. Rolling the patient ensures that the iodine covers the bladder mucosa.

9. The bladder mucosa appears covered with positive contrast, whereas the lumen appears dark, with a shadow of residual contrast material in the centre. This technique is used to evaluate the thickness of the bladder wall, the presence of lesions such as tumours, and the presence of calculi.

10. This procedure does not require anyone to remain in the room, so in the interests of radiation safety normal procedures should be followed.

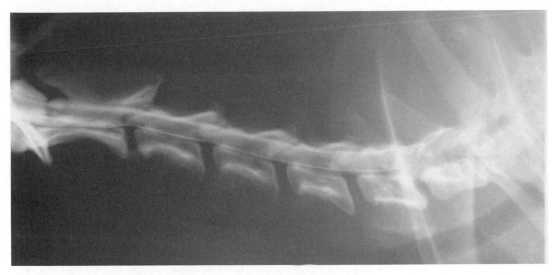

Figure 10.21 Lateral radiograph of the spine showing the effects of myelography.

PROCEDURE: MYELOGRAPHY—CISTERNAL AND LUMBAR PUNCTURE (FIG. 10.21)

ACTION

1. Administer a general anaesthetic to the patient.

2. Place the patient in lateral recumbency and take plain radiographs of the area under investigation.

3. Clip the neck caudal to the skull (cisternal) or over the lumbar spine (lumbar) and prepare the site as for a surgical procedure.

4. Select the non-ionic contrast material Omnipaque (200–300 mg/ml iodine) and gently warm it. The dose rate is 0.3–0.45 ml/kg depending on size.

5. For cisternal puncture: raise the table to about 10° tilt, with the patient's head at the raised end.

6. Flex the head to an angle of 90° so that the chin touches the sternum.

RATIONALE

1. This procedure is potentially painful and requires accurate placing of a spinal needle in the subarachnoid space. Any sudden movements could have serious consequences.

2. This will provide preliminary indications as to the diagnosis and enables exposure factors to be set.

3. Care must be taken to prevent the introduction of infection into the spinal cord.

4. Non-ionic iodine provides the least amount of irritation to the spinal cord. Warming reduces the viscosity of the liquid, making it easier to inject.

5. This ensures that contrast medium does not flow up into the ventricles of the brain, which may cause pain due to a rise in cerebral pressure, also this may result in fitting.

6. The needle is to be inserted into the cisterna magna, which is the cranial end of the subarachnoid space just behind the skull. Flexing the neck opens up access to this space.

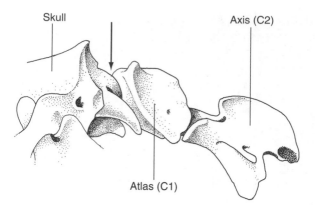

Figure 10.22 Myelography: site for cisternal puncture. Adapted, with permission, from *Veterinary Nursing*, p. 671, 2nd edn, by Lane and Cooper (1994). Butterworth Heinemann, UK.

7. Insert a spinal needle of a suitable length, depending on the patient's size, between the skull and the atlas (Fig. 10.22). Advance it until cerebrospinal fluid (CSF) drips from the needle. Collect a sample of CSF.

8. Inject the required amount of contrast medium slowly. Remove the needle and extend the neck. Take radiographs.

9. For lumbar puncture: flex the vertebral column by pulling the hindlegs forward.

10. Insert a spinal needle of a suitable length into the appropriate junction and note the twitch of the legs and anus.

11. Little or no CSF will appear through the needle. If this is the case, inject a small amount of contrast medium.

12. A test radiograph, centred over the needle, may be taken in lateral recumbency.

13. Inject the remainder of the contrast medium. Remove the needle and straighten the spine. Keep the head raised. Take the radiographs.

14. In either technique, once the contrast medium has been introduced take lateral views of the spine, starting at the site of injection and moving caudally. In the area of the cervical spine, remove the endotracheal tube from the larynx.

7. The presence of CSF indicates that the needle is in the correct position. Analysis of the sample of CSF may be an added diagnostic aid.

8. Slow injection prevents a sudden increase in pressure.

9. The site used is at the level of the L4–5 junction, or L5–6. This position should not be used if there is any indication of spinal instability.

10. This twitch indicates that the needle has passed through the spinal cord.

11. Lack of CSF does not indicate incorrect needle placement. A small amount of contrast material is injected to test for correct needle placement.

12. This will show whether the small amount of contrast medium has reached the correct site.

13. If the needle is left in position, it may damage the spinal cord. Keeping the head raised prevents the flow of contrast material towards the brain.

14. The entire spine should be examined, as additional lesions may be found. The endotracheal tube will lie over the spinal cord and make interpretation more difficult.

15. When the contrast medium has reached the main point of interest, take ventrodorsal and oblique views.
16. During recovery, the patient must be placed in its kennel with its head raised.

15. Lateral, ventrodorsal and oblique views allow accurate identification and location of the lesion.
16. This prevents flow of contrast medium into the ventricles of the brain, causing a painful rise in pressure and the risk of fits.

TECHNIQUES FOR PROCESSING RADIOGRAPHS

PROCEDURE: MANUAL PROCESSING (FIG. 10.23)

ACTION

1. Put on a pair of rubber gloves and a plastic apron.

2. Check that the levels and the temperatures of the developer and fixer tanks are correct. If appropriate check the temperature of the surrounding water bath.

3. Turn off all lights except the safelight.

4. Lock the door to the darkroom.

5. Unload the cassette and place the film in a hanger of a suitable design and size.

RATIONALE

1. Processing chemicals can be irritant and you should protect your hands and your clothes. Goggles will also protect your eyes from splashes.

2. If the levels of chemicals in the tanks are low, the upper parts of the film will not be processed. The temperature of the developer should be 20°C and the fixer 20–21°C. Temperatures that are too low will result in underdevelopment, and those that are too high result in overdevelopment (always check the label for accurate temperatures as they may vary).

3. White light will fog the film. The safelight must have the correct filter for the type of film.

4. Accidental opening of the door will allow light into the room, with subsequent fogging of the film.

5. Hangers minimise handling of the film during processing. There are two designs:

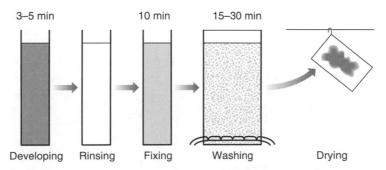

Figure 10.23   Routine for manual processing. Adapted with permission, from *Veterinary Nursing*, p. 657, 2nd edn, by Lane and Cooper (1994). Butterworth Heinemann, UK.

6. Place the film in the developer tank, moving it gently to remove bubbles and to coat the emulsion evenly. Set the timer and leave in the developer for the recommended time.

7. Take the film out of the developer tank, allowing any excess fluid to drip back into the tank. Replace the lid of the developer tank.

8. Place the film in the rinse tank and agitate it gently.

9. Place the film in the fixer tank and leave for 10 minutes.

10. Place the film in the wash tank for at least 30 minutes.

11. The room light can now be switched on.

12. Hang the film up to dry or place it in a drying cabinet.

13. Cassettes should always be reloaded in the dry area of the darkroom after use and stored ready for use. This may be done while you are waiting for the developing process to work.

channel and clip hangers. The size of the hanger must match that of the film.

6. Uneven coating of the film will cause uneven development. The recommended time for development is usually 4 minutes. Removing the film too soon causes a pale or underdeveloped film; leaving it for too long causes a dark or overdeveloped film.

7. If developer is allowed to mix with the rinse water, the water will become contaminated over a period of time. The lid of the developer tank prevents oxidation of the chemicals by air when it is not in use.

8. The water stops the action of the developer and rinses the film clean.

9. Fixer hardens the emulsion and fixes the image so that it can be viewed in white light. You may look at the image after the milky appearance on the film has disappeared (clearing). It must be replaced in the tank for the full time. Timing is not critical but should be a minimum of 8 minutes. If the fixing process is not complete, the film will turn brown when stored.

10. The wash tank should be filled with running water and is used to remove any residual chemicals. If chemicals remain on the film it becomes yellow with time.

11. The film is no longer sensitive to white light after 30 seconds in the fixer but if you can wait longer there will be no risk of light fogging.

12. The film must be thoroughly dried before storage. Viewing the radiograph for the final interpretation is best done using a dry radiograph, as swelling of the emulsion during processing may cause distortion of the image.

13. Loading must be done in the dark or under the safelight to prevent fogging. Avoid any splashing of chemicals in the wet area of the darkroom.

PROCEDURE: STARTING UP AN AUTOMATIC PROCESSOR

ACTION	RATIONALE
1. Check the levels of water and chemicals in the processor and the replenisher tanks. Check the position of the rollers.	1. The levels of the chemicals will fall with use. Other users may displace the rollers.
2. Turn on the water supply valve.	2. Water is needed to wash the films and to maintain the constant temperature necessary for processing.
3. Turn on the mains supply to the machine and the processor's power switch.	3. An electricity supply is essential.
4. Replace the lid of the processor.	4. The lid should be removed when not in use, but must be replaced to prevent fogging when in use.
5. Check the temperature of the processor.	5. A low temperature will result in underdevelopment of the films. The machine may take about 20 minutes to reach its recommended temperature.
6. Feed two or three old clean films through the processor.	6. These will remove dried chemicals from the rollers.
7. At the same time check that the replenishment pumps are working.	7. These work whenever a film is in the processor.

PROCEDURE: AUTOMATIC PROCESSING

ACTION	RATIONALE
1. Switch the processor on in the prescribed manner and check that the temperature is correct.	1. If the temperature is too low, the films will be underdeveloped. If the recommended set-up procedure is not followed, vital stages may be missed, resulting in fogging of the film or a lack of water to the processor.
2. Lock the door of the darkroom and switch the lights off.	2. Accidental opening of the door will allow light in, causing fogging of the film.
3. Remove the film from the cassette and place it on to the tray or entry roller of the processor.	3. The film should be placed in the correct orientation for entry to prevent damage.
4. Allow the film to be taken into the processor.	4. Restricting the movement of the film will cause scratching of the emulsion.
5. Wait for the audible or visible indicator before leaving the darkroom, inserting the next film or switching the light back on.	5. If a second film is put in before the first film has moved into the processor, the two may stick together.
6. Reload the cassette and place it in the storage area ready for use.	6. Loading must be done in the dark or under the safelight to prevent fogging. Avoid any splashing by chemicals or water.

PROCEDURE: SHUTTING DOWN THE AUTOMATIC PROCESSOR

ACTION

1. Make sure that there are no films in the processor.

2. Turn off the power switch on the processor and the mains isolator switch.
3. Turn off the water supply.

4. Remove the processor cover or lid.
5. Remove any chemical residue from inside the processor.

6. Place an antifungal tablet into the wash tank.
7. Ensure that the lid or cover is left in a slightly raised position.

RATIONALE

1. If the processor is switched off with films still passing through, they may be irreparably damaged.
2. Power should never be left on when the processor is not in use.
3. Water should never be left running unnecessarily.
4. The lid can be removed to give easy access.
5. Daily removal of any residue reduces damage that may occur if chemicals are left on the working parts for long periods of time.
6. This reduces the build-up of fungi and algae in the wash water.
7. Air circulation through the processor reduces the build-up of condensation.

PROCEDURE: CLEANING AN AUTOMATIC PROCESSOR

ACTION

1. Switch off the electricity supply to the machine.
2. Drain the water tank by opening the valve.

3. Remove the crossover rollers between the tanks and wash them in fresh water.

4. Place a splashguard between the fixer and the developer tank.
5. Remove the rollers from the developer tank. Wash in fresh water, remove any residual chemicals and check their movement.
6. Replace the developer racks after draining, taking care not to splash developer into the fixer.
7. Remove the rollers from the fixer tank. Wash in fresh water, remove any residual chemicals and check their movement.
8. Replace the fixer racks after draining, taking care not to splash fixer into the developer.
9. Remove the rollers from the wash tank and clean in fresh water.

RATIONALE

1. The combination of electricity and water could be fatal!
2. Draining the water allows proper cleaning to be carried out.
3. The crossover rollers collect chemical residues, which dry on them. At most times these rollers are out of the liquids.
4. This prevents cross-contamination between the tanks.
5. Dried developer on the rollers will scratch the emulsion, giving rise to 'roller marks', and prevent their free movement.
6. This prevents cross-contamination between the tanks.

7. Dried fixer on the rollers will scratch the emulsion, giving rise to 'roller marks', and prevent their free movement.
8. This prevents cross-contamination between the tanks.
9. The effect of heat, emulsion residue and water creates a build-up of sludge and algae. This reduces the quality of the image produced and the function of the processor.

10. Clean the empty tank with a sponge and fresh water.
11. Replace the wash tank racks.

12. Close the valve to the wash tank to allow refilling.
13. Replace the crossover racks.

14. Replace the lid of the processor and switch the power back on.
15. Pass a few old clean films through the processor.

10. Care should be taken to remove any algae that has built up on the tank sides.
11. The racks should be replaced carefully and seated in their correct positions.
12. Without water, the processor will not wash the films and may overheat.
13. These must be replaced last as they sit over all the other rollers.
14. The lid provides a light-tight seal to prevent fogging of the films.
15. These will pick up any residue that has been dislodged during cleaning. It is also a means of checking for correct function before clinical radiographs are processed.

MAINTENANCE OF RADIOGRAPHY EQUIPMENT

PROCEDURE: CARE OF INTENSIFYING SCREENS

ACTION

1. Moisten a soft cloth with a screen cleaning detergent or a small amount of commercial detergent and water.

2. Wipe the screen gently.

3. Do not wet the screen, and avoid spilling anything on the back of the screen.

4. Wipe the screen clean with a fresh dry cloth or piece of gauze.
5. Stand the cassette upright and leave it slightly open to dry.

6. Record when the cleaning was done and by whom.

RATIONALE

1. Intensifying screens are delicate and expensive pieces of equipment: any damage will appear on the radiograph and the screen may be rendered useless. Avoid the use of any material that will scratch the screens. Do not use cotton wool as this leaves small pieces of lint on the screen.
2. The detergent should be used sparingly and only just touch the screen.
3. Moisture damages the grains within the screen, affecting their efficiency, and will also cause the cardboard backing to disintegrate.
4. All detergent and moisture must be removed to prevent damage to the screen.
5. This prevents pooling of the detergent and allows air to circulate, reducing condensation.
6. Regular cleaning of the screens improves image quality. Any damage can be traced.

PROCEDURE: CHECKING SAFELIGHT FUNCTION

ACTION

1. Enter the darkroom and switch off the white light.
2. Do not switch on the safelight.

3. Select two films of the type commonly used in the practice but of the smallest size available.
4. Take one (film A) out of any protective covering and place your hand on it for 30 seconds.
5. Repeat this process with the other film (B), with the safelight switched on.

6. Process both films.

7. Compare the two films.

RATIONALE

1. White light will always fog the film.

2. This film will be used to provide a baseline for your assessment.
3. Keep the cost of this assessment to a minimum.

4. If the darkroom is truly lightproof, there will no image on this film.

5. If the safelight is leaking light of the wrong wavelength, it will produce an image of your hand. If the safelight is in working order, there will be no image on the film.
6. The image cannot be seen without processing.
7. This technique can also be used to assess the degree of light-proofing of the darkroom.

PROCEDURE: CHECKING FOR LIGHT LEAKAGE IN A CASSETTE

ACTION

1. Load the cassette to be investigated with a piece of new film and close it securely.
2. Expose each edge of the cassette to high-intensity light (100 W) for about 15 minutes.

3. Process the film and look at it on a viewer.

RATIONALE

1. A new film is used to make sure that no fogging is present.
2. High-intensity light simulates the type of light to which the cassette may normally be exposed.
3. If the edges of the cassette are leaking light, the processed film will show a dark border. Any border greater than 3 mm wide should be assumed to have resulted from leakage of light.

PROCEDURE: CHECKING THE X-RAY TUBE FOR LEAKAGE OF X-RAYS

ACTION

1. Set up the X-ray machine for a low exposure.

2. Close the light beam diaphragm.

3. Place a series of non-screen films around the X-ray tube head. Make sure each one is labelled with its position in relation to the tube.

4. Make an exposure.

5. Process the films and look at them on a viewer.

RATIONALE

1. The tube should be set up for normal use to make the test as realistic as possible.

2. This will reduce the exposure of the environment and the risk of scattered radiation.

3. Non-screen film is flexible and can be used to cover the entire head.

4. X-rays will barely escape as the primary beam, but if there is leakage from the head it will affect the films around the head.

5. Signs of leakage appear as grey areas on the radiograph and may correspond to joints in the tube head. **The machine should not be used until a further professional assessment has been made**.

PROCEDURE: CHECKING FOR THE ACCURACY OF THE LIGHT BEAM DIAPHRAGM

ACTION

1. Place a loaded cassette on the table under the X-ray tube head, keeping the standard film–focus distance.

2. Switch on the light beam diaphragm and collimate it to produce an area of approximately 10 cm^2.

3. Place a row of paper clips along the perimeter of the illuminated square.

4. On each corner, place an unfolded paper clip, with one end towards the corner.

5. Using a low exposure, expose the film.

6. Process and assess the radiograph.

RATIONALE

1. Use a small piece of film to reduce costs.

2. A small area prevents unnecessary contamination of the immediate environment and reduces the risk of scattered radiation.

3. The paper clips mark the edges of the irradiated square once the light beam diaphragm is switched off.

4. The pointed end of the clip accurately delineates the corners.

5. A low exposure reduces the risk of scattered radiation.

6. If the light beam indicates the area exposed by the primary beam accurately, the border of paper clips will be on the edge of the exposed film and the points of the unfolded clips will point to the corners. If the light beam diaphragm is inaccurate, an engineer should be called to correct the fault.

PROCEDURE: CHECKING A CASSETTE FOR POOR FILM–SCREEN CONTACT

ACTION

1. Place a piece of zinc or copper netting or metallic material with small holes cut out inside a small loaded cassette.

2. Collimate the beam to cover most of the cassette, leaving a minimal border around the edge.

3. Expose the cassette, using a low exposure.

4. Process and assess the radiograph.

RATIONALE

1. A specific test tool is available but any metal sheet with holes cut out will do as well. The holes must be present to provide a sharp edge as a means of assessment.

2. All radiographs should have at least a small border around the edge to indicate that the beam has been restricted to some degree.

3. A low exposure prevents unnecessary contamination of the immediate environment and reduces the risk of scattered radiation.

4. Areas of poor film–screen contact will show as darker blurred areas. Even film–screen contact will produce a sharp uniform image. If the cassette is affected it will be due to compression and ageing of the pressure pad underneath the back intensifying screen or warping of the screens. The cassette should be replaced.

DIAGNOSTIC ULTRASOUND

PROCEDURE: PREPARING THE PATIENT FOR AN ULTRASOUND EXAMINATION

ACTION

1. Administer a sedative to the patient.

2. Place the patient on an examination table in a position that provides sufficient access to the area under examination.

RATIONALE

1. Ultrasonography is a non-invasive painless procedure that is well tolerated by most animals. In some cases it may be easier to place a sedated patient in the correct position, and procedures such as biopsy or fine-needle aspiration may require deeper sedation or a general anaesthetic.

2. This may mean that the patient can remain standing or lie in lateral or dorsal recumbency. If the patient feels comfortable and secure, it will be unlikely to struggle. Avoid using areas where underlying bone and gas may block the movement of the ultrasound waves.

3. Clip the area and apply spirit.

3. Fur must be removed to provide good contact between the skin and the transducer of the ultrasound machine. Spirit is used to remove any remaining dirt and grease on the skin surface.

4. Apply coupling gel to the transducer and the skin.

4. Coupling gel ensures good contact between the skin and the transducer. Trapped air will create an artefact, which may affect the final diagnosis.

5. Apply the transducer to the skin within the prepared area.

5. When the transducer is applied to the skin, high-frequency sound waves pass through the patient's soft tissues as pressure waves. At interfaces between organs or between different tissues, some sound waves are reflected and return to the transducer. Here they are detected by the ultrasound equipment, which produces a cross-sectional image of the internal structure of the tissues.

PROCEDURE: CARE OF THE ULTRASOUND MACHINE

ACTION

1. The ultrasound machine should be plugged into the mains and switched on just before use. It should be switched off immediately after use.
2. The transducers should be stored in a suitable holder.

3. The transducer should be attached to the operator throughout the examination.

4. Select the correct mode before the examination.

RATIONALE

1. The machine may overheat if left on for long periods. Where the machine is only used occasionally, leaving it switched on wastes electricity.
2. All machines are equipped with a holder for the transducers, which will prevent damage. There are two types of transducer: the linear array transducer, which produces a rectangular field; and the sector transducer, which produces a fan-shaped field.
3. Transducers are very fragile and should not be dropped or banged. Using a wristband to attach the transducer to the user can prevent this.
4. This ensures that the procedure is carried out quickly and efficiently. There are three types of image display modes. Most ultrasonography is performed using B-mode ('brightness' mode); M-mode is used to show movement of structures on the frozen image and is used in echocardiology; A-mode was the first type and is rarely used.

5. Clean the transducer thoroughly after use.

5. Gel and hair affect the function of the transducer and may be a method of cross-infection.

FURTHER READING

Burns F, Whelehan P, Latham C 1997 Understanding radiography 3. Veterinary Practice Nurse **9**(2): 15–21

Bushong S 1997 Radiological Science for Technologists, 6th edn. Mosby, London

Dennis R 1987 Radiographic examination of the canine spine. Veterinary Record **121**(2): 31–35

Ford G 1999 Processing radiographs. Veterinary Nursing **14**(5): 187–188

Latham C 1996 Radiographic film faults and how to avoid them. Veterinary Practice Nurse **8**(3): 17–22

Care of laboratory equipment
- Care and use of autoclaves
- Care and use of the balance
- Care and cleaning of glassware
- Care and use of the centrifuge
- Care and cleaning of the incubator
- Care and use of the microscope
- Use of the Vernier scale
- Care of glass pipettes
- Use of volumetric and automatic pipettes
- Decontamination and disposal of laboratory waste
- Care of the water bath

Practical laboratory techniques
- Preparation of a smear using samples, e.g. fine-needle aspirate biopsies, thoracic fluid, etc.
- Preparation and storage of faeces for examination
- Worm egg count—modified McMaster method
- Trypsin digest test
- Iodine stain
- Sudan 3 stain
- Packed cell volume
- Total white blood cell count using a haemocytometer
- Total red blood cell count using a haemocytometer
- Preparation of a blood smear
- Reticulocyte count
- Giemsa stain
- Leishman's stain
- Diff-Quik stain
- Differential white cell count
- Preparation of tissue for histological examination
- Preparation of bacterial smears
- Gram's stain—rapid method
- Methylene blue stain
- Bacterial culture
- Culture for ringworm fungus
- Use of a Wood's lamp to detect *Microsporum canis*
- Collection and examination of coat brushings
- Collection of a skin scraping
- Preparation of a smear to identify the presence of mites
- Urine preservation
- Gross examination of urine
- To test the specific gravity of urine by refractometer
- To test urine for various parameters using a dipstick
- Urine sediment examination

11

Diagnostic laboratory techniques

J. Davis

Introduction

Laboratory tests are used to aid or confirm the diagnosis made by the veterinary surgeon. Many of these tests may be sent away to commercial laboratories, but most practices have some form of small laboratory of their own where a range of basic diagnostic tests may be carried out. It is often one of the veterinary nurses who is designated, or volunteers, to run the laboratory and it is vital that she or he is adequately trained to produce consistent good-quality results in which the veterinary surgeon can have confidence. The methods described in this chapter have been in daily use in our practice laboratory. They are simple to carry out, require the minimum of equipment and are easily performed by both student and qualified veterinary nurses.

Biochemistry analyses have not been included as most practices use wet or dry biochemical analysers. Enzyme-linked immunosorbent assay (ELISA) tests for feline leukaemia virus (FeLV) and feline immunodeficiency virus (FIV) are now so commonly used and are so simple to perform that specific instructions have not been included.

Health and safety in the laboratory

While undertaking laboratory procedures, observe the following guidelines:

- Wear a long-sleeved laboratory coat, gloves, masks (where necessary) and eye protection at all times.

- Wear the minimum of jewellery.
- The use of nail varnish is not acceptable and nails must be kept short and clean.
- Do not lick gummed labels or your fingers or suck the ends of pencils, pens, etc.
- A wash basin reserved for handwashing should be available and equipped with antibacterial soap and paper towels.
- Hands should be washed on entry to the laboratory and on leaving the room.
- All work surfaces should be cleaned and disinfected daily and after every hazardous procedure.
- As soon as you have finished with equipment, store it away tidily to avoid accidents.
- Samples and contaminated equipment should be disposed of safely and correctly.

- Sharps containers and clinical waste bags must be available in the laboratory at all times.
- If hazardous chemicals are used, take note of warning labels and act accordingly.
- Many bacteria are potential pathogens and should be handled in a contained environment such as a safety cabinet.
- Avoid mouth pipetting.
- Know where the first aid kit is stored and what action to take in an emergency; be familiar with the accident book.
- It is a good idea to list all procedures in a laboratory manual so that all staff members use the same methodologies.
- The use of external quality assurance or quality control schemes ensures confidence in your results.

CARE OF LABORATORY EQUIPMENT

PROCEDURE: CARE AND USE OF AUTOCLAVES

ACTION

1. Autoclaving is the most reliable method for sterilising culture media and laboratory equipment.

2. Before use check that there is sufficient water to cover the element.
3. Load the items.
4. Place an indicator strip near to the middle of the load.
5. Do not overfill the chamber.

6. Check that the steam discharge tap is open.
7. Adjust the safety valve to the required pressure.

8. Allow steam and air mixture to escape until all air has been eliminated from the chamber.
9. Close the discharge tap.

RATIONALE

1. When water is boiled within a closed vessel and at increased pressure, steam is formed and the temperature rises above 100°C. The high temperature will kill all micro-organisms and bacterial spores. (Some spores may survive a 15 minute programme.)
2. Autoclaves must not be allowed to boil dry.

4. These strips change colour to indicate when full sterilisation has taken place.
5. Items in the middle of the load may not be completely sterilised if the chamber is overloaded.

7. Each type of object has a specific required temperature, e.g. culture media are usually autoclaved at 121°C for 15 minutes.
8. You will see the steam escaping.

10. When pressure reaches the required level the safety valve will open: at this point, start to time the load.
11. When the time is complete, turn off the heater and allow the autoclave to cool.
12. Open the discharge tap.
13. Unload the items.
14. Pour out any water left in the chamber and wipe clean with a soft cloth.

10. A minute timer is useful.

11. When cool, the pressure gauge is calibrated to read zero.

PROCEDURE: CARE AND USE OF THE BALANCE

ACTION

1. Always make sure that the balance is placed on an even and stable surface.
2. Items placed on the top pan must be centred for accurate weight distribution.
3. Instrument accuracy can be checked using calibrated weights.

4. Before weighing zero the balance using the 'tare' button.
5. Weigh the item under test.
6. Record the result.
7. Carefully remove the item from the pan.
8. Turn off the power supply to the balance.
9. Clean the pan using a damp soft cloth (if spillage has occurred) or a soft clean lint-free tissue.

RATIONALE

1. Balances are extremely delicate instruments and can be damaged by excessive vibration.
2. Use forceps to place items carefully into the middle of the pan.
3. Use a suitable weight in the middle of the balance range to check the accuracy. This will depend on the number of decimal places to which your balance measures.
4. If using a balance boat, place the boat on the balance before zeroing the machine.

7. Use forceps for small items.

9. More detailed maintenance should be carried out by a trained engineer at an annual service.

PROCEDURE: CARE AND CLEANING OF GLASSWARE

ACTION

1. Important: if the glassware contains hazardous material, autoclave the glassware with the contents intact at 121°C for 45 minutes prior to discarding the contents.
2. If autoclaving is not required, proceed as follows: rinse the glassware immediately after use and place in a solution of non-toxic commercial laboratory detergent.
3. Using disposable gloves and a soft bush, remove any material present on the glassware.
4. Transfer glassware to a fresh solution of detergent and leave to soak for 20–30 minutes.

RATIONALE

1. Health and safety precautions must be observed when pathogens are likely to be present. Spore-forming organisms may withstand 15 minutes in an autoclave.
2. Detergents designed for laboratory use are available: harsh detergents are too abrasive and will damage glass.

3. Use a test-tube brush for narrow tubes: hard brushes scratch the surface of the glass.
4. Heavy soiling may require a longer soaking.

5. Once the glassware is visibly clean, rinse in tap water two or three times.
6. Transfer to a container of distilled/deionised water and rinse.
7. Allow to drain.

6. Two or three changes of distilled water are recommended.
7. Water runs off clean glass evenly: if any dirt remains, areas with a 'greasy' appearance will be visible.

8. Dry in drying oven at 160°C for 1 hour or allow to air dry.
9. If glassware is to be used for sterile procedures, sterilise in an autoclave at 121°C for 15 minutes.

8. If air drying, the atmosphere must be dust-free.
9. Bottles should be autoclaved with the lids screwed loosely to allow for the escape of expanding hot air. Tighten the lids after autoclaving; this prevents contaminated air being sucked in by the cooling air. Plug test-tubes with cotton wool.

10. Always cool glassware slowly. Do not put hot glassware on to a cold surface.
11. Check for cracks and chips and store in a dust-free atmosphere until required.

10. Glass will crack if it is subjected to sudden temperature changes.
11. Cracks or chips reduce thermal strength, leading to sudden breakage.

PROCEDURE: CARE AND USE OF THE CENTRIFUGE

ACTION

1. Always ensure that the centrifuge is placed on an even and stable surface.

2. Only use tubes recommended by the manufacturer.

3. The top of the centrifuge tube must not protrude above the top of the bucket. When using a microhaematocrit centrifuge, ensure that the plasticine end of the capillary tube is against the outer ring of the instrument.
4. Vacutainer tubes may be spun with their stoppers in place.

5. Lock the lid of the centrifuge securely.

6. Set the spin speed as appropriate.

7. After use, turn off the power supply.
8. Take out the buckets.
9. Wipe the rotor and buckets with a soft cloth and mild disinfectant solution.
10. Replace the buckets and close the lid.

RATIONALE

1. Slight vibration occurs when the machine is in motion and an uneven surface may cause the machine to move around.
2. Centrifuge tubes often have a tapered bottom and are designed to withstand centrifugal force.
3. Centrifugal force pushes material outwards. The plasticine end prevents material escaping from the tube.

4. If the tube is opened or broken, aerosol contamination of the environment could occur.
5. Most machines will not allow you to use them without locking the lid first. If you do not, the lid may fly open during use.
6. For example, urine requires a lower speed than heparinised blood for biochemistry.

9. To prevent contamination of the next sample.

PROCEDURE: CARE AND CLEANING OF THE INCUBATOR

ACTION

1. Remove all media from the incubator.

2. It is sensible to clean the instrument when workload is low but it should be done at least once a week.
3. Remove all the shelves and racks.

4. Using a mild detergent and soft cloth, wipe all the incubator surfaces and the shelves.

5. Allow to dry.
6. Using a disinfectant solution and fresh cloth, wipe all the incubator surfaces and shelves.
7. Allow to dry.
8. Replace the shelves.
9. Place a thermometer in glycerol in the middle of the incubator. Check that the bulb is covered. Switch on the incubator.
10. Read the thermometer after 1 hour.

11. Every month check on the door seal, electrical wiring and thermostat.

RATIONALE

1. If you take too long to clean out the incubator, the agar plates have to stand at room temperature, slowing the growth of the bacteria.
2. Incubators are used to culture bacteria so the risk of contamination of samples is high.

3. These are more easily cleaned out of the incubator.
4. Take care not to touch any electrical parts. If in doubt, switch off the power supply before cleaning.

6. The disinfectant used must be bactericidal and fungicidal to be effective.

9. The temperature of the glycerol alters slowly and allows the thermometer to be read without rapid fluctuations.
10. Most incubators run at $37°C \pm 1°C$. It is essential to check that the incubator reaches the correct temperature to ensure efficient incubation of the agar plates.
11. If in doubt about any component inform the practice or laboratory manager.

PROCEDURE: CARE AND USE OF THE MICROSCOPE (FIG. 11.1)

ACTION

1. Always ensure that the microscope is placed on an even and stable surface.
2. Before use, clean the eyepieces, condenser and objective lenses with lens tissue.
3. Clean the oil immersion lens with cleaning fluid.
4. Turn the light control to a minimum.

5. Turn on the instrument.
6. Adjust the eyepieces.

7. Place the slide on the stage. Some instruments have clips to hold the slide.

RATIONALE

1. Slight vibration will make it difficult to view the object.
2. Lens tissue is lint-free and prevents bits being left on the surfaces.
3. Isopropanol is most commonly used.

4. This prevents a sudden power surge, which may break the bulb when the microscope is switched on.

6. Use both eyepieces and position them so that both fields converge as one.
7. The slide should remain firmly in place to avoid unintentional loss of a particular field.

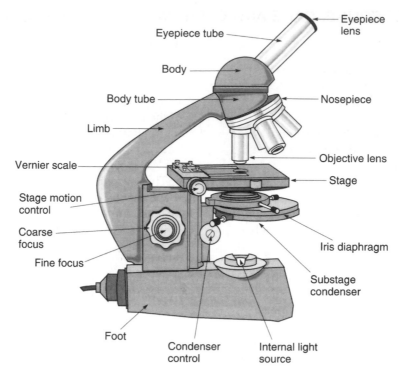

Figure 11.1 A light microscope. Reproduced, with permission, from *Preveterinary Nursing Textbook*, p. 224, by Masters and Bowden (2001). Butterworth Heinemann, UK.

8. Move the slide by using the knobs on the mechanical stage.

9. Examine the slide using the ×10 objective lens.

10. Focus first with the coarse and then the fine adjustment knobs.

11. If using oil immersion, place a drop of oil on to the slide.

12. Rotate the nosepiece until the ×100 objective lens is above the slide.

13. Lower the objective lens into the drop of oil. Always watch what you are doing: do not look at it through the eyepiece, as you will find it impossible to judge distances and may smash through the slide.

14. Focus using the fine control.

15. After use, remove the slide from the stage.

16. Reduce the light and turn off the power.

8. This allows the whole slide to be examined smoothly and accurately without touching the slide with your fingers.

9. At this stage the light can be adjusted using the light source knob or by repositioning the condenser.

10. Always focus upwards from the slide to prevent accidental damage to the slide.

11. Oil immersion provides increased magnification and is used for examination of bacteria and blood smears.

13. The lens must be lying in the oil to avoid distortion of the image. Avoid contaminating the dry lenses.

14. You may need to adjust the light to improve your view.

15. Move the clips before trying to remove the slide.

17. Turn the objective lenses on the nosepiece until the lowest power is in position above the stage.

17. Ready for use next time.

18. Remove any oil from the objective lenses using lens tissue and, if necessary, lens cleaning fluid.

18. Ready for use next time.

19. Cover the instrument when not in use.

19. This will prevent the build-up of dust on the objective and eyepiece lenses.

PROCEDURE: USE OF THE VERNIER SCALE (FIG. 11.2)

ACTION

1. The Vernier scale is a graduated device attached to the stage of the microscope.

2. One scale lies along a vertical edge and another along a horizontal edge.

3. Place the slide on the microscope stage and fix it with the clips, if present.

RATIONALE

1. It allows the position of an object on a slide to be accurately recorded so that you can find it again.

2. Use both position numbers to give a grid reference, similar to that on a map.

3. The slide must not move around as this will invalidate your scale references.

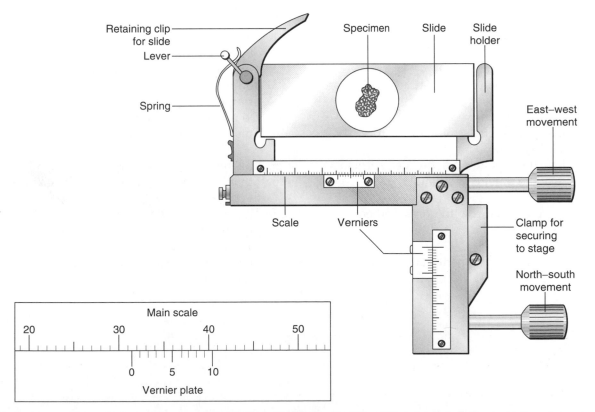

Figure 11.2 The Vernier scale. The zero on the Vernier plate is between 31 and 32 on the main scale, and it is mark number 6 on the Vernier plate that is exactly opposite a division on the main scale. The reading is therefore 31.6.

4. Locate the object you wish to identify.
5. Look at the scale on the vertical axis.
6. Record the number where the zero mark on the Vernier plate meets the main scale.

7. Make a note of which of the marks on the Vernier plate is exactly opposite a division on the main scale.
8. Record this reading, placing it after the decimal point.
9. Repeat steps 6–8 using the horizontal axis.

10. You now have a grid reference for that object on that slide, provided the slide is placed in the same position on the stage.
11. Record your grid reference, using the horizontal reading followed by the vertical reading.

5. See Figure 11.2.
6. Record the lower number if it falls between two divisions. In Figure 11.2 the zero mark falls between 31 and 32.
7. In Figure 11.2, mark number 6 is exactly opposite a division on the main scale.

8. In Figure 11.2 this will give a reading of 31.6.
9. You now have two readings, e.g. 31.6 and 90.1.
10. By tradition, slides are placed on the stage with the label to the right.

11. In this example, the reference would be 90.1 × 31.6. You may now remove the slide and go back to the same location later on.

PROCEDURE: CARE OF GLASS PIPETTES

ACTION

1. After use, place the pipette in a jar of disinfectant.
2. Soak for 1 hour.
3. Rinse the pipette several times in tap water.

4. Rinse the pipette several times in distilled water.
5. Rinse the pipette in methylated spirits.
6. Rinse the pipette in ethanol.

7. Plug the pipettes with non-absorbent cotton wool.

8. Pack into metal pipette canisters for autoclaving at 121°C for 15 minutes.

RATIONALE

1. Hypochlorite solution containing 1000 mg/l of free chlorine is most commonly used.
2. This removes bacterial contamination.
3. You may need to use a 'rubber policeman' or pipette filler to fill and empty the pipette. **Do not use your mouth**.
4. This leaves a clean surface on the glass.

5. This removes any grease.
6. Ethanol evaporates and leaves the inside of the pipette dry.
7. This prevents fluid being sucked up into the pipette filler and reduces cross-contamination.
8. The pipettes are sterilised ready for aseptic procedures.

PROCEDURE: USE OF VOLUMETRIC AND AUTOMATIC PIPETTES

ACTION

1. Using a soft cloth, clean the external parts of the pipette with a weak solution of commercial laboratory detergent.
2. Allow to dry.
3. Wipe the barrel end of the pipette (not the plunger) with isopropanol.
4. Some pipettes require the seals to be greased regularly: refer to the manufacturer's instructions.
5. When needed for use, attach a disposable tip.
6. Depress the plunger, place the tip in the solution and slowly release the plunger.
7. Transfer the tip to your next vessel, e.g. a test-tube, and place against the inner side of the vessel. Depress the plunger slowly.
8. Discard the tip.

9. The accuracy of your dispensing may be checked using a weight and balance.
10. Pipettes should be stored in a pipette rack or in the box provided when not in use.

RATIONALE

1. This removes grime accumulated by daily handling.

3. Wiping with spirit disinfects the part of the pipette that is attached to the tip.
4. Special grease is usually included in the maintenance kit supplied with the pipette.

6. The fluid will be aspirated into the tip.

7. The fluid will run down the side of the vessel.

8. Tips should not be used more than once, to avoid cross-contamination.
9. Calibrate the pipette by weight, e.g. 1 ml of distilled water weighs 1 g.
10. If pipettes are not stored properly the dispensing end may be damaged.

PROCEDURE: DECONTAMINATION AND DISPOSAL OF LABORATORY WASTE

ACTION

1. If possible, samples and contaminated agar plates should be placed in autoclave bags and autoclaved in a steam autoclave at 121°C for 45 minutes.

2. It is good practice to include an indicator, e.g. TST strip, to confirm that complete sterilisation has taken place.
3. Once sterilised, place the unopened autoclave bag into yellow hazardous waste bags and send away for incineration by a licensed waste disposal firm.
4. Sharps and other disposable items must be placed within a yellow commercial sharps bin, which is sealed and sent for incineration.
5. Metal items may be cleaned using non-hypochlorite disinfectants.

RATIONALE

1. Some spore-forming bacteria will survive a 15 minute run. Make sure that the autoclave has enough water to last a prolonged run. Contaminated laboratory waste should not leave the laboratory in a potentially harmful form.
2. If this device fails, the load is still unsafe and it must be reprocessed.

3. This further reduces the risk of contaminating the environment with the waste material.

4. This ensures that objects such as needles or scalpel blades sticking through will not injure anyone handling the bin.
5. Hypochlorite disinfectants will react with metal.

6. Some equipment may need special cleaning and disinfection.

6. Always follow the manufacturer's instructions, as there may be delicate parts that may be damaged by incorrect treatment.

7. Clean all work surfaces with disinfectant after every procedure.

7. Disinfectants must contain a bactericide, a fungicide and a virucide to be fully effective.

8. At the end of each working day leave the laboratory clean and tidy.

8. Untidy work areas lead to accidents.

PROCEDURE: CARE OF THE WATER BATH

ACTION

1. Turn off the power supply.
2. Remove the thermometer and shelf.

3. Pour away the water.
4. Wipe all the surfaces with detergent.

5. Replace the water.

6. Replace the thermometer.

7. Switch on the power.
8. Reduce heat loss by using the lid. This should not be used for open test-tube work.
9. Check that the correct temperature has been reached.
10. Put the items in a rack inside the bath and set the timer.
11. After the incubation time is complete, remove the items.
12. Turn off the water bath and allow to cool.

RATIONALE

2. The bath should have a thermometer to monitor the temperature; do not rely entirely on the dial.

4. If there are excessive deposits of calcium, soak the internal surfaces in a solution of Calgon for 2–3 hours.
5. The base tray must be covered; never run a water bath when it is empty.
6. Holders sited on the side of the bath should hold thermometers in place.

8. Condensation accumulates on the lid and drips into the fluid in the test-tubes.
9. Allow 20–30 minutes for the bath to warm up.
10. Always use a rack: bottles and tubes may float if free-standing.
11. Always use tongs to remove very hot bottles and tubes.

PRACTICAL LABORATORY TECHNIQUES

Cytology

PROCEDURE: PREPARATION OF A SMEAR USING SAMPLES FROM FINE-NEEDLE ASPIRATE (FNA) BIOPSIES, THORACIC FLUID, ETC.

Equipment. Microscope slides (degreased in methanol and dried), centrifuge tubes, centrifuge, Pasteur pipette.

ACTION

1. Place the sample/fluid in a centrifuge tube and centrifuge at 1500 r.p.m. for 3–5 minutes. Sediment can also be produced in the bottom of the tube by leaving it to stand for about 30 minutes.

RATIONALE

1. Centrifugation is used to spin down the cells and concentrate them at the bottom of the tube. Some samples, such as thoracic fluid, may contain very few cells.

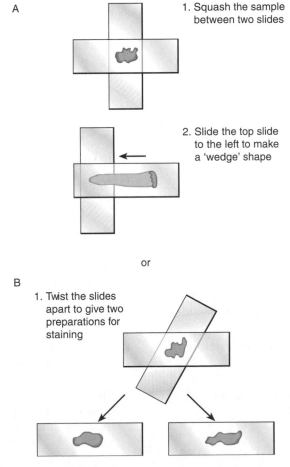

A

1. Squash the sample between two slides

2. Slide the top slide to the left to make a 'wedge' shape

or

B

1. Twist the slides apart to give two preparations for staining

Figure 11.3A, B 'Squash prep' used for cytology.

2. A smear may be made by touching a slide against a lesion.
3. FNAs may be prepared without centrifugation if sufficient cells have been harvested. Deposit cells on the slide by pushing the plunger of the syringe.
4. Decant the supernatant liquid from the centrifuge tube and discard. This leaves the sediment in the bottom of the tube.
5. Resuspend the cells by flicking the tube with your finger.

6. Using a pipette, place one or two drops on to the centre of a microscope slide.
7. Make two smears using the 'squash' method (Fig. 11.3).

8. Allow the smears to air dry.

9. Stain the smear with Leishman's, Gram's or Sudan 3 as appropriate.

2. Cells stick to the slide and can be used for the examination. This is known as a 'touch prep'.
3. FNAs are usually rich in cells.

4. The use of a conical tube helps in the separation of the sediment from the supernatant.
5. This remixes the cells with any remaining liquid and ensures a more even spread of cells on the slide.

7. This is used when there are few cells present in the sample. A 'wedge' method will spread the cells too thinly.
8. The use of artificial heat will damage the cells.
9. Gram's stain is used for bacterial examination, Leishman's stain is used for blood cells and Sudan 3 is used to stain fat in a lipoma, etc.

Faecal examination

PROCEDURE: PREPARATION AND STORAGE OF FAECES FOR EXAMINATION

ACTION

1. Faeces may be collected from the ground immediately after defecation.

2. Faeces may be collected using a gloved finger inserted through the anal sphincter into the rectum.
3. Place the sample in a sterile container. There should be sufficient faeces to fill the container.
4. Store the faeces in the refrigerator before examination.

5. Bacterial tests must be carried as soon as possible after collection.

RATIONALE

1. Old samples may have deteriorated, parasite eggs may hatch, and larvae may crawl away. Grass, soil or bacteria may contaminate the sample.
2. This ensures a fresh uncontaminated sample but care must be taken not to damage the rectal wall.
3. Too much air in the container encourages parasite eggs to hatch prior to examination.
4. Bacterial growth is slowed down in a cool temperature and the sample is preserved for longer.
5. More fastidious organisms such as *Campylobacter* spp. may be overgrown by more predominant species such as *Escherichia coli* and will be lost on culture.

PROCEDURE: WORM EGG COUNT—MODIFIED MCMASTER METHOD

Equipment. McMaster worm egg counting chamber, measuring cylinder, saturated sugar solution, Pasteur pipette, balance, balance boat, microscope, two glass beakers, tea strainer or sieve, spatula.

ACTION

1. Weigh 3 g of faeces into a beaker.
2. Measure 45 ml of saturated sugar solution using the measuring cylinder and pour it into the beaker.
3. Mix the solution with a spatula.
4. Pour the solution through the sieve into a second beaker.
5. Discard the debris remaining in the sieve.
6. Mix the solution in the beaker gently.
7. Allow the solution to stand at room temperature for 5–10 minutes.
8. If using a single-chamber type of McMaster slide, prepare it by placing the coverslip grid-side down.
9. Withdraw approximately 2 ml of the solution using a Pasteur pipette.

10. Fill the counting chamber and apply the coverslip (Fig. 11.4).

RATIONALE

1. The faeces should be fresh and moist.

4. This removes large particles but allow the eggs to go through.

7. This allows the worm eggs to float to the top of the saturated sugar solution.
8. Some slides have only one chamber and use a coverslip grid, while other have two chambers with integral grids (Fig. 11.4).
9. Make sure that you have enough liquid to fill the chamber of the slide completely. This stops bubbles forming over the grid.
10. The coverslip must make contact with the solution to avoid inclusion of air bubbles and avoid distortion of the image.

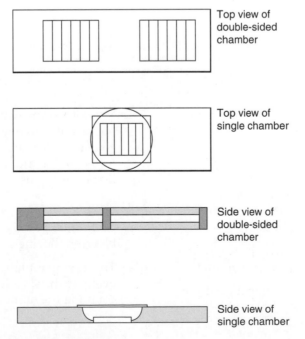

Top view of double-sided chamber

Top view of single chamber

Side view of double-sided chamber

Side view of single chamber

Figure 11.4 McMaster worm egg counting chambers.

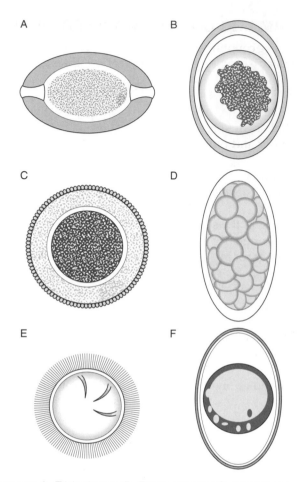

Figure 11.5 Worm eggs and oocysts: A, *Trichuris* spp.; B, *Toxascaris* spp.; C, *Toxocara* spp.; D, *Uncinaria* spp.; E, *Taenia* spp.; F, *Isospora* spp. Adapted, with permission, from *Veterinary Nursing*, p.355, 2nd edn, by Lane and Cooper (1994). Butterworth Heinemann, UK.

11. Leave the counting chamber on the bench for 5–10 minutes.

11. This allows the worm eggs and coccidial oocysts time to float to the top of the chamber. They are then visible when you focus on the grid. Note: tapeworm segments do not float—use a direct smear.

12. Examine the counting chamber using the ×10 objective on the microscope.
13. Count all the eggs seen over the grid (Fig. 11.5).

13. Count those on the lines as well as those between the lines.

14. Calculate the number of eggs as follows:
    - For a single counting chamber, multiply the number of eggs by 100.

14. This is a quantitative method and is used to evaluate the severity of an infection by counting the number of eggs in 1 g of

- For a double-chambered slide, multiply the total number of eggs on the slide by 50.

This gives the number of eggs per gram of faeces.

faeces. (A qualitative analysis tells you whether there are parasites present but does not indicate the severity of the infection.)

PROCEDURE: TRYPSIN DIGEST TEST

To detect the presence of faecal trypsin.

Equipment. X-ray film (unused), eight test tubes, Pasteur pipettes, incubator at 37°C, timer, balance, 5% sodium bicarbonate solution, test-tube rack.

ACTION

1. Place eight tubes in the test-tube rack and add 1 ml of sodium bicarbonate to each—apart from the first one.
2. Cut a portion of the X-ray film into eight strips.
3. Place 9 ml of sodium bicarbonate in the first test tube and add 1 g of faeces.
4. Take 1 ml of this solution and transfer it to the next tube. Mix well.
5. Take 1 ml of the solution and transfer it to the next test-tube. Mix well.
6. Continue in this manner until all the test-tubes have a solution in them.
7. Remove 1 ml from the last tube and discard.
8. Place a strip of X-ray film into each tube.

9. Incubate the tubes for 35 minutes at 37°C in the incubator.
10. When the time is complete, examine each strip in the area that was submerged in the solution.

11. Record the highest dilution at which digestion has taken place.

In dogs, this test has been superseded by the serum trypsin-like immunoreactivity test, which is more accurate.

RATIONALE

2. The strips must be able to fit into the test-tubes lengthways.
3. This gives a dilution of $1:10$.

4. This procedure is called a doubling dilution. It gives a dilution of $1:20$.
5. This gives a dilution of $1:40$.

6. The last one will have a dilution of $1:1280$.

8. Trypsin, a digestive enzyme which acts on protein and is normally present in the small intestine, will digest the gelatin layer on the film, leaving a clear area.
9. This reproduces the conditions in the body.

10. A clear area indicates the presence of trypsin in the faecal sample. A watermark or an area of partial digestion indicates insufficient trypsin in the sample.
11. If clearing has only occurred in the stronger solutions, e.g. $1:10$, but not in the weaker solutions, e.g.$1:320$, the patient may have exocrine pancreatic insufficiency (EPI).

PROCEDURE: IODINE STAIN

To detect the presence of starch and muscle fibres in faeces.

Equipment. Microscope slide, 2% Lugol's iodine or Gram's iodine solution, Pasteur pipettes, cover-slip, microscope, staining rack, saline, loop or swab, tap water.

ACTION

1. Using a pipette place 1–2 drops of saline on to the centre of a microscope slide.
2. Dip a swab or loop into the faeces sample and place a little into the saline on the slide. Mix well.
3. Allow the mixture to dry for 1 minute.
4. Place the slide on the staining rack and flood with iodine solution.
5. Leave the stain on for 3 minutes.
6. Wash gently with tap water
7. Place a coverslip over the smear.

8. Examine using the × 10 and × 40 objective lenses of the microscope.

RATIONALE

1. Saline emulsifies the faeces and helps to spread it evenly over the slide.

3. This fixes the faeces on the slide.

5. Iodine binds with the starch in the sample.
6. This stops further staining by the iodine.
7. The smear is best examined when wet. A coverslip prevents the objective lens from becoming contaminated.
8. Starch granules will be stained black; muscle fibres have squared ends and stain reddish brown.

PROCEDURE: SUDAN 3 STAIN

To detect the presence of fat in faeces.

Equipment. Microscope slide, Sudan 3 stain, normal saline, coverslip, swab or loop, Pasteur pipette, staining rack, microscope.

ACTION

1. Using a pipette, place 1–2 drops of saline on to the centre of the microscope slide.
2. Dip a swab or loop into the faeces sample and place a little into the saline on the slide. Mix well.
3. Allow the mixture to dry for 1 minute.
4. Place the slide on the staining rack and flood the slide with Sudan 3.
5. Leave the stain for 3 minutes.
6. Wash gently with tap water.

7. Place a coverslip over the smear.

8. Examine using the ×10 and × 40 objective lenses of the microscope.

RATIONALE

1. Saline emulsifies the faeces and helps to spread it evenly over the slide.

3. This fixes the faeces on the slide.

5. Sudan 3 stain binds with the fat in the sample.
6. This stops the action of the stain and removes any surplus.
7. The smear is best examined when wet. A coverslip prevents the objective lens from becoming contaminated.
8. Fat globules will stain orange-red.

Haematology

For haematological ranges in the dog and cat, see Table 11.1.

Table 11.1 Haematology ranges for the dog and the cat

Blood parameter	Dog	Cat
Red blood cells ($\times 10^{12}$/litre)	5.0–8.5	5.5–10.0
Packed cell volume (% of whole blood)	37–57	27–50
Total white blood cells ($\times 10^9$/litre)	6–15	4–15
Mature neutrophils ($\times 10^9$/litre)	3.6–10.5	2.5–12.5
% of all blood cells	60–70	45–75
Band neutrophils ($\times 10^9$/litre)	0–0.3	0–0.45
% of all blood cells	0–2	0–3
Eosinophils (% of all blood cells)	2–10	4–12
Basophils (% of all blood cells)	Rare	Rare
Monocytes (% of all blood cells)	3–10	0–4
Platelets ($\times 10^9$/litre)	200–500	200–600

PROCEDURE: PACKED CELL VOLUME (PCV)

Equipment. Blood sample in EDTA tube, capillary tube (plain), microhaematocrit reader, microhaematocrit centrifuge, soft plasticine or Cristoseal.

ACTION

1. Collect a blood sample in an EDTA tube.

2. Gently agitate the sample and place the end of a capillary tube in the blood.
3. Hold the tube at a 45° angle and allow the tube to fill until it is three-quarters full.
4. Place the opposite end of the tube into the plasticine pad.
5. Twist the capillary tube two or three times and take it out of the plasticine.
6. Wipe the tube with soft tissue.

7. Place the tube in one groove of the centrifuge with the plasticine plug facing outwards against the outer rim.

8. Place a similar tube on the opposite side of the centrifuge.

9. Screw the safety plate down over the tubes and close the lid.

10. Centrifuge for 5 minutes at 10 000 r.p.m.

RATIONALE

1. Sodium ethylene diamine tetra-acetic acid (EDTA) is an anticoagulant and prevents the blood from clotting. It is used to preserve most blood samples used for haematology.

3. Blood will be drawn up the tube by capillary action.
4. If you use the end containing the blood you will contaminate the plasticine.
5. This creates a plug which will prevent blood running out of the tube.
6. To remove excess blood, which could be a source of infection.
7. Centrifugal force causes the fluids to spin outwards. The sealed end prevents blood escaping as it is forced towards the perimeter.
8. This balances the tube under test and reduces vibration and subsequent damage to the centrifuge.
9. The safety plate prevents the tubes spinning out of position. Both plate and lid are essential for safety.

11. When the machine stops, remove the lid, safety plate and tube.
12. Place the tube into the groove on the microhaematocrit reader.

13. Line up the top of the plasticine plug with the line on the bottom of the reader (Fig. 11.6).

11. Never attempt to open the centrifuge while it is still running.
12. The blood will have separated into three layers (Fig. 11.6); from the top downwards:

   1. plasma
   2. buffy coat—white blood cells
   3. red blood cells.

13. The top of the plug marks the lowest point of the blood column.

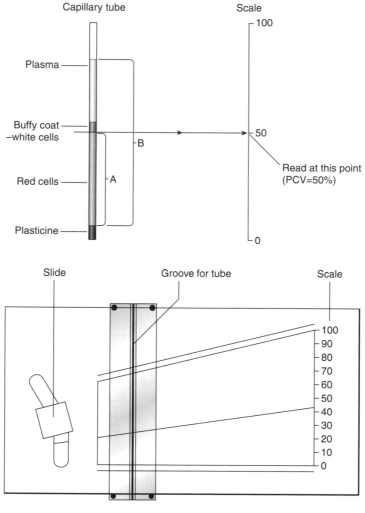

Figure 11.6 Measuring packed cell volume. A is the length of tube occupied by red cells; B is the total length of the column of blood.

14. Line up the top of the plasma with the diagonal line at the top of the reader (Fig. 11.6).
15. Move the slide so that the middle line is level with the top of the red cells (Fig. 11.6).
16. Read the measurement from the scale on the right side of the reader.

17. The PCV is the percentage of whole blood that consists of red blood cells.

14. The bottom of the plasma meniscus is used as the measuring point.

16. The scale is marked 1 to 100; the reading can be expressed as a percentage, i.e. 45 becomes 45%, etc.
17. PCV can also be calculated by measuring the length of tube occupied by red cells (A) and the total length of the blood column (B):

$$PCV\% = A/B \times 100.$$

Table 11.2 Leucocyte and erythrocyte counting fluids

	Leucocyte counting fluid	Erythrocyte counting fluid (Gowers' solution)
Contents	2 ml glacial acetic acid 1 ml gentian violet (1% aqueous) 100 ml distilled water	12.5 g anhydrous sodium sulphate 33.3 g glacial acetic acid 200 ml distilled water
Method	Filter through filter paper before use and shake well until mixed. Store in a dark glass bottle	Filter through filter paper before use and shake well until mixed. Store in a dark glass bottle
Use	Destroys red cells, leaving only white cells in the blood sample. Used for total white cell count by means of a haemocytometer	Destroys white cells, leaving only red cells in the blood sample. Used for red cell count by means of a haemocytometer

PROCEDURE: TOTAL WHITE BLOOD CELL COUNT USING A HAEMOCYTOMETER

Equipment. Blood sample in EDTA tube, haemocytometer and coverslip (Fig. 11.7), 2000 µl (2 ml) and 100 µl (0.1 ml) volumetric pipettes and tips, sterile container, tissue, white cell counting fluid (glacial acetic acid, Table 11.2), microscope.

ACTION

1. Using a 2 ml volumetric pipette, place 2 ml of white cell counting fluid (glacial acetic acid) in a sterile container.
2. Mix the blood in an EDTA tube by gentle agitation. Add 0.1 ml of the blood to the white cell counting fluid and mix well.
3. Leave to stand at room temperature for 5–10 minutes.

4. Place the coverslip on the haemocytometer and press firmly until Newton's rings can be seen.

RATIONALE

1. Particles of dust from a dirty container may be mistaken for cells when counting.

2. This is a 1:20 dilution.

3. The addition of glacial acetic acid to whole blood results in lysis of the red cells, leaving only the white cells to be counted.
4. Newton's rings appear as coloured rings and indicate that close contact has been made between the coverslip and the counting slide. Close contact ensures that the area filled with blood is an accurate volume.

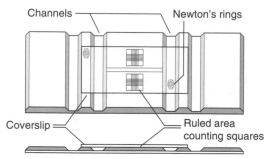

A Improved Neubauer haemocytometer

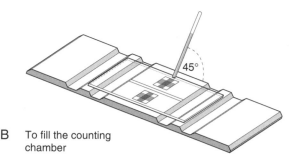

B To fill the counting chamber

Figure 11.7A, B To prepare a red or white cell count.

5. Using a capillary tube, draw up some of the treated blood and fill one side of the counting chamber. Do not allow fluid to flow into the well surrounding the plinth on which the grid is situated (Fig. 11.7).

6. Wait for 2 minutes.

7. Place the counting chamber on the microscope stage, being careful to keep it horizontal. Using the ×10 objective lens, count the white cells in all four large corner squares (Fig. 11.8, marked W).

8. Count only the white cells in the spaces and those on the top and right-hand lines of each square.

9. To calculate the number of white cells:

No. white cells in all four large squares = A

No. cells per litre of blood = A/20 × 10⁹.

5. If the end of the capillary tube is placed at the outside edge of the coverslip, fluid will run under the coverslip and across the grid. Removing the capillary tube just before the fluid reaches the end of the grid will halt the flow.

6. At first the white blood cells float around and are impossible to count. Wait for 2 minutes and they will settle.

7. Each large corner square is made of 16 smaller squares. You will count the white cells in (16 × 4) 64 small squares (Fig. 11.8).

8. If you count all the cells on all the lines you will count some cells twice.

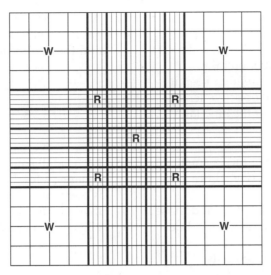

Figure 11.8 Image of a haemocytometer viewed under the microscope. Count the squares labelled R to calculate a red blood cell count. Count the squares labelled W to calculate a white blood cell count.

PROCEDURE: TOTAL RED BLOOD CELL COUNT USING A HAEMOCYTOMETER

Equipment. Blood sample in EDTA tube, haemocytometer and coverslip (Fig. 11.7), 20 ml and 0.1 ml volumetric pipettes and tips, sterile container, tissue, red cell counting fluid (Gowers' solution, Table 11.2), microscope.

ACTION

1. Using a pipette, dispense 20 ml of red cell counting solution into a clean sterile container.
2. Mix the blood in an EDTA tube by gentle agitation. Add 0.1 ml of the blood to the red cell counting fluid and mix well.
3. Leave to stand at room temperature for 5–10 minutes.

4. Place the coverslip on the haemocytometer and press gently until Newton's rings appear.

5. Using a capillary tube, draw up some of the treated blood and fill one side of the counting chamber. Do not allow fluid to flow into the well surrounding the plinth on which the grid is situated (Fig. 11.7).

RATIONALE

1. Particles of dust in a dirty container may be mistaken for cells when counting.
2. This gives a dilution of 1 : 200.

3. Red cell solution (Gowers' solution) destroys white cells so that only the red cells remain.
4. Newton's rings appear as coloured rings and indicate that close contact has been made between the coverslip and the counting slide. Close contact ensures that the area filled with blood is an accurate volume.
5. If the end of the capillary tube is placed at the outside edge of the coverslip, fluid will run under the coverslip and across the grid. Removing the capillary tube just before the fluid reaches the end of the grid will halt the flow.

6. Wait for 2 minutes.

7. Place the counting chamber on the microscope stage, being careful to keep it horizontal. Using the ×10 objective lens, locate the central square of the nine large squares (Fig. 11.8).

8. Change to the ×40 objective lens.

9. Count all the cells in five of the 25 small squares in the central area (Fig. 11.8, marked R).

10. Count only the cells in the spaces and those resting on the top and the right-hand lines of each square.

11. To calculate the number of red cells:

Total number of cells = A

$A/100$ = no. of red cells $\times 10^{12}/l$.

6. At first the red blood cells float around and are impossible to count. Wait for 2 minutes and they will settle.

9. Each small square is divided into 16 smaller squares: a total of (16×5) 80 small squares is counted.

10. If you count the cells on all the lines you will count some cells twice.

PROCEDURE: PREPARATION OF A BLOOD SMEAR

Equipment. Blood sample in EDTA tube, microscope slides previously soaked in methanol and dried, capillary tube, glass cutter, marker pen.

ACTION

1. Keep EDTA blood sample at room temperature. If it has been previously refrigerated, allow time for it to warm up.

2. Mix the sample thoroughly by gently rolling it between your hands for about a minute.

3. Prepare a spreader by chipping one corner off a glass slide. If necessary use a glass cutter.

4. Take a clean microscope slide that has been soaked in methanol and dried.

5. Using a capillary tube, place a small drop of blood on the right-hand end of the slide.

6. Place the spreader to the left of the blood drop at an angle of 45° to the horizontal and draw backwards to 'pick up' the blood.

7. Push the spreader forward with even pressure towards the left-hand end of the slide. The sides of the smear should be parallel and there should be a 'feathery tail' (Fig. 11.9).

8. Label the slide with a marker pen.

9. Dry the smear in the air.

10. Stain the smear with an appropriate stain.

RATIONALE

2. This suspends the cells evenly. Overvigorous mixing will damage the cells.

3. The use of a spreader stops the smear overlapping the edges of the slide.

4. Methanol removes grease from the slide and stops gaps appearing in your smear.

5. Too large a drop makes the smear too thick; too small a drop gives too short a smear and/or hesitation lines.

6. The blood will run along the spreader as it makes contact.

7. The smear should take up two-thirds of the slide and should be bullet-shaped. Straight edges are needed for the 'battlement' technique of counting cells.

8. This is important because if you make several slides at once they will all look the same.

9. The use of heat will damage the cells.

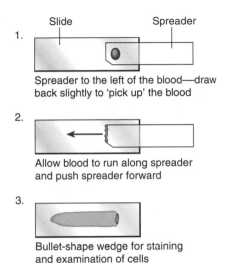

1. Slide | Spreader

Spreader to the left of the blood—draw
back slightly to 'pick up' the blood

2.

Allow blood to run along spreader
and push spreader forward

3.

Bullet-shape wedge for staining
and examination of cells

Figure 11.9 Preparing a blood smear.

PROCEDURE: RETICULOCYTE COUNT (FIG. 11.10)

Equipment. Blood sample in EDTA tube, new methylene blue stain, centrifuge, centrifuge tube, Pasteur pipettes or volumetric pipette, incubator at 37°C, microscope.

ACTION

1. Using a pipette, dispense 2 ml of methylene blue stain into a centrifuge tube.

2. Using a pipette, add 4–5 drops of well-mixed EDTA blood.
3. Mix gently and place in the incubator at 37°C for 30 minutes.
4. Remove from the incubator and place in the centrifuge.

5. Spin at 1000 r.p.m. for a minute.

6. Remove and discard the supernatant fluid using a pipette.

RATIONALE

1. Check that the stain is new methylene blue; you should not use McFadyean's methylene blue as this is used for identification of anthrax bacilli.
2. A heparinised sample is not suitable for haematology.
3. The sample can be incubated at room temperature if no incubator is available.
4. Make sure that you balance the centrifuge with a tube of a similar weight to avoid vibration and damage to the machine.
5. Spinning for faster or for longer will damage the cells.

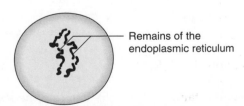

Remains of the
endoplasmic reticulum

Figure 11.10 A reticulocyte. An immature circulating red cell, it can be stained with a supravital stain, e.g. new methylene blue.

7. Gently flick the tube with your fingers.

8. Use this material to prepare a blood smear, as previously described.

9. Place the slide under the microscope and, using first the × 10 and then × 40 objective lens, look for red blood cells containing strands stained dark blue.

10. Count a total of 500 cells, noting the number of reticulocytes.

11. Calculate the number of reticulocytes as follows:

$$\text{Reticulocyte count} = \frac{\text{no. of reticulocytes}}{\text{total no. of cells counted}} \times 100\%$$

12. A correction factor is now applied to this number.

13. To calculate:

$$\text{Corrected reticulocyte count} = \frac{\text{reticulocyte count} \times \text{patient's PCV}}{\text{normal PCV for the species}}$$

7. This resuspends the cells in any remaining fluid.

9. These cells are the immature red blood cells known as reticulocytes (Fig. 11.10). The dark-blue strands are remains of the endoplasmic reticulum in the cytoplasm. The presence of reticulocytes indicates that new red blood cells are being formed by the bone marrow to replace those lost, e.g. by old age or haemorrhage.

10. Select an area where individual cells can be seen: this indicates that the smear is one cell thick (known as a monolayer).

12. In order to measure accurately the responsiveness of the bone marrow, the count takes the PCV of the patient into consideration.

PROCEDURE: GIEMSA STAIN

To demonstrate blood parasites.

Equipment. Prepared blood smear, Coplin staining jar, Giemsa stain—neat, Giemsa stain—diluted 1:3 parts with buffered water (pH 6.8), filter paper, distilled water (pH 6.8), Pasteur pipettes, staining rack, methanol, forceps, microscope, microscope oil.

ACTION

1. Prepare a blood smear as previously described and air dry. Place on the staining rack.
2. Using a pipette, flood the smear with methanol.
3. Leave for 3–5 minutes.
4. Drain off the methanol and allow the slide to dry in the air.
5. Flood the slide with neat Giemsa stain, pouring it through filter paper on to the slide. Leave it for 30 seconds.

RATIONALE

1. Do not use heat to dry the smear as this will damage the cells.

3. This fixes the smear.

5. Filtering the stain removes sediment, which may be mistaken for blood parasites.

6. Using forceps, transfer the slide to the Coplin jar containing Giemsa stain diluted 1 part to 3 parts with buffered water (pH 6.8). Leave for 15–20 minutes.
7. Remove the slide from the Coplin jar with forceps and rinse with buffered water.
8. Wipe the underside of the slide and allow to dry.
9. Place the smear on the microscope stage and examine under oil immersion (×100).

Note. Giemsa is a Romanowsky stain—one that uses a combination of two dyes, haematoxylin and eosin.

6. The slide is held vertically in the Coplin jar to prevent a build-up of stain sediment on the smear.
7. Avoid using tap water: an incorrect pH will alter the staining characteristics of the cells.
8. Do not touch the top of the slide—you will remove the blood smear!
9. This stain is used to identify the presence of blood parasites such as *Haemobartonella felis*. It is also useful for differential white cell counts.

PROCEDURE: LEISHMAN'S STAIN

Equipment. Prepared blood smear, Leishman's stain—neat, Leishman's stain—diluted 1:3 parts with buffered water (pH 6.8), buffered distilled water pH 6.8, Coplin jar, tissues or blotting paper, staining rack, filter paper, forceps, microscope, microscope oil.

ACTION

1. Prepare a blood smear, as previously described, and air dry. Place on the staining rack.
2. Flood the slide with neat Leishman's stain, pouring it through a piece of filter paper. Leave for 1 minute.
3. Using forceps, transfer the slide to the Coplin jar containing Leishman's stain diluted with buffered distilled water to a pH of 6.8. A gold film should be visible on the top of the liquid. Leave for 5 minutes.
4. Using forceps, remove the slide and rinse with buffered water.

5. Wipe the underside of the slide and air dry.

6. Examine under the microscope using oil immersion (×100).

Note. Leishman's stain is a Romanowsky stain—one that uses a combination of two dyes, haematoxylin and eosin.

RATIONALE

1. Do not use heat to dry the smear, as this will damage the cells.

2. Filtering the stain removes sediment, which may be mistaken for blood parasites.

3. The Coplin jar holds the slide in a vertical position to prevent the build-up of sediment. The gold film indicates that the stain is at the correct pH.

4. Do not use tap water: if the pH is incorrect it may change the staining characteristics of the cells.
5. Do not touch the top of the slide—you will remove the blood smear!
6. Leishman's is the stain most commonly used for differential white cell counts because it provides good cellular definition.

PROCEDURE: DIFF-QUIK STAIN

Equipment. Prepared blood smear, Diff-Quik stain, Coplin jars, forceps, distilled water buffered to pH 7.2, tissue, microscope, immersion oil.

ACTION

1. Prepare a blood smear, as previously described, and air dry.
2. Dispense the staining solutions into Coplin jars.
3. Dip the slide into the fixative solution for 1 second, five times. Allow excess to drip back into the jar.
4. Dip the slide into stain solution 1 for 1 second, five times. Allow excess to drip back into the jar.
5. Dip the slide into stain solution 2 for 1 second, five times. Allow excess to drip back into the jar.
6. Rinse the slide with buffered water.
7. Wipe the underside of the slide.

8. Allow the smear to air dry.

9. Place the slide on the microscope stage and examine using oil immersion (×100).

Note. Diff-Quik is a Romanowsky stain—one that uses a combination of two dyes. Although it

RATIONALE

1. Do not use heat to dry the smear, as this will damage the cells.
2. These glass jars with lids will prevent dust from falling into the stains.
3. Leaving the slide in the fixative for too long results in unsatisfactory staining.

4. This solution stains the cellular components red.

5. This solution stains the cellular components blue.

7. If you always keep the smear side facing towards you while staining, you will not be tempted to wipe the wrong side and lose your smear.
8. Do not use heat to dry the smear as this will damage the cells.
9. Stains must be renewed once a week to maintain their efectiveness.

is quick and easy to use it gives poor cellular definition.

PROCEDURE: DIFFERENTIAL WHITE BLOOD CELL COUNT

Equipment. Prepared blood smear, Leishman's or Giemsa stain, microscope, immersion oil.

ACTION

1. Prepare a blood smear and air dry, as described previously.
2. Stain using either Leishman's or Giemsa stain, as described previously.
3. Place the slide on the microscope stage and examine under ×10 objective lens.

4. Move out the ×10 objective and place a drop of oil on the slide. Move the ×100 objective into position making contact with the drop of oil.

RATIONALE

2. Leishman's stain provides good cellular definition and is quicker to do than Giemsa.
3. This enables you to select an area at least one-third from the end of the smear on the side edge.

4. Watch what you are doing from the side, not through the lens—this may damage the slide. The use of oil immersion provides increased magnification.

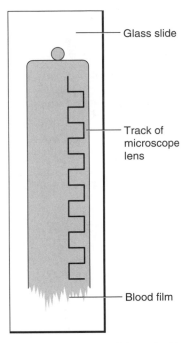

Figure 11.11 The battlement technique for differential blood films. Adapted, with permission, from *Veterinary Nursing*, p. 348, 2nd edn, by Lane and Cooper (1994). Butterworth Heinemann, UK.

5. Carefully focus on the selected field using the fine adjustment knob.

6. Move the slide following the line of a 'battlement' (Fig. 11.11) as follows: move two fields along the edge of the smear, two fields up, two fields along, two fields down. While you are doing this, count 100 white blood cells.

7. As you count, record the numbers of each cell type (Fig. 11.12).

8. Calculate the percentage of each cell type using these figures (Table 11.1).

5. Do not use the coarse focus as the incremental movements mean your view goes out of focus very quickly.

6. This enables you to cover a reasonable area of the smear and overcomes biased cell distribution on the slide. You may count more than 100—the greater the number of cells counted the greater the accuracy of the sample.

7. You may record your results manually on paper or by using some form of commercial differential counter.

8. For example, suppose you have counted 72 neutrophils among your 100 cells, then the percentage of neutrophils in the blood is 72/100 = 72%.

Histopathology

PROCEDURE: PREPARATION OF TISSUE FOR HISTOLOGICAL EXAMINATION

Equipment. Formol saline, wide mouthed sample container, scissors or scalpel.

ACTION

1. Make up 10% formol saline by diluting one part of formalin with nine parts of normal saline.

RATIONALE

1. 10% formol saline is the most commonly used fixative.

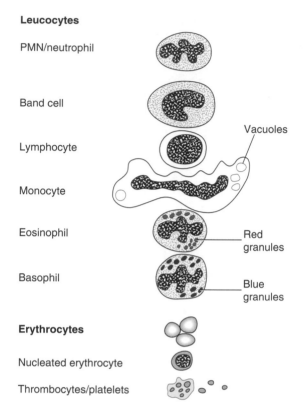

Leucocytes

PMN/neutrophil

Band cell

Lymphocyte

Vacuoles

Monocyte

Eosinophil

Red granules

Basophil

Blue granules

Erythrocytes

Nucleated erythrocyte

Thrombocytes/platelets

*Leishman's—nucleus = purple
cytoplasm = blue
erythrocytes = pink/grey
reticulocytes = blue/pale blue*

Figure 11.12 The range and Leishman's staining characteristics of blood cells visible in a blood smear. PMN, polymorphonuclear leucocyte. Adapted, with permission, from *Veterinary Nursing*, p. 6350, 2nd edn, by Lane and Cooper (1994). Butterworth Heinemann, UK.

2. Select a wide-mouthed container.

3. Select a piece of tissue no more than 1–2 cm thick. If the tissue sample is large, slice it into two or three pieces.

4. Add approximately 10 times the volume of the sample of formol saline.

5. If the sample is to be posted, avoid using any more than 60 ml of formol saline. If the sample will not be adequately fixed in 60 ml, fix it in a large pot, remove it and wrap it in formalin-soaked gauze and post in a plastic bag.

2. Tissue is soft when taken from a patient and hardens as it becomes fixed. Removing hardened tissue from a narrow-mouthed container is very difficult.

3. Diffusion through the tissue takes too long if the tissue is too thick.

4. The sample must be completely submerged in the formol saline.

5. Always check the postal regulations before sending samples through the post. Formalin is toxic and must not be allowed to leak out of the package.

6. Wrap the sample in absorbent material and place in a leak-proof polypropylene transport box.
7. Send it to the laboratory using 'next day' delivery.

6. Glass bottles should not be sent through the post.
7. Samples may deteriorate if left too long.

Microbiology

PROCEDURE: PREPARATION OF BACTERIAL SMEARS

Equipment. Platinum loop (may use a single use/disposable loop), Bunsen burner, glass microscope slide, sterile normal saline, agar plate containing bacterial growth.

ACTION

1. Heat the loop in the flame of a Bunsen burner. Allow it to cool.
2. Using the loop, place 2–3 drops of saline on to the centre of the microscope slide.
3. Flame and cool the loop again.
4. Using the loop, select an isolated bacterial colony and carefully remove it from the agar plate.
5. Mix the colony with the saline on the slide, spreading out the fluid to cover 1–2 cm.

6. Flame and cool the loop. Discard in the appropriate way.

7. Pass the smear gently over the Bunsen burner flame until it is dry.

8. Stain the smear using Gram's or methylene blue.

RATIONALE

1. Flaming the loop will sterilise it. Cooling prevents damage to the bacteria.
2. This is used to dilute and spread the bacterial colony.

4. If there is more than one type of organism on the plate you will need to make a smear for each type.
5. Mixing with saline results in a single layer of cells, allowing you to identify the shape of the cells.
6. The loop has been contaminated and must be sterilised before it is discarded to prevent the spread of disease.
7. This fixes the slide. If the smear is still wet when it is stained, some bacteria may float off, contaminating the stain and causing the loss of some areas of the smear.

PROCEDURE: GRAM'S STAIN—RAPID METHOD

Equipment. Prepared bacterial smear, crystal violet stain, Gram's or Lugol's iodine, acetone, carbol fuchsin (dilute) or safranine, staining rack, wash bottle containing tap water, blotting paper or tissue, microscope, timer, Pasteur pipettes.

ACTION

1. Place the prepared smear on the staining rack with the smear facing upwards.
2. Using a pipette, flood the slide with crystal violet for 30 seconds.

RATIONALE

1. You can also stain smears in Coplin jars.

2. At this stage the cell walls of Gram-positive organisms absorb the stain and become purple.

3. Wash the slide with tap water.
4. Flood the slide with iodine for 60 seconds.
5. Flood the slide with acetone for 2–3 seconds.

6. Wash the slide with water.
7. Flood the slide with carbol fuchsin for 30 seconds.
8. Wash the slide with tap water.
9. Wipe the back of the slide.

10. Pass the slide rapidly over the flame of the Bunsen burner to dry it.
11. Place the slide under the microscope and examine using oil immersion (×100).

3. To remove the crystal violet stain.
4. This fixes the smear.
5. This decolourises the smear and is a rapid stage.
6. To remove the stain.
7. This counterstains the bacteria: Gram-negative bacteria stain pink at this stage.
8. To remove the stain.
9. Do not wipe the front of the slide and lose the smear.
10. Do not overheat as the slide may shatter.

11. Bacteria range in size from 0.5 μm to 5 μm in length and are best viewed under high magnification. Gram-positive bacteria, e.g. *Clostridia* spp., *Staphylococcus* spp. and *Streptococcus* spp., stain purple; Gram-negative bacteria, e.g. *Escherichia coli* and *Salmonella* spp., stain pink. Gram's stain is used to identify the shape of bacteria and to classify them into Gram-positive or Gram-negative groups.

PROCEDURE: METHYLENE BLUE STAIN

Equipment. Prepared bacterial smear, staining rack, Llöffler's methylene blue, tissue or blotting paper, Pasteur pipette, wash bottle containing tap water, microscope.

ACTION

1. Place the prepared smear on the staining rack with the smear facing upwards.
2. Using a pipette, flood the slide with methylene blue stain and leave for 3 minutes.
3. Wash the slide with tap water.
4. Pass the slide rapidly over the flame of the Bunsen burner to dry it.
5. Place the slide under the microscope and examine using oil immersion (×100).

RATIONALE

1. You can also stain in Coplin jars.

2. This stains the bacterial cells.

3. To remove the stain.
4. Do not overheat as the slide may shatter.

5. Bacteria range in size from 0.5 μm to 5 μm in length and are best viewed under high magnification. The bacteria stain blue. Methylene blue stain is used to identify the shape of the bacteria.

PROCEDURE: BACTERIAL CULTURE

Equipment. Sample material, Petri dish containing agar gel, platinum loop (may use a single use/disposable loop), Bunsen burner, incubator, marker pen.

ACTION

1. Label the Petri dish with an appropriate laboratory code.

2. Flame the platinum loop in the Bunsen flame; heat until red hot from the handle end towards the loop and then bring up through the flame.

3. Cool the loop by waving it in the air for a few seconds.

4. Dip the loop into the sample.

5. Pick up the half of the Petri dish containing the agar and turn it over so that the surface of the agar is uppermost.

6. Smear the material on the loop over a small area on the left of the agar (Fig. 11.13).

RATIONALE

1. Use the client name, a number or the animal's name—develop your own system. It is important not to mix up samples: all agar plates look alike in the incubator.

2. This sterilises the loop and kills all bacteria, making it safe to use.

3. If the loop is too hot it will kill bacterial cells and produce no growth on the plate.

4. If it sizzles it is too hot!

5. Petri dishes have a base, into which the agar is poured and allowed to set, and a lid— they look similar.

6. This is known as the 'well' and is the start of your inoculation area.

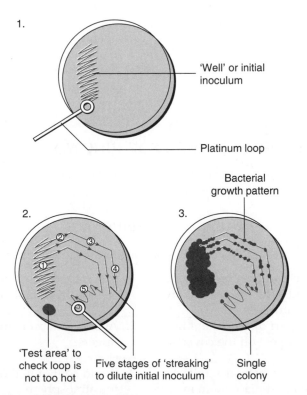

Figure 11.13 Technique for the inoculation of an agar plate.

7. Replace the Petri dish into its lid.

7. Do not leave agar plates open to the air for too long as they may become contaminated.

8. Flame and cool the loop as before. Remove the lid of the dish and check that the loop has cooled by placing it on a piece of the agar on one side of the plate.

8. If it sizzles it is too hot.

9. Pick up the Petri dish and, using the loop, make 3–4 short streaks all in the same direction from the 'edge' of the well (Fig. 11.13). Take care not to tear the agar.

9. This action begins to spread the contents of the sample evenly over the plate.

10. Continue to spread the sample over the plate, as shown in Figure 11.13.

10. The aim is to dilute the sample and so form single colonies of bacteria on the final stroke.

11. Place the lid on the dish and put it in the incubator with the agar side on top.

11. If the lid is uppermost, condensation will occur. The water droplets will drip down on to the surface of the agar, causing the bacterial colonies to spread.

12. Do not stack plates more than two or three high inside the incubator.

12. Air must be able to circulate freely and overcrowding will prevent this.

13. Incubate at 37°C for 18–24 hours.

13. Most pathogenic bacteria are described as normothermic and will grow at normal body temperature.

14. Remove from the incubator and examine for signs of bacterial growth.

14. Colonies of bacteria appear as round, often slightly raised 'lumps'; the colour may be characteristic of the species. They are distributed along the streak lines.

15. If there is no visible growth, incubate the plate for another 18–24 hours.

15. Some bacteria take longer to grow than others.

Parasitology

PROCEDURE: CULTURE FOR RINGWORM FUNGUS

Equipment. Sabouraud's agar or commercial ringworm agar, e.g. Dermatofyt, forceps, Bunsen burner, marker pen, microscope slide, coverslip, inoculation loop, saline, Pasteur pipette.

ACTION

RATIONALE

Remember ringworm fungi are zoonotic—always wear gloves when handling samples!

1. Place the forceps in the flame of the Bunsen burner for a few seconds. Remove and allow to cool to room temperature.

1. The forceps must be sterilised before use to reduce the risk of bacterial contamination.

2. Remove the lid of the Petri dish containing the Sabouraud's agar or peel off the cover of the commercial agar.

2. Avoid contaminating the agar with your fingers.

3. Using the forceps, take 6–8 hairs from the sample to be examined and place them in the centre of the agar. Replace the lid or seal the cover of the commercial agar.

3. Avoid contamination by microorganisms in the atmosphere.

4. Incubate at room temperature for up to 28 days.

5. When fungal growth is visible, examine and identify.

6. To make a smear of the fungus, use a pipette to place 2–3 drops of saline in the centre of a glass microscope slide.

7. Sterilise a platinum loop by passing it through the flame of the Bunsen burner and allow to cool.

4. Ringworm fungus grows very slowly, although some species may grow within 4 days.

5. On Sabouraud's medium, growth appears as a white fluffy colony. On a commercial agar, an indicator placed in the agar results in a red coloration. Some contaminants may also create a colour change: it is important to identify the fungus under the microscope.

6. Saline helps to spread the colony over the slide.

7. To prevent contamination of the fungus.

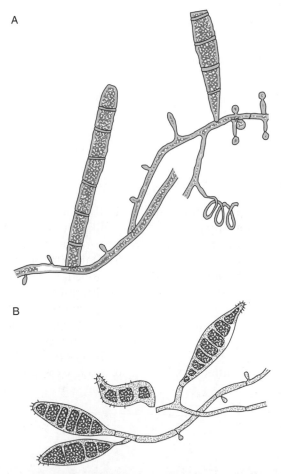

A

B

Figure 11.14 Microscopic appearance of ringworm fungus. A, *Trichophyton* spp.: look for septate hyphae, micro- and macroconidia; the latter are thin-walled and cylindrical. B, *Microsporum* spp.: look for septate hyphae, micro- and macroconidia; the latter are thick-walled, long, spindle-shaped or distorted. Adapted, with permission, from *Veterinary Nursing*, p. 377, 2nd edn, by Lane and Cooper (1994). Butterworth Heinemann, UK.

8. Using the loop, pick up a small amount of the fungal colony and mix with the saline in the slide. Sterilise and discard the platinum loop.

8. To prevent contamination by any remaining fungus on the loop.

9. Place a coverslip over the material.

9. The use of a coverslip provides a uniform layer for examination.

10. Place the slide under the microscope and examine using the ×10 objective and then the ×40 objective lenses. The addition of lactophenol cotton blue or Quink ink may enhance the appearance.

10. Ringworm is caused by dermatophytes such as *Trichophyton* and *Microsporum* spp. Look for the typical micro- and macroconidia (Fig. 11.14). Lactophenol cotton blue can be used to stain the background and the spores to aid visualisation of the fungus.

PROCEDURE: USE OF A WOODS' LAMP TO DETECT *MICROSPORUM CANIS*

Equipment. Wood's lamp, eye protection.

ACTION

RATIONALE

Remember ringworm fungi are zoonotic—always wear gloves when handling samples or suspected cases!

1. This is best performed in a darkened room.

1. A darkened room will intensify the fluorescent effect.

2. Put on the eye protectors.

2. Ultraviolet light is potentially dangerous and can damage the conjunctiva of the retina.

3. Switch on the lamp and allow to warm up for 5 minutes.

4. Ask an assistant (also wearing eye protectors) to restrain the patient on a non-slip examination table.

4. If the animal feels secure, it will be less likely to try to escape.

5. Hold the lamp over the affected areas and look for signs of apple-green fluorescence.

5. Only 60% of cases of *Microsporum canis* infection show this fluorescence. Lack of fluorescent areas does not rule out ringworm infection. Other particles in the coat, e.g. skin flakes, dirt, detergent and paraffin oil, may fluoresce a non-specific blue-white.

6. Turn off the lamp immediately after use.

6. Long exposure to ultraviolet rays will burn the skin.

PROCEDURE: COLLECTION AND EXAMINATION OF COAT BRUSHINGS

To demonstrate the presence of surface-living ectoparasites.

Equipment. Flea or nit comb, Petri dish.

ACTION

1. Comb through the patient's fur and collect the superficial debris and hairs in a Petri dish.
2. Examine with a hand lens or low-powered microscope.

3. If the presence of fleas is suspected, take a sample of hair containing black specks and cover with a few drops of water.

RATIONALE

1. The fur may contain parasites, eggs and faeces as well as skin scales and dirt.

2. This is used to demonstrate the presence of the surface-living ectoparasites, such as *Cheyletiella* spp., fleas and lice (Fig. 11.15).
3. Flea dirt appears as gritty black specks in the coat. These are made of partially digested blood, which forms a pink-stained solution when dissolved in water.

PROCEDURE: COLLECTION OF A SKIN SCRAPING

To demonstrate the presence of burrowing ectoparasites.

Equipment. Sterile sharp scalpel blade, clippers, clean collecting pot, suitable antiseptic powder or ointment.

ACTION

1. Select a suitable area of the patient for sampling and gently clip. If many areas are affected, take samples from several of them.

2. Hold a sharp sterile scalpel blade at right angles to the skin and draw repeatedly across the area until it bleeds.

3. Place the scalpel blade and all the skin debris into a clean collecting pot.

4. Dress the scraped area with a suitable antiseptic.

RATIONALE

1. This reduces the amount of hair in the sample. The technique is used to demonstrate the presence of burrowing mites such as *Sarcoptes* and *Demodex* spp., which will not be present on superficial hair (Fig. 11.15).
2. The presence of blood indicates that the deeper layers of the skin have been reached. Use of a sharp blade makes the whole procedure easier and less painful for the patient.
3. This need not be sterile as identification of mites will not be confused with the appearance of contaminating micro-organisms.
4. This prevents the development of secondary bacterial infection.

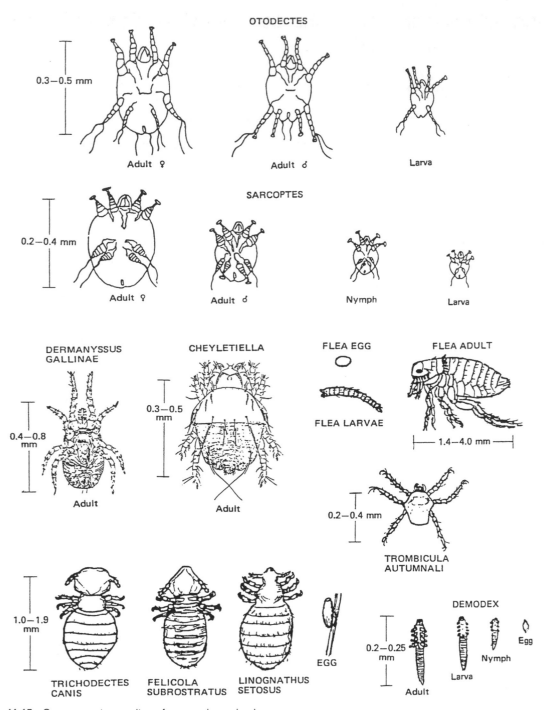

Figure 11.15 Common ectoparasites of companion animals.

PROCEDURE: PREPARATION OF A SMEAR TO IDENTIFY THE PRESENCE OF MITES

Equipment. Scraped skin sample, 10% potassium hydroxide, glass slide, coverslip, Pasteur pipette, microscope, Bunsen burner, forceps.

ACTION

1. Place some of the material collected by skin scraping on to the centre of a microscope slide.
2. With a pipette, add 2–3 drops of 10% potassium hydroxide.
3. Place a coverslip over the sample.

4. Holding the slide with forceps, warm it gently over a Bunsen burner—do not boil it.
5. Allow the slide to cool.
6. Place the slide under the microscope and examine under the ×4 objective and then the ×10.

7. You may have to prepare several slides from your sample to be certain of the result.

RATIONALE

1. Do not use too much material as the parasites may be masked by skin debris.

2. This solution is caustic—take care!

3. This provides a uniform layer for examination and prevents the lens from becoming contaminated.
4. Warming breaks down and clears the debris, making the parasites easier to see.

6. Larger parasites such as *Sarcoptes* may be seen under ×4 magnification, but *Demodex* will only be seen under a higher magnification (Fig. 11.15).
7. Parasites may only be present in low numbers and may easily be missed if only one smear is made.

This technique may be used to demonstrate the presence of ear mites, *Otodectes cynotis* (Fig. 11.15). Brown discharge is collected from the ear and treated in the same way before microscopic examination.

Urine examination

PROCEDURE: URINE PRESERVATION

Equipment. Collecting containers.

ACTION

1. Samples may be collected by catheterisation, midstream free flow or cystocentesis. (For catheterisation techniques see Chapter 3.)

2. Collect the sample into a clean, preferably sterile container.

RATIONALE

1. Free-flow samples can be collected by the owner and are the most commonly used. A midstream sample is more representative of the bladder contents, as the first part of the stream may contain contaminants from the urethra.
2. Owners may use clean jam jars, plastic containers or commercially designed collecting equipment. For cats use any empty clean litter tray or commercially prepared urine collecting litter. If the sample

3. Transfer the urine into a boric acid tube and a plain sample tube.

4. If the sample cannot be dispatched or tested immediately, store it in the refrigerator.

is to be used for bacteriology the container must be sterile.

3. Boric acid is used to preserve samples for bacteriology. The bacterial numbers remain unchanged in the boric acid solution until it is tested. Plain tubes are used for specific gravity estimation, dipstick tests and sediment examination. They may also be used for bacterial examination, if within 20 minutes of collection.

4. Refrigerated urine should be tested within 24 hours of collection.

PROCEDURE: GROSS EXAMINATION OF URINE

Equipment. Urine sample in clean sample pot.

ACTION

1. Collect sample in a clean transparent pot, as described previously.
2. Look at the colour of the sample.

3. Hold the sample up to the light and examine its clarity.

4. Remove the lid of the container and smell the sample.

RATIONALE

1. You must be able to examine the urine easily.
2. Normal urine is yellow but it may vary in intensity. Deep yellow urine will be more concentrated than pale yellow urine; a browny-yellow colour may indicate the presence of bilirubin; red may indicate the presence of blood or haemoglobin. Some drugs may change the colour of urine.
3. Normal urine is clear. Increased turbidity indicates the presence of sediment, e.g. crystals, bacteria, pus or blood cells.
4. Normal urine has a smell that is characteristic of the species, e.g. tomcat urine is instantly recognisable and is different from that of the queen. The smell of ammonia may be caused by stale urine; the smell of pear drops is due to the presence of ketones.

PROCEDURE: TO TEST THE SPECIFIC GRAVITY OF URINE BY REFRACTOMETER

Equipment. Urine sample, refractometer, Pasteur pipettes, distilled water, lint-free tissue.

ACTION

1. To calibrate the refractometer, wipe the glass prism (Fig. 11.16) with a piece of lint-free tissue; using a pipette, place two drops of distilled water on to the prism. Place the plastic cover over the prism.
2. Hold the refractometer up to the light and look at the scale through the eyepiece. Note the point on the scale that marks the boundary between the light and dark areas.
3. If the reading is not exactly 1.000, adjust the refractometer using the screw on the top of the instrument until the reading is 1.000.

4. Wipe off the distilled water with a piece of dry tissue.
5. Using a fresh pipette place two drops of the test urine on to the prism. Close the plastic cover.
6. Hold the refractometer up to the light and read the scale as before. Record your result.

RATIONALE

1. The refractometer must be calibrated before use to ensure that it measures accurately.

2. For distilled water, this should read 1.000.

3. Note: some refractometers may have a different method of adjustment—check the instructions. The refractometer will now read accurately.

5. If you use the same pipette you may dilute the urine sample with water remaining in the pipette.
6. Normal specific gravity of dog urine is 1.018–1.045. Normal specific gravity of cat urine is 1.020–1.040. Urine shows a higher

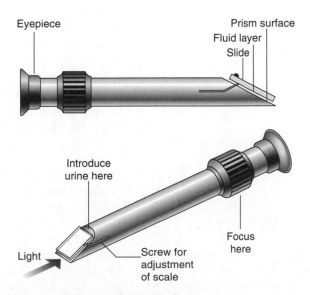

Figure 11.16 Refractometer—for measuring the specific gravity of urine

specific gravity in cases of dehydration, reduced water intake and shock and a lower specific gravity where water intake is increased, as is seen in cases of pyometra and chronic renal failure.

7. Rinse off the urine with distilled water and wipe with lint-free tissue.
8. Replace in the case.

7. Do not leave the urine sample to dry on the prism.
8. The refractometer must be stored in its case to prevent accidental damage and keep it dust-free.

PROCEDURE: TO TEST URINE FOR VARIOUS PARAMETERS USING A DIPSTICK

Equipment. Fresh urine sample, minute timer, dipstick test.

ACTION

1. Select the correct type of dipstick test. The sticks are presented in a screw-top container containing large numbers of sticks. The instructions are printed on the label.

2. Check the expiry date.

3. Remove the lid of the dipstick container and take out one stick. Replace the lid.
4. Dip the stick in the fresh urine sample until all the pads are wet.

5. Remove the stick from the urine and tap gently on the side of the sample pot.
6. Using the timer, make sure that you keep to the time intervals stated on the side of the bottle.
7. Check that you read the results from the correct end of the stick.
8. Hold the dipstick container in one hand and the dipstick in the other and compare the colour of each pad with the correct one on the side of the container.

RATIONALE

1. Commercial reagent dipsticks consist of a series of test reagent pads mounted on a plastic strip. The tests vary in number and in type, e.g. some may test only glucose, while others may have as many as ten tests, including those for pH, protein, blood and bilirubin. Make sure that the tests you need are included on the stick and that the tests are validated for animals: some are validated for humans and may give irrelevant results.

2. Out-of-date dipsticks may give unreliable results.

3. Do not contaminate the remaining dipsticks with urine.
4. Results are more accurate if the sample is fresh. Never use on a preserved sample. Stale samples may have bacterial growth or be contaminated by faeces or blood, which may affect the results.

5. To remove any surplus urine.

6. Each test pad requires a specific time in contact with the urine before it reacts appropriately.

7. If you read from the wrong end you will get results that are incorrect for that test pad.
8. Each reagent pad will change colour; the range of colour changes is illustrated on the label, accompanied by the appropriate result.

9. Record your results.

10. Dispose of the dipstick in the clinical waste.

9. Do not rely on your memory: the results may need to be kept for some time.

10. Pathogens may be present on the stick.

PROCEDURE: URINE SEDIMENT EXAMINATION

Equipment. Fresh urine sample, microscope, glass slide, coverslip, Pasteur pipettes, urine centrifuge tube, centrifuge, Sedistain (optional).

ACTION

1. Using a pipette, place 3–5 ml of urine in a centrifuge tube.
2. Place the tube in the centrifuge.
3. Place a similar tube on the opposite side of the centrifuge.
4. Spin at 1–2000 r.p.m. for 2–3 minutes.

5. Using a pipette, remove and discard most of the supernatant, being careful not to disturb the sediment.
6. Flick the test-tube with your fingers.

7. If you wish, add 1–2 drops Sedistain to the sediment in the tube, but this is optional.

RATIONALE

1. A conical tube will help to separate the sediment from the supernatant.

3. The machine must be balanced to prevent vibration and damage.
4. Spinning for a longer time will damage any cells present in the urine.
5. Only the sediment is required for this procedure.

6. This resuspends the sediment in any remaining liquid and makes a more even smear on the slide.
7. Sedistain may make the material in the sediment easier to identify.

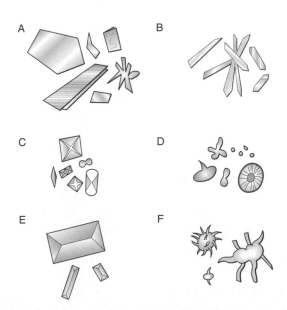

Figure 11.17 Urine crystals: A, urates; B, hippuric acid; C, calcium oxalate; D, Calcium carbonate; E, struvite; F, ammonium urate. Adapted, with permission, from *Veterinary Nursing*, p. 359, 2nd edn, by Lane and Cooper (1994). Butterworth Heinemann, UK.

8. Using a pipette, place 1–2 drops of the sediment on to the centre of a glass slide and add a coverslip.

8. This provides a uniform layer for examination and protects the lens from contamination.

9. Place the slide under the microscope and examine using the ×10 and ×40 objective lens.

9. Look for evidence of casts, red and white blood cells, epithelial cells, spermatozoa, mucin threads, bacteria and crystals (Fig. 11.17).

FURTHER READING

Benjamin M 1974 Outline of Veterinary Clinical Pathology, 2nd edn. Iowa State University Press, Ames, IA

Cooper B, Lane DR (eds) 1999 Veterinary Nursing. Butterworth-Heinemann, Oxford

Davidson M, Else R and Lumsden J 1998 Manual of Laboratory Techniques. BSAVA, Gloucester

Simpson G (ed) 1996 Practical Veterinary Nursing. BSAVA, Gloucester

The rabbit
- To restrain a rabbit
- To sex a rabbit
- To administer fluids or liquid medication
- To place a naso-oesophageal feeding tube
- Subcutaneous injection
- Intramuscular injection
- Intravenous injection
- Intraperitoneal injection
- To place an intra-osseous catheter
- Induction of anaesthesia
- Maintenance and monitoring of anaesthesia
- Post-operative care

Small rodents
- To restrain a chinchilla
- To sex a chinchilla
- To restrain a gerbil
- To sex a gerbil
- To restrain a guinea pig
- To sex a guinea pig
- To restrain a hamster
- To sex a hamster
- To restrain a mouse
- To sex a mouse
- To restrain a rat
- To sex a rat
- To administer fluids or liquid medication
- To administer medication by parenteral routes
- To collect a blood sample
- Induction of anaesthesia
- Maintenance and monitoring of anaesthesia
- Post-operative care

The ferret
- To restrain a ferret
- To sex a ferret
- To administer fluids or liquid medication
- Subcutaneous injection
- Intramuscular injection
- Intraperitoneal injection
- Intravenous injection
- Induction of anaesthesia
- Maintenance and monitoring of anaesthesia
- Post-operative care

Cage and aviary birds
- To capture and restrain a bird
- To capture a bird using the towel method
- To administer fluid via a crop tube
- Intramuscular injection
- Intravenous injection
- Intra-osseous injection
- To collect a blood sample
- Induction of anaesthesia
- Maintenance and monitoring of anaesthesia
- Post-operative care

Reptiles
- To restrain a snake
- To administer fluids or liquid medication
- Intravenous injection or blood sampling
- To restrain a tortoise or terrapin
- To administer fluids or liquid medication
- Intravenous injection or blood sampling
- To restrain a lizard
- To administer fluids or liquid medication
- Intravenous injection or blood sampling
- Induction of anaesthesia
- Maintenance and monitoring of anaesthesia
- Post-operative care

12

Treatment of exotic species

R. Mowbray

Introduction

The presentation of various exotic species of animal to the veterinary surgeon for treatment is rapidly becoming an everyday occurrence. The care and handling needed by these animal differs from that required by dogs and cats in the following ways:

- Response to human contact. Most exotic species have an innate fear of humans and any form of human contact is likely to induce a degree of distress. Certain individual animals, e.g. some rabbits, guinea pigs and ferrets, may tolerate or actively seek human company but to most the instinct is to run or, in some cases, to attack. This must be taken into consideration when providing nursing care: observe the patient unobtrusively, avoid unnecessary physical contact and be aware that most 'exotics' do not appreciate the sound of the human voice.
- Methods of restraint. Some species are small and agile and can be easily injured by inept handling, while others have wings, providing a different means of escape. Reptiles are cold-blooded; they depend on their environment for heat and energy and may suddenly become very active in the warmth of your hands. All are capable of causing injury to the ill-prepared handler.
- Reaction to anaesthesia. The term 'exotics' covers a wide range of species showing an equally wide range of differing responses to anaesthetic agents. It is not the brief of this

chapter to describe the action of each anaesthetic agent but the veterinary nurse must ensure that she or he is familiar with the clinical parameters and the reflexes that can be used to monitor the level of anaesthesia

By understanding that the nursing care required by exotic species is different from that normally given to dogs and cats, the veterinary nurse can significantly increase the chances of recovery and survival of the exotic patient.

THE RABBIT – *ORYCTOLAGUS CUNICULUS*

For biological data see Table 12.1.

Handling and restraint

PROCEDURE: TO RESTRAIN A RABBIT

ACTION	RATIONALE
1. Observe the rabbit before handling.	1. To assess the nature and condition of the rabbit: if it is aggressive you may need to ask for assistance. Restraint may cause respiratory arrest in dyspnoeic animals. Severe stress and fear may lead to cardiac arrest.
2. Rabbits should be handled gently but firmly.	2. Rabbits have an innate fear of humans, who they perceive as predators.
3. Talk quietly to the rabbit and approach from behind the head.	3. The eyes of the rabbit are placed on each side of the head, providing good lateral vision but very poor backwards vision. There is no need to offer a hand for the rabbit to sniff—it may be mistaken for food.
4. If the animal is fractious, grasp by the scruff and support the weight with one hand under the hindquarters (Fig. 12.1).	4. **Never** pick a rabbit up by the ears! The hindlegs must be supported at all times. Rabbits have a fragile skeleton and large lumbar muscles. By struggling or kicking, rabbits can easily break their hindlegs or dislocate or fracture their spine, resulting in paralysis. They also have large claws, which may injure you.
5. More docile rabbits may be restrained by placing one hand under the thorax, gripping the forelegs between the thumb and forefingers of that hand. Support the hind end with your other hand.	5. Some rabbits may resent being scruffed. The back should be kept in a normal curved position to avoid spinal fracture.
6. To carry the rabbit, tuck the head and front feet under your upper arm and support the body along your forearm (Fig. 12.2).	6. Keeping the rabbit close to your body avoids the risk of it kicking and scratching you. Keeping its head in the dark makes the rabbit relax.
7. A large towel can be used as an additional means of restraint. Place the rabbit on the	7. Covering the feet protects the handler from injury, while the head is available for

Table 12.1 Biological data relating to rabbits and small rodents

	Chinchilla	Gerbil	Guinea pig	Golden hamster	Mouse	Rat	Rabbit
Life span (years)	10–12	3–4	4–8	2–3	2–3	3–4	5–12
Adult weight	400–600 g	50–60 g	750–1000 g	80–120 g	20–40 g	400–800 g	1–8 kg
Body temperature (°C)	38–39	37.4–39	38.6	36.2–37.5	37.5	38.0	38.3–39.4
Respiratory rate (breaths/min)	40–80	90–140	90–150	70–80	100–250	70–150	35–60
Pulse rate (beats/min)	100–150	250–500	130–190	280–412	500–600	260–450	130–325
Oestrus cycle (days)	41 Seasonally polyoestrous	4–6	15–17	4	4–5	4–5	No regular cycle Induced ovulator
Age at puberty	8 months	10 weeks	M 8–10 weeks F 4–5 weeks	6–10 weeks	6–7 weeks	8–10 weeks	4–6 months
Gestation period (days)	111	24–26	63	16	19–21	20–22	28–32
Development of young at birth	Precocial	Altricial	Precocial	Altricial	Altricial	Altricial	Altricial
Weaning age	6–8 weeks	24–27 days	2–3 weeks	3–4 weeks	3–4 weeks	3–4 weeks	4–6 weeks
Type of diet	Herbiverous Coprophagic	Omniverous Coprophagic	Herbiverous Need vitamin C	Omniverous Coprophagic	Omniverous Coprophagic	Omniverous Coprophagic	Herbiverous Coprophagic
Natural behaviour	Nocturnal Social	Nocturnal Monogamous	Diurnal Social	Nocturnal Solitary	Nocturnal Social	Nocturnal Social	Crespuscular Social

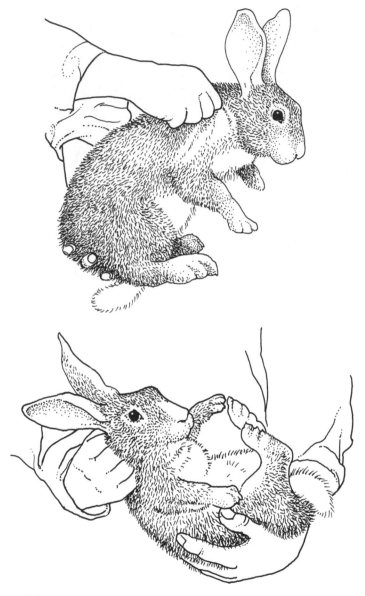

Figure 12.1 Restraining a rabbit.

opened towel with its head projecting from one side. Wrap the towel around the body, covering the feet and leaving the head exposed (Fig. 12.3).

8. Excessively aggressive rabbits may be removed from a cage by throwing a towel over the animal and covering it completely. The rabbit can be unwrapped when it is safely on the examination table.

examination and administration of medicines.

8. Care must be taken to avoid injuring the rabbit or being injured yourself.

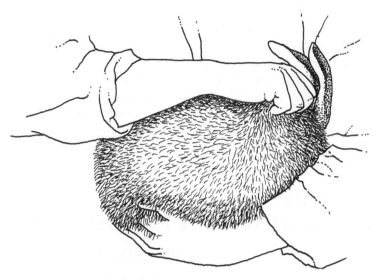

Figure 12.2   Carrying a rabbit with the head tucked under your arm.

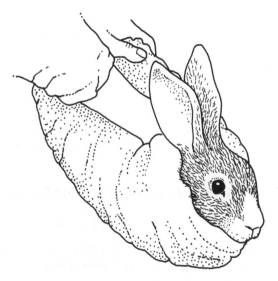

Figure 12.3   A large towel wrapped securely around the rabbit can be very helpful for restraint.

PROCEDURE: TO SEX A RABBIT

ACTION

1. Hold the scruff of the rabbit and support its weight by placing one hand under its hindquarters.
2. Gently lower the rabbit on to an examination table so that it lies in dorsal recumbency. Maintain your hold on the scruff.

RATIONALE

1. The rabbit must be held firmly to avoid possible injury to itself or to you.

2. This position provides easy access to the genitalia.

3. With your free hand, part the fur in the area around the genitalia. It may be easier for the examination to be carried out by an assistant while you maintain a firm hold on the rabbit.
4. Apply gentle pressure on either side of the genital opening.

Note. Young rabbits are very difficult to sex. Adult male rabbits have large scrotal sacs which are visible lateral and cranial to the penis. Adult

3. The buck (male) has a pointed protruding opening to the penis; the doe (female) has a slit-like opening to the vulva.

4. In the buck, pressure should cause the penis to be extruded; in the doe, pressure exposes the mucosal surface of the vulva.

females often have a prominent fur-covered dewlap under the chin.

Administration of medicines

PROCEDURE: TO ADMINISTER FLUIDS OR LIQUID MEDICATION

ACTION

1. Place the rabbit in sternal recumbency on an examination table and wrap it in a towel, as previously described.
2. Take the head in one hand and tilt slightly to one side.
3. Using a syringe of an appropriate size containing the liquid medication, place the nozzle into the uppermost corner of the mouth.
4. Apply gentle pressure to the syringe and give the medication. Allow time for the rabbit to swallow.

PROCEDURE

1. Using this method the legs are restrained but the head is exposed, providing access to the mouth.
2. In this position, one corner of the mouth is uppermost.
3. Avoid using large syringes as they are difficult to control.

4. Give fluid in boluses of 0.25–0.5 ml. If the fluid is given too fast the rabbit will choke or the liquid may escape from the mouth.

PROCEDURE: TO PLACE A NASO-OESOPHAGEAL FEEDING TUBE

ACTION

PROCEDURE

Rabbits always breathe through their noses, so this procedure is not recommended for rabbits showing signs of respiratory distress.

1. Select a 5–8F feeding tube.
2. Lay the tube along the outside of the rabbit's body, from the external nares to the caudal end of the sternum. Mark the point of the external nares with a tape or ballpoint pen.

3. Restrain the rabbit in sternal recumbency and wrap in a towel, as previously described.
4. Apply local anaesthetic spray to one of the rabbit's nostrils. Wait for 3–5 minutes.

1. The size depends on the size of the rabbit.
2. As the tube is passed through the nasal cavity and down the oesophagus, the pen or tape mark reaches the opening to the nasal cavity and indicates that the end of the tube has reached the distal oesophagus, close to the entrance to the stomach.
3. In this position the body is restrained but there is access to the head.

4. This desensitises the opening to the nasal cavity and facilitates tube placement.

5. Apply lidocaine (lignocaine) gel to the end of the tube.

5. This lubricates the passage of the tube so that it can be inserted without resistance.

6. Raise the rabbit's head and place the tip of the tube into the selected nostril at the ventral meatus. Gently advance the tube medially and ventrally. Return the head to a normal position as the pharynx is approached. Continue until the mark on the tube lies at the entrance to the nasal cavity.

6. This ensures that the tube passes down into the distal oesophagus.

7. Take a radiograph of the lateral thorax and abdomen.

7. It is important to check that the tube is in the oesophagus and not in the trachea. Introducing a small volume of saline down the tube is a simple means of monitoring, but rabbits do not always cough when this is done. The use of a lateral radiograph is a more reliable method. The rabbit will be conscious and must be restrained. Make sure that correct radiological protection measures are carried out.

8. Pass the external part of the tube over the bridge of the nose and between the ears. Fix in place using superglue, tape or sutures at the external nares and at the base of one ear.

8. It is important that the tube is not dislodged by patient interference.

9. If necessary, use a Buster collar.

Note. This technique can be used to administer liquid oral medication or for feeding hospitalised rabbits.

PROCEDURE: SUBCUTANEOUS INJECTION

ACTION

1. Place the rabbit in sternal recumbency on a suitable examination table with a non-slip surface.

2. Select a sterile 21 or 23G needle and a syringe of an appropriate size. Draw up the drug to be administered.

3. Grasp the loose skin of the scruff and inject the drug into the subcuticular space.

4. Withdraw the needle and gently massage the site.

RATIONALE

1. If the rabbit feels secure it will be less likely to struggle and injure itself. Minimal restraint is needed but the rabbit must be prevented from leaping off the table.

2. Large volumes can be given by subcutaneous injection.

3. You may draw back on the syringe before injecting of the drug to check that a vein has not been penetrated, but this is not usually necessary with a subcutaneous injection.

4. To aid dispersion of the drug. Absorption of a drug from this area takes about 30–40 minutes.

PROCEDURE: INTRAMUSCULAR INJECTION

ACTION	**RATIONALE**
1. Place the rabbit in sternal recumbency on a suitable examination table with a non-slip surface.	1. If the rabbit feels secure it will be less likely to struggle and injure itself.
2. Select a 23G needle and a syringe of appropriate size. Draw up the drug to be administered.	2. 0.5–1.00 ml can be given by this route. Large volumes will cause pain and damage to muscle tissue.
3. Grasp the scruff of the rabbit with one hand.	3. This prevents the rabbit from moving or leaping off the table.
4. Inject into the lumbar muscles.	4. This is a large muscle mass, which is easily accessible. The procedure can be performed single-handedly in docile rabbits. Assistance may be required if the patient is more active.
5. Alternatively the quadriceps group of muscles on the cranial aspect of the thigh may be used. Restrain the rabbit in sternal recumbency and extend a hindleg towards the veterinary surgeon.	5. This position provides easy access to the muscle group.
6. The veterinary surgeon will hold the muscle between the finger and thumb of the left hand and introduce the needle into the muscle with the right hand.	6. Assume that the veterinary surgeon is right-handed.
7. Draw back on the syringe to check that a vein has not been penetrated.	7. Muscle tissue is well supplied with blood vessels and there is a danger of accidental venepuncture. Care must also be taken to avoid the sciatic nerve, which runs behind the femur.
8. If no blood appears in the hub of the needle, inject the drug into the muscle.	
9. Withdraw the needle, applying gentle pressure over the site.	9. To aid dispersion of the drug. Absorption from this area takes approximately 15–20 minutes.

PROCEDURE: INTRAVENOUS INJECTION

ACTION	**RATIONALE**
1. Place the rabbit in sternal recumbency on an examination table with a non-slip surface.	1. If the rabbit feels secure it will be less likely to struggle and injure itself.
2. Wrap the rabbit in a towel with the head uncovered, as previously described.	2. This restrains the body while providing access to the head.
3. Clip the fur lying over the marginal ear vein of one ear. Clean the site but avoid the use of spirit.	3. The marginal ear vein runs down the side of each ear. The use of spirit can collapse the vein, making sampling and injection more difficult.

4. Apply local anaesthetic cream to the site. Wait for 10 minutes.

5. Place a ball of cotton wool soaked in hot water under the ear.
6. Apply pressure to the base of the selected ear.

7. Maintain the pressure while the veterinary surgeon inserts a 23G needle through the overlying skin into the marginal ear vein.
8. The veterinary surgeon will draw back on the syringe.
9. If blood appears in the hub of the needle, release the pressure on the vein a little, while the veterinary surgeon injects the drug to be given.
10. When the procedure is complete, the veterinary surgeon will slowly withdraw the needle while you apply pressure over the injection site for a few seconds.

Note. If repeated injections are to be given, use an intravenous or a butterfly catheter held firmly in place with superglue or tape. If collecting a

4. This desensitises the area so that the rabbit is less likely to shake its head when the needle is introduced.
5. This causes the vein to dilate, making it easier to see.
6. This pressure acts as a tourniquet, preventing blood returning from the ear pinna to the heart, so dilating or 'raising the vein' and making it more visible.
7. The vein should be clearly visible.

8. If blood appears in the hub of the needle, the vein has been penetrated.
9. Do not inject more than 1.5 ml, as larger volumes may cause damage to the vein.

10. This prevents haemorrhage into the surrounding tissues.

blood sample, use the saphenous, the cephalic or the jugular veins. The maximum volume that can be collected at one time is 2.5 ml.

PROCEDURE: INTRAPERITONEAL INJECTION

ACTION

1. Place the rabbit in sternal recumbency on an examination table with a non-slip surface.
2. Grasp the scruff with one hand and the hindlegs with the other hand.
3. Pick the rabbit up and hold it in dorsal recumbency with its spine against your chest (Fig. 12.4).
4. The veterinary surgeon will introduce a short needle at a point midway between the xiphisternum and the pubis.

5. Draw back on the syringe and examine the contents.

6. If there is nothing in the syringe, gently inject the contents of the syringe.
7. When the procedure is complete, withdraw the needle.

RATIONALE

1. If the rabbit feels secure it will be less likely to struggle and injure itself.
2. The rabbit must be held firmly to prevent it struggling during the procedure.
3. This position exposes the abdomen for injection, but care must be taken with dyspnoeic patients.
4. This position should avoid accidental penetration of the bladder or stomach. Rabbit skin is thin and a short needle easily penetrates the abdominal wall.
5. If blood, urine or gut contents appear, reposition the needle. If nothing appears in the hub of the needle, it is safe to proceed with the injection.
6. Up to 50 ml of fluid can be given by this route.

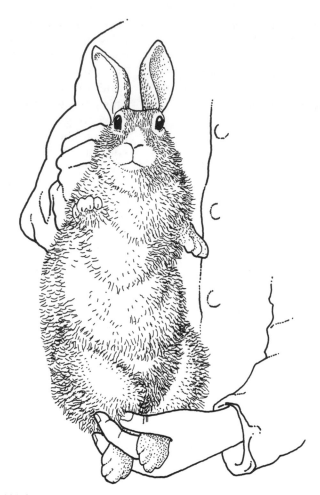

Figure 12.4 Restraining a rabbit for an intraperitoneal injection.

Note. This technique can be used to collect samples of fluid from the peritoneal cavity and urine from the bladder.

PROCEDURE: TO PLACE AN INTRA-OSSEUS CATHETER

ACTION

1. Select an appropriate site.

2. Prepare the site aseptically.
3. Infiltrate the area with local anaesthetic.

RATIONALE

1. In the rabbit the proximal femur and the proximal tibia provide ease of access and a medullary cavity from which fluid can be rapidly absorbed.
2. To prevent the introduction of infection.
3. To desensitise the tissues. The rabbit may be under a general anaesthetic but this depends on the nature and condition of the individual patient.

4. Select a spinal needle or plain needle of an appropriate size and insert it into the bone.

5. Flush the needle with heparinised saline.

6. Fix the needle in place with tissue glue or by suturing.
7. Attach a short length of tubing and a syringe or attach a fluid giving set to the needle.

8. If the needle is to be left *in situ*, bandage the area. You may need to use a Buster collar.

9. When giving further fluid or drugs through the needle, maintain an aseptic technique.
10. Flush with heparinised saline before each use.
11. Keep the needle patent by flushing with heparinised saline at least three times daily even if it is not being used.

Note. This route is useful for small animals whose veins are often fragile and easily damaged by needles and catheters. If the needle is

4. The needle must be of a size that will enter the medullary cavity: use a radiograph of the leg or previous experience to assess the size.
5. The needle may become blocked with tissue fragments. Heparinised saline will ensure that it is patent.
6. It is important that the needle does not become dislodged.
7. This procedure may be used to give a bolus of fluid or a slow infusion. Absorption from this site is as rapid as from the intravenous route.
8. To prevent the risk of infection, to reduce limb mobility and to prevent patient interference. A Buster collar will also prevent interference but intra-osseus catheters are usually well tolerated.
9. To prevent the introduction of infection.

10. To flush out any blood clots.

11. To maintain patency.

dislodged, haemorrhage from the site is unlikely to occur.

General anaesthesia

General considerations are listed in Table 12.2.

PROCEDURE: INDUCTION OF ANAESTHESIA

ACTION

1. Weigh the rabbit.

2. During the induction process the rabbit must be handled gently and calmly.

3. If using an injectable agent, e.g. fentanyl/ fluanisone or ketamine/medetomidine, give by the appropriate route, restraining the patient as described previously (Table 12.3).

4. Supplement with oxygen by mask or by intubating the patient.

RATIONALE

1. To calculate the correct dose of anaesthetic. It is important not to overdose the patient.
2. This process easily distresses a rabbit and it may contribute to cardiac or respiratory arrest.
3. Injectable agents provide a rapid and stress-free induction. Use small syringes for more accurate dosing.

4. This should be done even when using injectable agents.

Table 12.2 Points to be considered during anaesthesia of the rabbit

Action	Rationale
1. There is no need for preoperative starvation of rabbits	1. Rabbits are unable to vomit. Starvation may cause a fatal hypoglycaemia, especially in smaller individuals. The stomach is never completely empty as rabbits exhibit coprophagia
2. Avoid dehydration by giving fluids intravenously, subcutaneously, intraperitoneally or intra-osseously	2. This is not usually necessary in routine operations but can be particularly important in rabbits that are in a poor state of health or anorexic
3. Keep the patient warm at all times using a heat pad or by wrapping in 'bubblewrap' but check regularly for signs of hyperthermia	3. Hypothermia may be a problem in small animals, particularly during anaesthesia and post-operatively, as they have a large surface area in relation to their bodyweight. Anaesthetics depress temperature regulation and may cause vasodilation. If viscera are exposed during surgery, heat loss will be increased
4. Apply an ophthalmic lubricant to protect the eyes	4. Rabbits have bulging eyes, which are prone to drying out during anaesthesia. If ketamine is used in any anaesthetic combination, the eyes will remain central and fixed
5. Make sure that the tongue is pulled forward if the patient is not intubated	5. A rabbit's tongue is large and may obstruct the airway

5. If using inhalation anaesthesia, e.g. isoflurane, induce using a mask or an induction chamber.

5. Using a mask is easier if the rabbit has been given a premedicant. An induction chamber of a suitable size for the patient may take several minutes to fill. Induction by either of these methods is not recommended as the rabbit may hold its breath or may struggle violently, injuring its back. The most commonly used anaesthetic, isoflurane, is irritant to mucous membranes.

6. Give 100% oxygen for 1–2 minutes before attempting to intubate the rabbit.

6. To increase the oxygen concentration in the anaesthetic mixture. Intubation is more difficult than in the dog and cat and may take longer, as the glottis and larynx are not visible.

7. Intubate the rabbit by placing it in sternal or dorsal recumbency with the head and neck extended. Use a laryngoscope to illuminate the area and an 'introducer', such as that found inside a cat urinary catheter, to stiffen the endotracheal tube. Slide the tube over the introducer into the trachea and remove the introducer.

7. The glottis of the rabbit is small and obscured by the tongue. A fatal laryngospasm may occur if care is not taken.

8. Alternatively, intubation may be performed 'blind'. Estimate the position of the larynx externally and advance the endotracheal tube until it lies in the correct position. Check for correct positioning.

8. The larynx may be palpated externally. Listen for respiratory sounds through the tube to check positioning. A transparent tube may show evidence of condensation from the moisture in the exhaled breath.

9. Attach the endotracheal tube to the anaesthetic circuit.

9. The circuit must be appropriate to the species, e.g. Ayr's or Jackson Rees modified T-piece.

Table 12.3 Anaesthetic agents used in small rodents and rabbits

Drug	Species, dose rate and route of administration					Comments
	Mouse	Rat	Guinea pig	Rabbit		
Acepromazine	0.5–1.0 mg/kg i.m.	0.5–1.0 mg/kg i.m.	0.5–1.0 mg/kg i.m.	0.75–1.00 ml/kg—sedation		Sedation only
Atipamezole (Antisedan)	1.0–2.5 mg/kg i.p.	1.0–2.5 mg/kg i.p.	1.0–2.5 mg/kg i.p.	0.001 mg/kg s.c., i.p., i.v.		Used to reverse the effects of medetomidine Effects last for 45–60 minutes
Fentanyl/fluanisone (Hypnorm)/diazepam	0.4 ml/kg–5 mg/kg i.m.	0.3 ml/kg–2.5 mg/kg i.m.	1 ml/kg–2.5 ml/kg i.m.	0.3 ml/kg i.m. 2 mg/kg i.p.		Sedation. Dilute 1:10 to reduce inflammation at the site
Fentanyl/droperidol (Innovar-Vet)	0.06–0.30 ml/kg i.m.	0.1–0.5 ml/kg i.m.	0.22–0.88 ml/kg i.m.	0.15–0.44 ml/kg i.m.		
Isoflurane	2–5% induction; 0.25–4.0% maintenance	2–5% induction; 0.25–4.0% maintenance	2–5% induction; 0.25–4.0% maintenance	3–5% induction; 1.5–1.75% maintenance		Anaesthetic of choice for all species
Ketamine (K): medetomidine (M)	50–75 mg/kg (K): 10 mg/kg (M) i.p.	50–75 mg/kg (K): 10 mg/kg (M) i.p.	50–75 mg/kg (K): 10 mg/kg (M) i.p.	5 mg/kg (K) i.v.: 0.35 mg/kg (M) i.m.		Minor procedures. Use higher doses of ketamine for females. Reverse effect of medetomidine with atipamazole
Propofol (Rapinovet)	12–26 mg/kg i.v.	7.5–10.0 mg/kg i.v.	—	2–3 mg/kg i.v.		Rapid induction and anaesthesia. Lasts for 5 minutes

10. Take appropriate steps to keep the rabbit warm at all times.

10. Heat loss can be reduced by wrapping in 'bubblewrap' or a 'space blanket' or by use of a heat pad.

PROCEDURE: MAINTENANCE AND MONITORING OF ANAESTHESIA

ACTION

1. Make sure that you are familiar with the reactions of the rabbit under general anaesthesia.
2. Pay particular attention to the rate and depth of respiration.

3. Monitor the tension of the jaw.
4. Pinch the ear.

5. Assess the pedal reflex.

6. The corneal and palpebral reflexes can also be used to assess depth of anaesthesia.

RATIONALE

1. Rabbits are not as relaxed as dogs and cats.

2. This is the most reliable method of monitoring the depth of anaesthesia. Laboured breathing and pauses between breaths indicates deep anaesthesia.

4. Absence of a headshake indicates an acceptable level of surgical anaesthesia.
5. This reflex remains for longer than in the dog and cat and is only lost under deep anaesthesia.
6. These are similar to those in the dog and cat.

PROCEDURE: POST-OPERATIVE CARE

ACTION

1. The rabbit must be monitored until it is completely conscious and behaving normally.
2. Place the rabbit in a cage in a room that is warm, quiet and dimly lit.
3. Ensure that the rabbit is kept warm using a heat pad or Vetbed, or blankets or towels placed under and over the body. Avoid the use of shavings or hay, etc.
4. Monitor the core temperature until completely conscious.

5. If necessary, be prepared to give oxygen.
6. If the rabbit shows signs of pain, e.g. tooth grinding, grunting, lack of appetite or if the condition warrants it, provide analgesia.

RATIONALE

1. Avoid too much direct attention, e.g. talking to the rabbit, as this will increase the levels of stress. Observe from a discreet distance.
2. Bright lights and noise will distress the rabbit during recovery.
3. Hypothermia can be fatal or will prolong the recovery period. Loose bedding such as shavings may clog the mouth and nose.

4. Use a rectal thermometer but try to avoid excessive manipulation of the recovering rabbit.
5. This will increase the rate of recovery.
6. Any procedure that would cause pain in any other species should be considered to cause pain in the rabbit and would warrant the use of analgesics. Correct use of analgesics, e.g. carprofen or buprenorphine will do no harm.

7. If the rabbit does not eat or drink soon after recovery, consider providing fluid therapy— either intravenously or intraperitoneally; this should include glucose.

8. Monitor urine and faeces output.

7. Lack of fluid may rapidly cause serious dehydration. Lack of food may lead to a fatal hypoglycaemia. Both will compromise recovery.

8. General anaesthesia and surgery may impair both kidney and intestinal function. Overhandling of the intestine may cause paralytic ileus, which is indicated by a lack of faeces.

SMALL RODENTS

For biological data see Table 12.1, page 309.

Handling and restraint

It is the natural response of a frightened rodent to bite. This can be avoided by knowing how to handle each species correctly, but if you are bitten:

- Replace the rodent in its cage with your finger still in its mouth. As the rodent feels its feet on a firm surface it should let go!
- Do not attempt to pull your finger from the rodent's mouth, as the injury will be made worse by the backward-pointing curved teeth.
- Do not shake the rodent off your finger, as this will cause serious injury to the rodent.
- Wash the bite thoroughly under running water, apply antiseptic ointment and cover for as long as you are working with the animals.
- Consult your doctor if it becomes excessively painful or swollen.
- Keep your tetanus vaccination up to date.

The chinchilla—Chinchilla laniger

PROCEDURE: TO RESTRAIN A CHINCHILLA

ACTION

1. If the chinchilla is tame, pick it up by placing one hand around its shoulders.

2. Avoid grasping hold of the fur.

3. Once removed from the cage, most chinchillas will sit quietly on your forearm, gently restrained by the base of the tail.

RATIONALE

1. Chinchillas are relatively easy to handle: most are not aggressive and rarely bite. Be aware of the pressure you are putting on the chest, as this can restrict normal breathing.

2. Rough handling can cause patches of fur to come away in your hand—a condition known as 'fur slip'. In the wild this mechanism enables the chinchilla to escape from predators. New fur may take several months to grow back and may be of a different shade.

3. If the animal feels supported and secure it will be unlikely to try to escape.

4. More nervous or active animals can be lifted by the base of the tail with your other hand supporting the body.

5. To restrain for any clinical procedure, hold the base of the tail with one hand and place the other around the shoulder and chest.

4. Only lift by the base of the tail, as further down may injure the tail. Do not leave the animal unsupported for any longer than is necessary.

5. This can be used to hold the animal firmly for such procedures as injection and examination.

PROCEDURE: TO SEX A CHINCHILLA

ACTION

1. Grasp the base of the tail with one hand and support the body around the shoulders.
2. Hold the chinchilla in dorsal recumbency, moving the tail to expose the genital area.

RATIONALE

1. If the animal feels supported and secure it will be unlikely to try to escape.
2. This can be done single-handedly unless the chinchilla struggles.

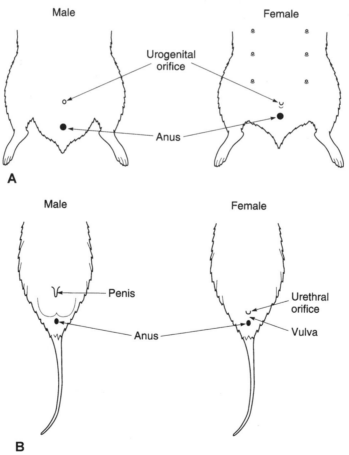

Figure 12.5 General method of sexing rodents: A, hamsters; B, mice. Reproduced, with permission, from *Preveterinary Nursing Textbook*, p. 113, by Masters and Bowden (2001). Butterworth Heinemann, UK.

3. Examine the genital area and measure the anogenital distance.

3. This is the distance between the anus and the opening of the vulva (female) or the penis (male) and is longer in the male than in the female (Fig. 12.5). The female chinchilla has a large, cone-shaped clitoris, which may be mistaken for the penis of the male. Adult male chinchillas have a pair of large testes which are very obvious during the breeding season of November–March.

The gerbil—Meriones unguiculatus

For biological data see Table 12.1, page 309.

PROCEDURE: TO RESTRAIN A GERBIL

ACTION

1. If the gerbil is tame and used to being handled, scoop it into your cupped hands.
2. If the gerbil is less tame, immobilise it by placing your hand over it.
3. Move your hand to grasp the scruff and lift the animal clear of the cage.

4. Further restraint can be achieved by using your other hand to hold the base of the tail.

RATIONALE

1. Gerbils are extremely active creatures and can jump horizontally and vertically.
2. This will prevent it escaping. The darkness will temporarily calm it.
3. Most gerbils are not aggressive, but some will try to bite: make sure that you grasp enough scruff to prevent it turning around to bite.
4. Do not hold the tip of the tail as the skin may be shed, leaving a raw and painful tail.

PROCEDURE: TO SEX A GERBIL

ACTION

1. Restrain the gerbil by grasping the scruff as described previously.

2. Examine the ventral surface of the gerbil.

3. Examine the genital area and measure the anogenital distance (Fig. 12.5).

RATIONALE

1. If the gerbil feels secure and comfortable it will be less likely to struggle or to attempt to bite you.
2. Male gerbils have no teats; females have four pairs of teats arranged along the ventral body wall of the thorax and the abdomen.
3. The anogenital distance is the distance between the anus and the opening of the vulva (female) or the penis (male) and is longer in the male than in the female (Fig. 12.5). Adult male gerbils have a pair of testes lying in the inguinal region.

The guinea pig—Cavia porcellus

For biological data see Table 12.1, page 309.

PROCEDURE: TO RESTRAIN A GUINEA PIG

ACTION

1. Guinea pigs should be brought to the surgery in small covered boxes.

2. Open the box in a dim light if possible.

3. Pick up the animal by placing one hand around its shoulders and chest (Fig. 12.6).
4. Lift the guinea pig clear of the cage or box, supporting its weight with your other hand.
5. Move your thumb from around the shoulders and place it under the mandible (Fig. 12.6).
6. If further restraint is needed, place the guinea pig in dorsal recumbency and extend the hindlegs.

PROCEDURE

1. Guinea pigs are nervous animals and a box provides security and darkness, which will calm them.
2. This will reduce stress, but you must be able to examine the patient.
3. Guinea pigs are generally non-aggressive and can be handled gently but firmly.
4. This is important if the animal is pregnant or heavy.
5. This prevents the animal from lowering its head to bite.

6. The animal will be unable to move.

PROCEDURE: TO SEX A GUINEA PIG

ACTION

1. Restrain the guinea pig in dorsal recumbency, as previously described.

RATIONALE

1. This provides good exposure of the genital area.

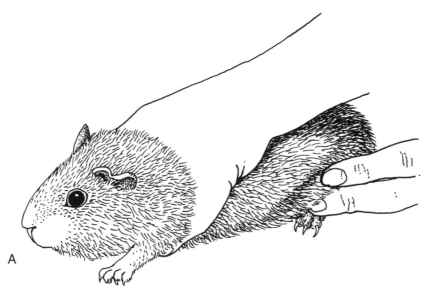

Figure 12.6 Restraining a guinea pig for examination. A, Initial restraint is achieved by grasping the animal around the shoulders. B, The hindquarters should be supported if the animal weighs more than 200–300 g.

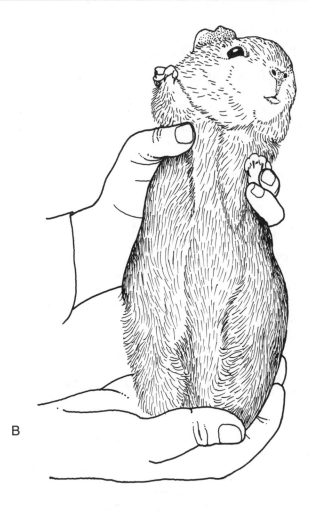

Figure 12.6 *Continued*

2. Examine the inguinal region.

2. Both male (boar) and females (sow) have a single pair of nipples in the inguinal region. Adult males have a pair of large testes.

3. Examine the genital opening.

3. Females have a Y-shaped opening; males have a slit-shaped opening.

4. Apply gentle pressure on either side of the genital opening.

4. In the male, the penis will extend and protrude. Female guinea pigs have a pale-coloured clitoris, which may protrude, but it is much less obvious than the male penis.

Note. Guinea pigs can be sexed as early as 1–2 days old.

The Hamster—Mesocricetus auratus (Syrian or golden hamster)

PROCEDURE: TO RESTRAIN A HAMSTER

For biological data see Table 12.1, page 309.

ACTION

1. Waking a sleeping hamster can provoke an aggressive response.
2. As the hamster runs around on the floor of the cage or box, grasp a large section of the scruff (Fig. 12.7).

3. Lift the hamster upwards.

4. Draw the scruff tight to prevent the hamster from moving around.

5. If the hamster does not need to be examined or injected, you can pick it up in your cupped hands or allow it to run into a small cup or jug.

RATIONALE

1. Allow the hamster time to wake up before attempting to pick it up.
2. Hamsters are unpredictable and often aggressive. It is important to take a large area of scruff to prevent the animal turning around to bite you.
3. Hamsters are not very heavy and can be lifted with one hand.
4. In this position you can inject the animal and examine the teeth and the oral pouches. If the scruff is too tight the eyes will bulge.
5. The hamster can be moved from cage or box to an induction chamber but is not sufficiently restrained for any clinical procedure.

PROCEDURE: TO SEX A HAMSTER

ACTION

1. Restrain the hamster in one hand using the scruff, as previously described.

RATIONALE

1. Make sure you are holding enough of the scruff to prevent the hamster turning around and biting you.

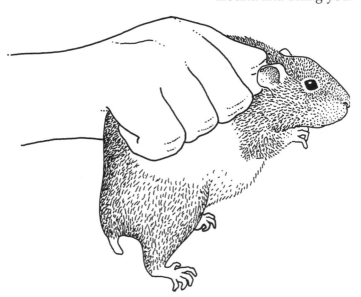

Figure 12.7 Picking a hamster up by the scruff of the neck.

2. Examine the genital area and measure the anogenital distance (Fig. 12.5).

2. Adult males have a pair of large testes. These are visible from the dorsal surface as the hamster runs around. The anogenital distance is the distance between the anus and the opening of the vulva (female) or the penis (male) and is longer in the male than in the female (Fig. 12.5).

3. Examine the ventral surface of the hamster.

3. The male hamster has no teats; the female has six pairs arranged along the ventral body wall of the thorax and abdomen.

4. If the hamster is mature, examine the region of the hips.

4. Male hamsters have a scent gland over each hip. This becomes pigmented as the animal ages. The gland is not present in the female.

Note. The much smaller Chinese and Russian hamsters are also popular children's pets. The techniques for handling and sexing these species are exactly the same as described for the Syrian hamster.

The mouse—Mus musculus

For biological data see Table 12.1, page 309.

PROCEDURE: TO RESTRAIN A MOUSE

ACTION

1. If the mouse is tame and used to being handled, scoop it into your cupped hands.

2. If the mouse is not used to being handled, pick it up by the base of the tail.

3. Lift the mouse clear of the cage and place it on a rough surface such as a towel, your sleeve or the top of the wire cage.
4. Pull the mouse gently backwards (Fig. 12.8).

5. With your other hand, grasp a large amount of scruff between your finger and the base of your thumb while keeping control of the tail.
6. Lift the mouse up and transfer your hold on the tail to between the third and fourth fingers of that hand (Fig. 12.8).

RATIONALE

1. This works well for tame mice, but many mice are very nervous and may attempt to bite: a careful approach is essential.
2. Do not pick it up by the tip of the tail as the outer skin may be shed, leaving the tail raw and painful.
3. Mice are light enough to be lifted by the tail without the need to support the body.

4. The mouse will grip the surface and is sufficiently restrained for an initial examination.
5. If you do not take enough of the scruff the mouse will be able to turn round and bite you.

6. The mouse is restrained securely and as it is held in one hand only your other hand is free to examine or inject it.

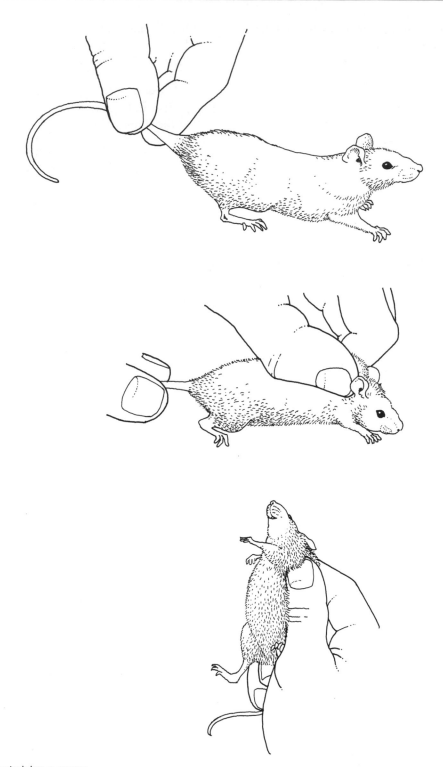

Figure 12.8 Restraining a mouse.

PROCEDURE: TO SEX A MOUSE

ACTION

1. Restrain the mouse by the scruff and tail as previously described.
2. Examine the ventral surface of the body.

3. Examine the genital region and measure the anogenital distance (Fig. 12.5).

RATIONALE

1. Mice can easily struggle and escape if not held securely.
2. Male mice do not have teats; females have seven pairs arranged along the ventral body wall of the thorax and abdomen.
3. The anogenital distance is the distance between the anus and the opening of the vulva (female) or the penis (male) and is longer in the male than in the female (Fig. 12.5). Adult males have a pair of large testes lying in the inguinal region.

The rat—Rattus norvegicus

For biological data see Table 12.1, page 309.

PROCEDURE: TO RESTRAIN A RAT

ACTION

1. With one hand, grasp the body around the shoulders and lift clear of the cage.

2. Position your thumb so that is lies under the lower jaw (Fig. 12.9).

3. Alternatively, if the rat is aggressive or unused to being handled, pick it up by the base of the tail.
4. Place the rat on the cage lid or on a rough surface, maintaining your grip on the tail.
5. As the rat moves forward, place your other hand over the shoulders and chest.
6. Move your thumb and forefinger to lie behind the rat's elbows so that the forelegs are pushed forward to cross under the chin.
7. If the rat struggles when first restrained, allow it to rest on your sleeve with a minimum of restraint.

   Note. Rats do not like being picked up by the scruff and this may cause the animal to bite.

RATIONALE

1. Rats are intelligent, docile animals that rarely bite unless they are frightened or in pain. Be aware of how much pressure you are applying to the chest: too little will allow the animal to escape; too much will compress the chest and may make the animal bite you.
2. Use your thumb to apply pressure and to push the jaw up. This will prevent the animal from biting.
3. Do not pick up by the tip of the tail as the outer skin may be shed, leaving a raw and painful tail.
4. This provides something that the rat can grip.
5. Do not hold too tightly, as this will affect the rat's respiration and may cause distress.
6. The rat is held securely and it can be examined without the risk of being bitten.

7. After a short time, the rat will relax.

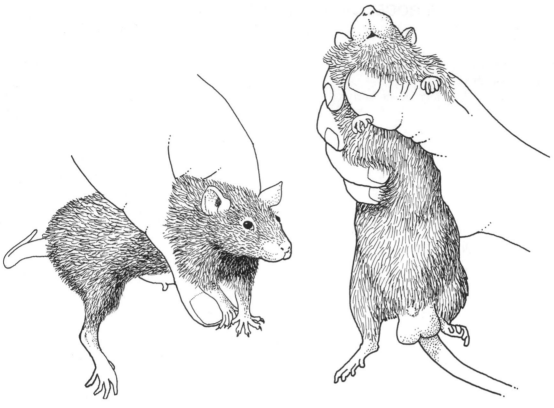

Figure 12.9 Restraining a rat.

PROCEDURE: TO SEX A RAT

ACTION

1. Restrain the rat by picking it up around the shoulders.
2. Lift it clear of the cage and hold it in dorsal recumbency.
3. Examine the ventral surface of the body.

4. Examine the genital area and measure the anogenital distance (Fig. 12.5).

RATIONALE

1. If the rat feels secure it will be less likely to struggle or to bite.
2. In this position you have access to the relevant parts of the animal.
3. Male rats do not have teats; females have five pairs arranged along the ventral body wall of the thorax and abdomen.
4. The anogenital distance is the distance between the anus and the opening of the vulva (female) or the penis (male) and is longer in the male than in the female (Fig. 12.5). Adult males have a pair of large testes lying in the inguinal region.

Administration of medicines

PROCEDURE: TO ADMINISTER FLUIDS OR LIQUID MEDICATION

ACTION

1. Medication such as antibiotics can be given to small rodents in the drinking water or in food.

2. If the animal is not drinking, liquid medication or replacement fluids can be given by inserting a syringe or pipette into the side of the mouth at the level of the diastema (space between the incisor and molar teeth).

3. The chinchilla, guinea pig and rat can be given liquid through a 3–4F catheter inserted into the pharynx, oesophagus or stomach. Make a mouth gag by drilling a hole crossways through a 1 ml syringe case. Place the 'gag' across the mouth of the patient and pass the catheter through the hole and down the pharynx. Ensure that the catheter is correctly placed before injecting any fluids by listening for respiratory sounds in the tube or by taking a lateral radiograph of the animal.

RATIONALE

1. Withhold all other sources of water or food, so that the animal has to take in the medication. This is not recommended as the animal may not be eating or drinking normal amounts—therefore the precise dose is unknown.

2. Use an unbreakable syringe to prevent the animal biting through the nozzle. Sweeten the liquid with fruit juice to increase acceptability.

3. This technique enables you to give volumes of up to 5 ml. The use of the gag prevents the patient biting through the catheter. It is vital to check that the catheter is not in the trachea, as the administration of fluid into the lungs may 'drown' the animal or cause aspiration pneumonia.

PROCEDURE: TO ADMINISTER MEDICATION BY PARENTERAL ROUTES

For details of injection sites see Table 12.4.
General points to be considered are as follows.

ACTION

1. For most procedures, use a 23 or 25G needle.

2. If giving small volumes of drugs use small syringes.

3. When using the intramuscular route, give small volumes.

4. When restraining an animal for an intraperitoneal injection, hold the animal with its head downwards.

RATIONALE

1. Small needles cause less damage to the tissues.

2. Larger sizes are more difficult to handle when restraining small struggling rodents.

3. Large volumes may cause tissue damage pain, irritation and possible self-mutilation at the site. This route is not recommended in very small rodents, e.g. mice.

4. This allows the intestines to fall cranially, making them less likely to be punctured by the needle. This is not recommended for debilitated or dyspnoeic animals—restrain them vertically.

Table 12.4 Parenteral routes for the administration of medicines in small rodents

Species of rodent	Subcutaneous	Intramuscular	Intraperitoneal	Intravenous
Chinchilla	Scruff or the flank. Avoid rough handling as this causes 'fur slip'	Quadriceps group on cranial thigh or semimembranosus/semitendinosus on caudal thigh. No more than 0.3 ml	Restrain with head lower than hindquarters. Insert needle in posterior quadrant to the right of the midline 2.5 cm in front of pubis	Use the cephalic, saphenous or jugular veins
Gerbil	Scruff. Up to 2 ml	Quadriceps group. No more than 0.3 ml. Not recommended	Restrain with head downwards. Insert needle into lower left quadrant. Give 3–4 ml	Not recommended
Guinea pig	Lift the skin between the scapulae. Up to 10 ml	Quadriceps group. No more than 0.3 ml	Restrain with head lower than hindquarters. Insert needle in posterior quadrant to the right of the midline 2.5 cm in front of pubis at 45°	Ear veins, but these are very small and fragile. Apply local anaesthetic cream to prevent head shaking when needle is introduced
Hamster	Scruff. Up to 3–4 ml	Quadriceps group. No more than 0.1 ml. Not recommended	Restrain with head downwards. Insert needle either side of midline in inguinal region, caudal to umbilicus, which avoids the caecum, at an angle of 45°. Aspirate before injecting	Not recommended
Mouse	Scruff. Up to 2 ml	Quadriceps group. No more than 0.05 ml. Not recommended	Insert needle into lower right quadrant to avoid caecum on the left at an angle of 20°. Aspirate before injecting—should be a vacuum. Give 2–3 ml	Lateral tail veins. Warm complete mouse or tail to dilate the veins. 0.2 ml can be injected
Rat	Scruff or flank. Up to 5–10 ml	Quadriceps group. No more than 0.3 ml	Insert needle into lower right quadrant to avoid caecum on the left at an angle of 20°. Aspirate before injecting—should be a vacuum. Give 10–15 ml	Lateral tail veins. Warm complete rat or the tail to dilate the veins. 0.5 ml can be injected

PROCEDURE: TO COLLECT A BLOOD SAMPLE

ACTION

1. The sample required may be as small as a drop of blood or may be a larger volume.

2. In any species, no more than 10% of the total blood volume may be taken at any one time.
3. Select the appropriate site for the species (Table 12.5).

4. Prepare the site aseptically.
5. Select a suitably sized needle and a 1 ml syringe.

6. Ask an assistant to restrain the animal appropriately and to apply pressure to the selected vein—known as 'raising the vein'.

7. Introduce the needle into the vein at an angle to the skin with the bevel uppermost. Once the needle is in the vein, advance it parallel to the skin.

RATIONALE

1. A drop of blood can be used to make a smear to examine the red or white cells. Larger volumes may be used for biochemical analysis.
2. For details of blood volumes see Table 12.5.

3. In all the small rodents, clipping a nail may yield a small volume of blood but this is not recommended unless really necessary as it causes pain and distress.
4. To prevent the introduction of infection.
5. Choose a size that is as large as is practicable for the species. The needle must be able to enter the vein and must not be so small that it impedes the flow of blood and damages the red cells, leading to haemolysis of the sample.
6. When collecting blood it will be necessary to have an assistant to restrain the animal to avoid injuring the animal and causing it distress. Pressure should be applied to the vein to dilate it, making it more obvious for venepuncture.
7. The body of the needle now lies within the lumen of the vein.

Table 12.5 Blood sampling in small rodents

Species	Adult blood volume (ml/kg)	Total adult blood volume (ml)	Maximum sample volume (ml)	Site for venepuncture	Comments
Rabbit	57–65	58.5–585	5–50	Cephalic, jugular	Large variation in size
Chinchilla	—	40–60	5.00	Cephalic, jugular	
Gerbil	66–78	8.00	0.5	Jugular, cardiac puncture	Cardiac puncture must only be performed under a GA. Risk of permanent heart damage
Guinea pig	69–75	50–60	5.00	Ear vein, cardiac puncture	Cardiac puncture must only be performed under a GA. Risk of permanent heart damage
Hamster	78	8.00	0.5	Cardiac puncture	Cardiac puncture must only be performed under a GA. Risk of permanent heart damage
Mouse	58.5	2.00	0.25	Lateral tail vein	Dilate the vein by warming the tail.
Rat	54–70	30	3.00	Lateral tail vein, jugular	Dilate the vein by warming the tail

8. Either allow blood to drip from the hub of the needle into a collecting pot, or attach the syringe and gently pull back the plunger.

8. Larger volumes can be collected by using a syringe. The vein will collapse around the needle if you try to withdraw the blood too quickly. The blood sample may also be haemolysed as a result of red cell damage.

9. Empty the syringe into an appropriate collecting pot and rotate gently.

9. If the sample is to be analysed, the pot must contain an appropriate anticoagulant, e.g. EDTA, lithium heparin. Gentle rotation will mix the blood with the anticoagulant; overenthusiastic mixing will damage the blood cells.

10. Ask your assistant to apply pressure over the site of venepuncture while you slowly withdraw the needle from the vein.

10. To prevent haemorrhage into the surrounding tissues and encourage clotting.

11. Dress the site appropriately.

11. To prevent infection and to prevent self-mutilation at the site.

General anaesthesia

PROCEDURE: INDUCTION OF ANAESTHESIA

ACTION

1. Many patients to be anaesthetised are geriatric.

2. The patient may already be debilitated, in poor condition or obese before it is presented to the veterinary surgeon.

3. The patient may be affected by a pre-existing illness.

4. The patient may be anorexic and dehydrated. Always assess the level of dehydration and delay anaesthesia until it has been corrected.

5. There is no need for preoperative fasting in small rodents.

6. Weigh the patient.

7. Anaesthetic induction may be performed in an induction chamber or by mask, using an inhalation anaesthetic agent such as 4% isoflurane.

RATIONALE

1. Small rodents have a short lifespan, which must be considered when undertaking anaesthesia.

2. These all increase the risk of anaesthesia.

3. Make a careful clinical examination to identify any risk factors, e.g. chronic respiratory disease.

4. Provide replacement fluid therapy by the appropriate route.

5. Fasting may lead to a fatal hypoglycaemia. Many species exhibit coprophagia so the stomach and intestines are rarely completely empty.

6. This enables accurate anaesthetic doses to be calculated and provides a baseline for clinical assessment during recovery, e.g. whether the animal is eating or drinking.

7. Induction chambers are preferred, as masks are often too big for small rodents. Induction by inhalation is stressful to the patient and there is a risk of injury, as the patient may struggle during the procedure.

8. Induction can be performed using injectable agents (Table 12.3).

The advantage is rapid recovery, which reduces the risk of hypothermia.

8. These provide a smooth stress-free induction but recovery rates may be longer, depending on the choice of drug.

PROCEDURE: MAINTENANCE AND MONITORING OF ANAESTHESIA

ACTION

1. Once the patient is anaesthetised, maintain using an inhalation anaesthetic agent, e.g. 2% isoflurane delivered by mask, or supplement injectable drugs with oxygen by mask.

2. Monitor body temperature and keep the patient warm at all times by using a heat pad, or wrapping in 'bubblewrap' or a 'space blanket'.

3. Prepare the surgical site carefully.

4. Apply ophthalmic ointment to the eyes.

5. Monitor the depth of anaesthesia using reflexes and monitoring equipment.

6. Monitor respiration.

RATIONALE

1. Small rodents are difficult to intubate. Inhalation anaesthesia delivered by mask may lead to fluctuations in depth.

2. Small rodents have a large surface area to bodyweight ratio, which means that they lose heat rapidly. Under anaesthesia the body's ability to regulate the core temperature is impaired, adding to the problem of hypothermia.

3. Rodent skin is thin and can be easily nicked by clippers. Avoid the use of spirit to sterilise the site as this will further cool the patient.

4. Rodents have prominent eyes, which can be dried by the heat of the operating light and the lack of a blink reflex, leading to keratitis and corneal ulceration.

5. Each species varies in its response to anaesthesia and it is important to become familiar with these variations. The use of electronic monitoring equipment may be difficult, as it is designed and calibrated for use in larger animals, such as the cat and the dog.

6. Respiratory depression or arrest can be overcome by oxygen delivered by mask or by the use of respiratory stimulants such as doxapram.

PROCEDURE: POST-OPERATIVE CARE

ACTION

1. After the surgical procedure is complete, place the patient in a secure warm cage in a quiet, warm and darkened room and cover with a towel, blanket, 'bubblewrap' or a 'space blanket', as appropriate.

2. Observe the patient quietly and unobtrusively.

3. Monitor the core temperature.

4. Monitor respiration.

5. If the patient shows signs of pain, e.g. tooth grinding, vocalisation, aggression, hunched position, provide analgesia.

6. Continue to monitor the patient after it has regained consciousness.

7. Instruct the owner of the warning signs to watch out for when the patient is taken home.

RATIONALE

1. Hypothermia during recovery can be fatal. Initially the temperature of the cage should be kept at 35°C, falling to 26–28°C as the animal regains consciousness. Any noise or bright light will overstimulate a recovering animal.

2. Rodents do not appreciate being touched or talked to as a dog would. Look at the animal from a distance and only interfere if it is really necessary.

3. To be aware of hypothermia before it becomes critical.

4. Respiratory depression or arrest may also occur during the recovery period.

5. Any procedure that would cause pain in any other species should be considered to cause pain in the rodent and warrants the use of analgesics. Correct use of analgesics, e.g. carprofen or buprenorphine, will do no harm.

6. Observe whether the animal is eating or drinking. Note the production of faeces and urine.

7. The owner should monitor the patient for at least 24 hours after the surgical procedure.

THE FERRET – *MUSTELA PUTORIUS FURO*

For biological data see Table 12.6.

Handling and restraint

PROCEDURE: TO RESTRAIN A FERRET

ACTION

1. Place one hand around the shoulders and neck (Fig. 12.10).

2. Lift the ferret clear of the cage and support the hind end with your other hand.

RATIONALE

1. Ferrets vary in temperament: some are quite tame and relax when handled, whereas others may be aggressive. The ferret has a well-muscled neck which must be held firmly.

2. Ferrets can be quite heavy and need to be supported. The body should not be stretched as this causes the animal to

Table 12.6 Ferrets—biological data

Parameter	Measurement	Comment
Life span	5–11 years	
Adult weight	Jill: 600–900 g	Weight fluctuates with the time of year—heavier in the winter
	Hob: 1–2 kg	
Body temperature	37.8–40°C	Rises to 40°C when the ferret is excited
Respiratory rate	30–40 breaths/min	
Pulse rate	200–400 beats/min	
Oestrous cycle	Seasonally polyoestrous. Induced ovulator	Season starts in March and continues until September. Female remains in oestrus until she is mated. Ovulation occurs 30–40 hours after mating
Age at puberty	Jill: 7–10 months	Puberty occurs in the spring after birth, so age varies
	Hob: 5–14 months	
Gestation period	38–44 days	Young are altricial. May be eaten by the jill if disturbed
Litter size	2–6	
Weaning age	6–8 weeks	
Diet	Carnivorous	Require 30% protein; 30% fat. Can be fed on tinned or dry cat food

3. Move your thumb so that it lies under the lower jaw. Place your forefinger around the neck, leaving the other fingers under the forelegs (Fig. 12.10).
4. Hold the ferret gently but firmly.

5. Tame ferrets may rest along the handler's forearm.

6. If a more secure hold is required, grasp a large portion of scruff and suspend the body.

struggle. Some ferrets like to be dangled by the front end while their knuckles are rubbed!

3. This prevents the ferret from moving its head to bite you.

4. Ferrets are very agile creatures, designed for going down holes, and they can wriggle free if not held firmly.
5. Gentle restraint is usually adequate for a physical examination. Handle ferrets that may be in pain with caution, as they may bite.
6. The ferret has a large area of scruff. Suspending the animal induces relaxation.

PROCEDURE: TO SEX A FERRET

ACTION

1. Restrain the ferret by the scruff or by holding around the shoulders, as previously described.
2. Examine the genital area.

RATIONALE

1. This position leaves one hand free to examine the ferret.

2. In the male (hob), the opening to the penis is situated on the ventral abdomen just caudal to the umbilicus, giving a long anogenital distance. Male ferrets have a pair of testes that enlarge during the breeding season. In the female (jill), the vulva lies close to the anus and becomes swollen when the female is in oestrus.

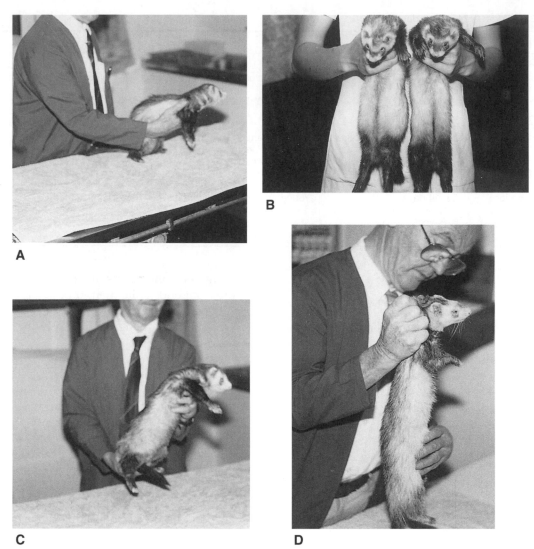

Figure 12.10 Restraining a ferret. A, Gentle restraint may be achieved by just raising the ferret off the table, using one hand under its chest. Do not squeeze. B, Picking up a ferret with a hand around the upper chest. With these two ferrets of the same size, the one on the left has an enlarged spleen, seen as a noticeable swelling on the left side of the abdomen. C, Supporting the heavy ferret—especially important with pregnant jills. D, 'Scruffing' a ferret to palpate the internal organs. Reproduced, with permission, from *Ferret Husbandry, Medicine and Surgery* by Lewington (2000). Butterworth Heinemann, UK.

Administration of medicines

PROCEDURE: TO ADMINISTER FLUIDS OR LIQUID MEDICATIONS

ACTION

1. Restrain the ferret by the neck and shoulders and support the hind end on a table or allow it to dangle.

RATIONALE

1. In this position you have control of the head. Supporting the hind end on a table may encourage the ferret to struggle. This will depend on the weight, temperament and condition of the ferret.

2. Using a small syringe filled with the liquid, place the nozzle into the side of the mouth.

3. Slowly deposit the liquid towards the back of the tongue.

2. Avoid using large syringes as they are difficult to manipulate while holding the patient. This procedure may be used to give liquid medication or replacement fluid.

3. Do not give the medication too fast as the ferret lacks a cough reflex and may aspirate the liquid.

PROCEDURE: SUBCUTANEOUS INJECTION

ACTION

1. Grasp a large section of the scruff of the ferret.

2. Select a sterile 23G needle and a syringe of an appropriate size, fill with the medication and introduce the needle into the scruff.

3. Apply pressure to the plunger and inject the drug.

4. Remove the needle from the scruff.

RATIONALE

1. Ferrets have a large scruff and this position both restrains the ferret and provides a suitable site for the injection.

2. A maximum of 5–10 ml can be given at this site.

3. There is no need to draw back on the syringe in a subcutaneous injection as the risk of penetrating a blood capillary is low.

4. Absorption of the drug from this site takes about 30 minutes.

PROCEDURE: INTRAMUSCULAR INJECTION

ACTION

1. Ask an assistant to restrain the ferret in sternal recumbency on the examination table, placing one hand behind the head and the other pinning the lumbar region to the table.

2. Locate either the quadriceps group on the cranial aspect of the thigh or the semimembranosus/semitendinosus group on the caudal aspect of the thigh.

3. Select a sterile 23G needle and a syringe of an appropriate size, fill with the drug and introduce the needle into the muscle.

4. Draw back on the syringe.

5. If no blood appears in the hub of the needle, gently inject the drug.

6. Apply gentle pressure over the injection site and withdraw the needle.

RATIONALE

1. This restrains the body firmly, preventing struggling and possible injury to the ferret and to the handler.

2. These muscles are relatively large and can be easily located between the finger and thumb. Do not use the lumbar muscles as these are thin, and penetration of a kidney is a risk if the ferret struggles.

3. The muscle mass is small, so only small volumes can be given by this route— maximum of 0.5 ml.

4. Muscle tissue has a good blood supply and there is a risk of penetrating a blood vessel.

5. Do not inject too rapidly as the pressure may cause the drug to spurt out of the hub.

6. This aids dispersion of the drug. Absorption from this site takes 15–20 minutes.

PROCEDURE: INTRAPERITONEAL INJECTION

ACTION

1. Ask an assistant to restrain the ferret by holding it around the shoulders and chest with the thumb under the chin and the fingers under the forelegs, as previously described (Fig. 12.10).
2. Use the other hand to support the hind end.

3. In this position the assistant should rest the body against his or her chest, presenting the ventral abdomen towards you.
4. Select a 21–23G needle and a small syringe and fill it with the drug to be administered.

5. Introduce the needle to one side of the midline and into one of the lower quadrants of the abdomen. The needle should be pointing cranially.
6. Draw back on the syringe.

7. If the hub of the needle is empty, inject the drug into the peritoneal cavity and withdraw slowly.

RATIONALE

1. This restrains the body firmly, preventing struggling and possible injury to the ferret and to the handler.

2. The hind end must be held firmly to prevent the ferret moving around and injuring itself during the procedure.
3. The ventral abdomen is the site of the injection.

4. This procedure may also be used to administer fluid therapy. A maximum of 8 ml can be given at any one time.
5. This will decrease the risk of entering one of the abdominal organs.

6. To check that you have not penetrated an organ. If urine, intestinal contents or blood appear in the syringe, reposition the needle.

PROCEDURE: INTRAVENOUS INJECTION

ACTION

1. Restrain the ferret in sternal recumbency by grasping a large section of the scruff and placing the legs firmly on a table.
2. Extend one of the forelegs towards the veterinary surgeon, with the elbow in the palm of your hand.
3. Place the thumb of this hand across the crook of the ferret's elbow and apply gentle pressure.
4. Gently rotate your thumb outwards.
5. The veterinary surgeon will clip a small area over the cephalic vein and prepare it aseptically.
6. The veterinary surgeon will select a 23G needle and a small syringe filled with the drug to be administered and insert the needle through the skin and into the vein.

RATIONALE

1. If the ferret feels secure it will be less likely to try and escape.

2. This is the same position as is used in the dog or the cat.

3. This pressure will cause the cephalic vein to dilate and become more obvious.

4. This completes the dilation of the vein.
5. To prevent the introduction of infection into the vein.

6. Use a small gauge needle as the vein has a narrow diameter.

7. The veterinary surgeon will draw back on the syringe.
8. If blood appears at the hub of the needle, inject the drug slowly into the vein.
9. When the procedure is complete, you should apply gentle pressure over the injection site while the veterinary surgeon slowly withdraws the needle.
10. Dress the site appropriately.

7. To check that the needle is in the lumen of the vein.
8. Drugs given by the intravenous route are instantly absorbed.
9. This pressure prevents haemorrhage into the surrounding tissues.

10. To prevent infection and self-mutilation of the wound.

Note. The lateral saphenous vein running over the lateral aspect of the hock may also be used. If fluid therapy is to be given, place a catheter into the cephalic, saphenous or jugular vein. Blood samples can also be collected from these veins.

General anaesthesia

PROCEDURE: INDUCTION OF ANAESTHESIA

ACTION

1. Starve the ferret for 6–12 hours before anaesthesia but allow free access to water.

2. Weigh and examine the animal before giving the anaesthetic.

3. Atropine given subcutaneously or intramuscularly can be used as a premedicant.
4. Induce anaesthesia by using an inhalation agent, such as isoflurane given by mask or by placing the ferret in an induction chamber.

5. Induction can also be achieved by using an appropriate injectable agent, e.g. ketamine, given by the correct route.
6. Once the ferret is anaesthetised, intubate with a 1.5–3.0 uncuffed endotracheal tube.

RATIONALE

1. Ferrets are able to vomit so it is important to ensure that the stomach is empty. Older ferrets should not be starved for longer than 4 hours, as there is a risk of an insulinoma precipitating a hypoglycaemic attack. Access to water should minimise dehydration.
2. This provides an accurate weight from which to calculate your dose and guarantees that there are no underlying problems that may affect the anaesthetic.
3. Atropine reduces salivation and gastrointestinal secretions and minimises cardiac arrythmias.
4. The response to inhalation anaesthesia is similar to that of the cat and the dog. Isoflurane provides rapid induction and recovery.
5. Do not use injectable agents in sick or debilitated patients.

6. This is an easy procedure, as the ferret is able to open its mouth wide for visualisation of the larynx. Ferrets do not seem to suffer from laryngospasm.

PROCEDURE: MAINTENANCE AND MONITORING OF THE ANAESTHETIC

ACTION	RATIONALE
1. To maintain the anaesthetic use a non-rebreathing circuit delivering isoflurane.	1. The type of circuit must be appropriate to the size of the animal.
2. During anaesthesia make sure that the ferret is kept warm by placing on a heat pad or wrapping in 'bubblewrap' or a 'space blanket'.	2. Hypothermia may be a problem, as the ferret has a large surface area in relation to its body weight so it loses heat very rapidly.
3. Monitor the hydration status of the patient.	3. Give intravenous fluids to sick or debilitated animals during surgery.
4. Monitor the depth of anaesthesia by assessing respiratory rate and depth, heart rate, jaw tone, withdrawal and palpebral reflexes.	4. Response to anaesthesia is similar to that of the cat.
5. If the procedure is painful or likely to be painful, provide analgesia, e.g. buprenorphine or flunixin.	5. Pre-emptive analgesia is the most effective, i.e. that given before the onset of pain. The use of analgesics reduces the dose of anaesthetic required and increases the rate of recovery post-operatively.

PROCEDURE: POST-OPERATIVE CARE

ACTION	RATIONALE
1. After the surgical procedure is complete, place the patient in a secure warm cage in a quiet, warm and darkened room and cover with a towel, blanket, 'bubblewrap' or a 'space blanket', as appropriate.	1. Hypothermia during recovery can be fatal. Any noise or bright light will overstimulate a recovering animal.
2. Observe the patient quietly and unobtrusively.	2. Ferrets do not appreciate being touched or talked to. Look at the animal from a distance and only interfere if it is really necessary.
3. Monitor the core temperature.	3. To be aware of hypothermia before it becomes critical.
4. Monitor respiration.	4. Respiratory depression or arrest may also occur during the recovery period.
5. If the patient shows signs of pain, e.g. vocalisation, aggression, hunched position, provide analgesia.	5. Any procedure that would cause pain in any other species should be considered to cause pain in the ferret and would warrant the use of analgesics. Correct use of analgesics, e.g. flunixin or buprenorphine will do no harm.
6. Continue to monitor the patient after it has regained consciousness.	6. Observe whether the animal is eating or drinking. Note the production of faeces and urine.

7. Instruct the owner of the warning signs to watch out for when the patient is taken home.

7. The owner should monitor the patient for at least 24 hours after the surgical procedure.

CAGE AND AVIARY BIRDS

Handling and restraint

PROCEDURE: TO CAPTURE AND RESTRAIN A BIRD

ACTION

1. Make sure that all doors and windows are closed and that the extractor fans are turned off.
2. Remove all movable objects from the cage, e.g. perches, feeding bowls, toys.
3. Turn the lights off or, if possible, dim them. Use a small hand-torch covered in a red or blue filter for illumination.

4. Tip the cage on its side.

5. Approach the bird slowly.

6. Quickly grab the bird around its neck or close your hands around the wings and body (Fig. 12.11).

7. Wear clean strong gloves if catching larger birds such as cockatoos and macaws (Fig. 12.12).

RATIONALE

1. If the bird escapes from its cage, it will not be able to get out of the room or be injured in the extractor fan.
2. This makes capture quicker and easier and therefore less stressful for the bird.
3. Most common species of cage and aviary birds are active in daylight. A dim light will simulate night and induce quiet behaviour. Birds do not see well in red or blue light.
4. This enables you to approach the bird from the bottom of the cage and provides more room for manoeuvre.
5. This avoids causing air movement, which will startle the bird.
6. It is important to catch the bird quickly, firmly and gently to avoid causing distress. Closing your hands around the body holds the wings closed and prevents them flapping and possibly breaking. This method can be used to catch small psittacine birds, e.g. budgerigars, lovebirds and others such as canaries and finches.
7. These birds have vicious beaks. The use of gloves reduces your sense of touch when handling small birds.

PROCEDURE: TO CAPTURE A BIRD USING THE TOWEL METHOD

ACTION

1. Select a suitable towel.
2. Drape the towel over one hand.
3. Advance your towelled hand towards the bird and trap it in a corner of the cage.

RATIONALE

1. A hand towel is about the right size.
2. This disguises your hand.
3. Trap the bird as quickly as possible. Making several attempts to catch the bird causes fear and distress and may damage the wings and plumage.

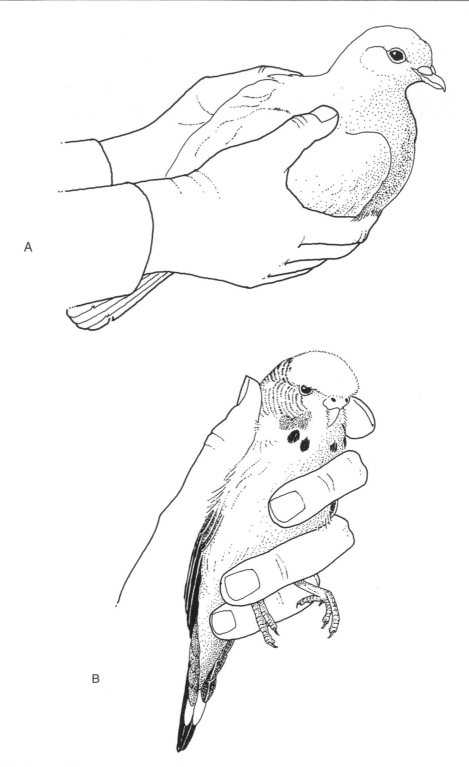

Figure 12.11 Handling small birds. A, A pigeon held in the hands. Note how the two hands encompass the wings and prevent the bird from flapping. B, A budgerigar in the hand. Note how the fingers form a 'net' around the bird: undue pressure must not be applied.

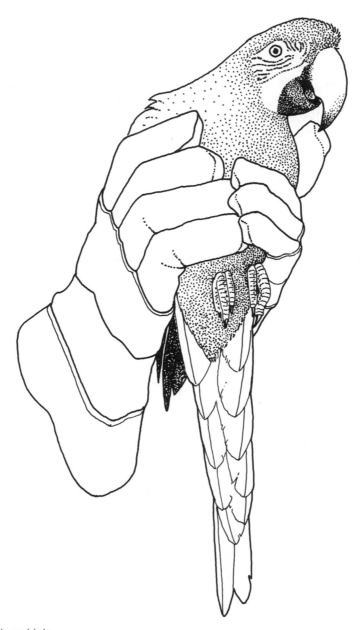

Figure 12.12 Handling large birds.

4. Catch hold of the bird by the neck.

4. The bird cannot bite you if the head and neck are controlled. There is very little chance of you strangling the bird because your hand is covered in the towel, which reduces the pressure you are able to apply.

5. Taking your hand out of the towel, place your thumb and forefinger over the temporo-mandibular joint on either side of the head.

5. This prevents the bird from biting you.

6. Take care with larger psittacines, e.g. macaws and cockatoos.

Note. If you are bitten you can try:

- Blowing on the bird's face.
- Squeezing the top of the bird's head.
- As a last resort, open the beak with whelping forceps—take care as you may damage the beak.

Avoid pulling your finger out of the beak as this is curved and you may lose a chunk of flesh!

6. These species can deliver a nasty bite.

It is often better if owners are not present during capture and treatment, as the more intelligent species will associate their experience with the owner.

Administration of medicines

PROCEDURE: TO ADMINISTER FLUID VIA A CROP TUBE

ACTION

1. Select some form of metal catheter or crop tube and attach to the end of a syringe filled with warmed fluid.
2. Place the crop tube against the bird and mark the approximate area of the crop with a felt or ballpoint pen.

RATIONALE

1. Metal crop tubing catheters are available, but a Spreull needle can be used. Plastic and rubber tubing may be bitten through.
2. This measures the length of crop tube that must be inserted down the oesophagus to reach the crop. Ingesta travels from the mouth down the oesophagus into the crop,

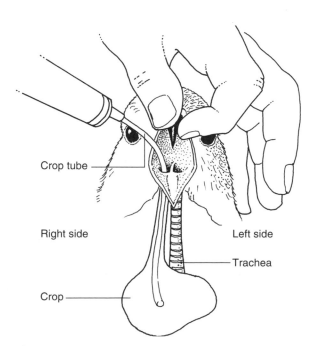

Crop tube

Right side

Left side

Trachea

Crop

Figure 12.13 Crop tubing a parrot.

3. Lubricate the crop tube.

4. Restrain the bird by the neck.

5. Insert the crop tube on the right side at the junction of the upper and lower beak (Fig. 12.13). Extend the neck as you advance the tube.

6. Direct the tube upwards towards the roof of the oropharynx and then down towards the oesophagus.

7. Advance the crop tube down the right dorsal side of the oesophagus until it enters the crop.

8. Slowly administer an appropriate volume of fluid.

9. Slowly withdraw the crop tube and observe the patient.

which is a diverticulum of the oesophagus, lying outside the body cavity in the ventral part of the neck (Fig. 12.13).

3. To facilitate the passage of the crop tube down the oesophagus. KY jelly is a suitable lubricant.

4. You may need an assistant to hold the wings close to the body.

5. Extending the neck stretches the oesophagus, making placement easier.

6. This ensures that the tube does not enter the glottis and trachea of the bird. Birds have a poor cough reflex and may asphyxiate or develop pneumonia if fluid enters the lungs or air sacs. Using a tube that is wider than the glottis may help to prevent incorrect positioning.

7. The crop lies on the right side of the neck. The end of the tube can be palpated when it enters the crop. In fledglings, the tube can be seen passing down the oesophagus.

8. Slow infusion prevents the fluid refluxing up the oesophagus.

9. Slow withdrawal prevents damage to the tissues. It is important to observe the patient for adverse reactions.

PROCEDURE: INTRAMUSCULAR INJECTION

ACTION

1. Restrain the bird so that it cannot struggle, holding its wings close to the body.

2. Identify the pectoral muscles forming the breast of the bird. Select an area in the caudal part of the muscle group.

3. Using a sterile 21–23G needle and a syringe of an appropriate size, part the feathers and introduce the needle into the muscle.

RATIONALE

1. Small birds such as finches can be restrained and injected single-handedly, but be aware of the pressure that you are applying around the chest as this may restrict respiration. You may need an assistant to restrain larger species while you inject.

2. The pectoral muscles form the largest area of muscle in the bird.

3. Feathers should never be plucked unless it is essential. They will only grow back at the next moult and this may take months. Lack of feathers may affect insulation, flight and appearance, depending on the site and the species.

4. Draw back on the syringe.

5. If no blood appears in the hub of the needle, inject the drug.

6. Withdraw the needle and apply pressure over the site.

4. To check that you have not penetrated a blood vessel.

5. Drugs are rapidly absorbed from this site. Absorption from subcutaneous injections is slow, so intramuscular injections are more commonly performed.

6. To prevent haemorrhage into the surrounding tissues. Birds bleed readily from injection sites.

PROCEDURE: INTRAVENOUS INJECTION

ACTION

1. Restrain the bird in the appropriate position to expose the vein. Ask an assistant to hold the head or hold the mask if the patient is anaesthetised.

2. Wet the feathers to enable the vein to be more easily visualised.

RATIONALE

1. The following veins may be used for venepuncture:

   • Brachial (or basilic) vein—on the medial side of the elbow within the wing.
   • Jugular vein—on either side of the neck. The right jugular vein is larger than the left.
   • Medial metatarsal—on the caudal aspect of the leg. Easily visualised in larger species.

2. Avoid plucking the feathers to expose the vein. New feathers will not grow back until the next moult. Loss of feathers may affect the bird's ability to fly or to keep warm. In show birds it may affect their appearance.

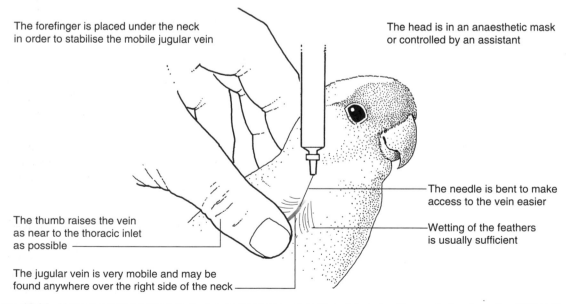

The forefinger is placed under the neck in order to stabilise the mobile jugular vein

The head is in an anaesthetic mask or controlled by an assistant

The needle is bent to make access to the vein easier

Wetting of the feathers is usually sufficient

The thumb raises the vein as near to the thoracic inlet as possible

The jugular vein is very mobile and may be found anywhere over the right side of the neck

Figure 12.14 Using the right jugular vein to give an intravenous injection. Adapted, with permission, from the *BSAVA Manual of Psittacine Birds*, edited by P. Beynon and N. Forbes (1996). BSAVA, Cheltenham.

<table>
<tr><td>

3. Prepare the site aseptically.
4. Raise the vein by applying pressure at the base of the right side of the neck (jugular), proximal to the injection site on the upper wing (brachial) or around the lower leg (median metatarsal).
5. Insert a small needle at an angle into the vein and draw back on the syringe. If using the jugular vein you may need to bend the needle (Fig. 12.14).
6. If blood appears in the hub of the needle, inject the drug slowly.

7. If the injection is to be repeated or if fluid is to be given intravenously, an indwelling 20G needle can be inserted into the jugular vein.
8. Suture or glue the catheter in place and cover with a light dressing.

</td><td>

3. To prevent the introduction of infection.
4. Veins carry blood towards the heart. Pressure applied between the chosen site and the heart will prevent venous return and cause the vein to dilate or be 'raised'.

5. To check that the needle has penetrated the vein. Bending the needle facilitates access to the jugular vein.

6. If the drug is injected too quickly, the pressure may cause it to spurt out of the hub of the needle.
7. This prevents damage to the vein by repeated injection.

8. It is important that the catheter does not become dislodged by the bird's movement or by self-mutilation.

</td></tr>
</table>

PROCEDURE: INTRA-OSSEOUS INJECTION

ACTION

RATIONALE

1. Restrain the bird with a wing or leg extended.

2. Prepare the site aseptically.

3. Select a 20–22G needle.
4. Introduce the needle into the bone and flush with heparinised saline.

5. Connect to a syringe or to a giving set and bag of fluid.
6. Calculate the fluid requirement:

   Maintenance volume =
   75 ml/kg bodyweight
   Fluid deficit of 4–10% = 40–100 ml/kg
   bodyweight replaced over 48 hours.
7. Set the fluid to run at the required drip rate.

1. The optimum site for an intra-osseous injection is the distal radius or the proximal tibiotarsus. These bones have a medullary cavity from which fluid can be rapidly absorbed.
2. To prevent the introduction of infection. Avoid plucking the feathers to expose the site. New feathers will not grow back until the next moult. Loss of feathers may affect the bird's ability to fly or to keep warm. In show birds it may affect their appearance.
3. This size will enter the medullary cavity.
4. The saline will flush out any blood or bony tissue that accumulates as the needle is pushed through the cortex of the bone.
5. This procedure can be used to administer a bolus of fluid or for continuous infusion.
6. The majority of ill birds are dehydrated. Birds that are dehydrated and anorexic may suffer from a metabolic acidosis: correct this with lactated Ringer's (Hartmann's) solution.

7. Volumes required are usually small.

8. Cover the site with a bandage.

8. It is important that the needle or catheter is not dislodged by the bird's movement or by self-mutilation.

PROCEDURE: TO COLLECT A BLOOD SAMPLE

ACTION

1. Restrain the bird on its back on a soft surface with one wing extended; if you are right-handed use the right wing.

2. Wet the feathers over the site.

3. Prepare the site aseptically.
4. Place the first and second finger of the left hand on the mid-distal humerus, with the palm on the carpus of the wing.
5. Raise the vein with the thumb of your left hand.
6. Select a 23–27G needle and a 1 ml syringe.

7. Flush the needle and syringe with dilute heparin (1:100) before use.
8. Introduce the needle into the vein and draw back on the syringe.

9. Collect the blood sample.
10. Withdraw the needle, applying gentle pressure over the site for 2–3 minutes as you do so.

   Note. The jugular vein can also be used for blood sampling.

RATIONALE

1. The site for collecting a reasonable sample of blood is the brachial vein, which lies on the ventral aspect of the wing, distal to the elbow. A small sample can be collected by clipping a toenail. Small samples can be used for sexing the bird but the cells are often distorted, which may affect haematological studies.
2. This enables you to see the vein more clearly. Avoid plucking the feathers to expose the vein. New feathers will not grow back until the next moult. Loss of feathers may affect the bird's ability to fly or to keep warm. In show birds it may affect their appearance.
3. To prevent the introduction of infection.
4. This keeps the wing extended and restrained.

5. Your right hand is free for sample collection.

6. The needle must be able to enter the vein but must not be so small that it impedes the flow of blood and damages the red cells, leading to haemolysis of the sample.
7. This prevents the blood from clotting if the sample collection is slow.
8. If blood appears at the hub of the needle, the needle is correctly positioned in the vein.

10. This prevents haematoma formation.

General anaesthesia

PROCEDURE: INDUCTION OF ANAESTHESIA

ACTION

1. Do not starve birds that are less than 120 g in weight. Large psittacines may be starved for 1–2 hours. Fruit-eaters and waterfowl should be starved for 4–10 hours.
2. Make sure that all equipment is ready before you start the procedure.

3. Handle the bird as little as possible.
4. Induce anaesthesia by using a mask and an inhalation agent, e.g. isoflurane, or by using an injectable agent, e.g. ketamine.
5. Intubate the bird. This should be done for all but very short procedures.

6. Attach to an appropriate type of anaesthetic circuit.

RATIONALE

1. Starvation in small birds may cause a fatal hypoglycaemia and increase the anaesthetic risk. Grain-eaters, e.g. psittacines, seldom regurgitate.
2. The procedure should run as smoothly and as quickly as possible to reduce stress to the patient, which might otherwise increase anaesthetic risk.
3. To reduce stress.
4. For dose rates see Table 12.7.

5. Use an uncuffed tube as birds have complete tracheal rings that may be ruptured by inflation of the cuff. Intubation protects the airway and allows IPPV to be performed if necessary. Psittacines have large fleshy tongues that obscure the view of the glottis making intubation difficult: use a tongue depressor.
6. The circuit should provide low resistance, particularly for small birds.

Table 12.7 Anaesthetic agents for use in cage and aviary birds

Anaesthetic agent	Dose rate and site of administration	Comments
Isoflurane	4–5% induction; 2.0–2.5% maintenance	Anaesthetic of choice for most species
Halothane	Induce at 1% increasing to 3%; maintain at 1.5–3%	Slow induction will reduce the chances of cardiac failure
Ketamine/diazepam (K/D)	Psittacines 10–50 mg/kg(K):0.5–2.0 mg/kg (D) i.m. Pigeons 10–25 mg/kg(K):0.5–1.0 mg/kg (D) i.m.	Use lower end of dose range if possible Provides good muscle relaxation Useful for oral procedures in pigeons
Ketamine/medetomidine (K/M)	Psittacines 3–7 mg/kg(K):75–150 mg/kg (M) i.m. Pigeons 1.5–2.0 mg/kg (K):60–85 mg/kg (M) i.v.	Reversed by atipamezole. Righting reflex regained within 3–10 minutes
Propofol (Rapinovet)	3–5 mg/kg i.v.	Very short duration. May cause cardiac and respiratory depression Not recommended for psittacines as duration is too short

PROCEDURE: MAINTENANCE AND MONITORING OF ANAESTHESIA

ACTION	RATIONALE
1. Maintain anaesthesia using an inhalation agent, e.g. 2% isoflurane (Table 12.7).	1. If an injectable agent has been used, supplement with oxygen via a mask or endotracheal tube.
2. The flow rate through the circuit should be three times the minute volume.	2. Flow rate is approximately 3 ml/g bodyweight and should not be less than 0.75 l/min. A high flow rate prevents hypercapnia.
3. At all times ensure that the patient is warm. Use a heat pad or wrap in 'bubblewrap' or a 'space blanket'.	3. Birds have a high core temperature of 40–44°C owing to their high metabolic rate.
4. Assess the need for fluid therapy. If necessary, give intravenously or by intra-osseous injection, as previously described.	4. Ill birds are often dehydrated and provision of fluid will increase the chances of recovery.
5. Monitor the depth of anaesthesia using appropriate reflexes.	5. Toe, cere and wing reflexes are lost on a medium plane; palpebral reflex is lost on a deeper plane; and the corneal reflex is lost when the bird is very deeply anaesthetised.
6. Monitor respiration.	6. The rate and depth of respiration decrease as anaesthesia deepens. The rate should not fall below half the normal resting rate. The respiratory pattern should remain stable.
7. Monitor the heart rate.	7. Use a cardiac monitor or an oesophageal stethoscope. Heart rate is a good indicator of pain: it increases when the bird feels pain.
8. Place ECG leads over the distal tarsometa-tarsus and carpal joints of each wing.	8. To monitor the rate and pattern of the heart.

PROCEDURE: POST-OPERATIVE CARE

ACTION	RATIONALE
1. After the surgical procedure is complete, remove the endotracheal tube and wrap the bird in a towel.	1. This keeps the bird warm and prevents the wings from flapping during recovery, causing possible damage. If isoflurane is used the bird can be allowed to recover slowly in your hands before being placed in its cage.
2. Place the bird into its own cage to recover in a warm quiet darkened room.	2. Remove all portable object such as toys, feeding bowls and perches to facilitate handling of the bird if necessary. If the bird is placed in a normal recovery cage, it will have to be caught to place it back into its own cage: this increases the stress to the bird.

3. Keep the bird under discreet observation.

4. Continue to monitor the bird's progress for a few days after the operation.

5. If necessary, feed the bird using a crop tube, as previously described.

3. Many problems can develop during the recovery period. Birds do not need to be talked to or touched.

4. It is important that the bird begins to eat and drink. Small birds cannot survive for long without a source of energy.

5. To prevent the onset of dehydration and hypoglycaemia.

REPTILES

Zoonoses. All species should be handled with care as many reptiles are known to carry zoonotic diseases. Salmonellosis is the most common disease. It is difficult to determine whether or not an individual is infected as the bacteria may be shed intermittently in the faeces and bacterial culture may not detect all species. *Salmonella* is spread by ingestion of the faeces, so, although careful handling is not a risk, you must wash your hands after touching any reptile species.

As a general rule, the species of reptile most commonly kept as pets can be handled safely; however, precautions should be taken when handling venomous species. Large constrictors such as pythons should not be handled on your own, as you might need assistance if they wind themselves around your arm or your neck.

Snakes

PROCEDURE: TO RESTRAIN A SNAKE

ACTION

1. Ask the owner if the snake is used to being handled.

RATIONALE

1. This gives an indication of the response the snake may make to being handled and examined.

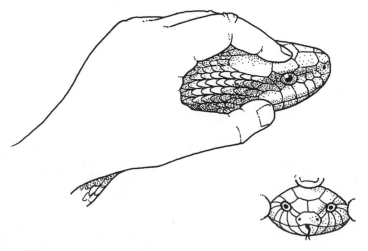

Figure 12.15   Restraining the head of a snake.

2. A snake should be transported in a soft bag, which is closed securely by doubling over the top and then tying it.

3. Open the bag or vivarium and look inside.

4. If the snake is tame, pick it up gently around the body and lift it from the bag or the vivarium.

5. Avoid making sudden movements or waving your hand in front of the snake.
6. As soon as possible, support the body and allow the snake to move around.

7. If further restraint is needed, place a finger and thumb on either side of the head and one finger on the top of the head (Fig. 12.15). Support the body with your other hand.
8. To handle more aggressive or vicious snakes use a towel. Move the towel towards the snake and catch the snake behind the head with your towel-covered hand.

2. Bumping against the hard surfaces of a cage or box can easily damage a snake. Snakes are very good at pushing through loosely tied knots. A pillowcase makes a good snake bag.
3. This helps you to locate the position of the snake's head.
4. Handle gently but positively. Snakes bruise easily but, as they have a slow metabolism, the injury may not show for several weeks. A snake may die from severe bruising.
5. This may cause the snake to strike.

6. Never suspend the body by the head: snakes have a single occipital condyle and the neck is easily broken. Use minimal restraint. Snakes do not like being held tightly or being stretched out.
7. In this position the snake is prevented from biting.

8. If the snake strikes it will hit the towel. Snake hooks can be used.

PROCEDURE: TO ADMINISTER FLUIDS OR LIQUID MEDICATION

ACTION

1. Select and lubricate a 5–8F catheter.

2. Lay the catheter along the outside of the snake. Mark the approximate position of the stomach on the catheter using a ballpoint pen.
3. Select an appropriate size of syringe and fill with fluid.

4. With the snake on a table, restrain the head and open the mouth uing a blunt metal spatula.

RATIONALE

1. The type used for dogs and cats is appropriate. Lubrication aids the introduction of the catheter.
2. The stomach lies approximately halfway down the length of the snake.

3. It is good practice to have all equipment ready before you begin to handle the snake as this reduces the stress caused by the procedure.
4. Snakes, teeth are very sharp and may point backwards in some species. They are also very dirty and any bite may become infected. Take steps to avoid being bitten.

5. Use a mouth gag if necessary.

5. Most snakes will open their mouths quite easily when gentle pressure is applied. Make a gag by folding a small piece of radiographic film and cutting a hole in the centre. The catheter is passed through the hole.

6. Support the weight of the body on the table or ask an assistant to help you.

6. Never suspend the body by the head: snakes have a single occipital condyle and the neck is easily broken.

7. Slowly insert the catheter into the back of the mouth and down the oesophagus.

7. The glottis, leading to the trachea and lungs, sits forward in the oral cavity to avoid asphyxiation when the snake is swallowing prey. It is easy to see and there is little risk of the catheter entering it.

8. Insert the catheter to the level of the stomach.

8. The ballpoint pen mark will lie at the level of the mouth.

9. Introduce the fluid in the syringe slowly.

9. If you introduce the fluid too quickly, the pressure applied may cause the fluid to spurt out of the junction with the syringe.

10. Gently withdraw the catheter and observe the snake.

10. To check that there are no adverse effects.

PROCEDURE: INTRAVENOUS INJECTION OR BLOOD SAMPLING

ACTION

1. Restrain the snake appropriately.

RATIONALE

1. The site for intravenous injection is the ventral venous sinus in the midline of the ventral tail. The jugular vein can be used but may require a surgical cut-down. The palatine veins can be seen when the mouth is open but the snake must be anaesthetised or sedated if these are used.

2. Prepare the site aseptically using povidone-iodine or 70% ethanol.

2. To prevent the introduction of infection.

3. Select a small needle and syringe.

3. The needle must be small enough to enter the vein.

4. Insert the needle between the paired caudal scales distal to the cloaca. Angle the needle at right angles to the tail. Draw back on the syringe.

4. In the male, care must be taken to avoid damaging the hemipenes, which lie here. If blood appears in the hub of the needle, the needle is correctly positioned in the vein.

5. Collect the sample into a lithium heparin tube.

5. EDTA lyses the cells.

6. A drop of blood can be used to make a blood smear.

6. This is useful for haematology.

7. If injecting intravenously, slowly give the drug into the vein.

8. Withdraw the needle.

Note. The total volume of blood is approximately 5–8% of bodyweight. This is about 70 ml/kg and, of this, 10% can be collected in one withdrawal.

Sites for the administration of parenteral drugs. These are:

- subcutaneous—under the loose skin over the ribs
- intramuscular—into the intercostal muscles.

Injections may be given into the tail, but snakes have a renal portal venous system in which blood flows from the hind end of the body to the kidneys before returning to the heart. Any drug injected into the hind end may be eliminated by the kidneys without being absorbed. Nephrotoxic drugs must not be injected into the hind end.

Chelonians

These are the shelled reptiles, e.g. tortoises and terrapins.

PROCEDURE: TO RESTRAIN A TORTOISE OR TERRAPIN

ACTION

1. Consider the species you are to handle.

2. Pick a tortoise up by placing both hands around the middle of the shell or carapace and support the whole body.

3. If handling a terrapin, wear plastic gloves.

4. Pick a terrapin up by placing your hands at the rear of the carapace just cranial to the hindlegs. To achieve a better grip, place your fingers into the inguinal area.
5. More aggressive individuals, e.g. snapping turtle, can be restrained in a towel while you move your hands towards the back of the carapace.
6. Soft-shelled terrapins should be handled wearing leather gloves.

RATIONALE

1. Most tortoises are non-aggressive and used to being handled. They may withdraw into their shells. Some species of terrapin, and particularly the snapping turtle, are aggressive and may bite, rather than withdraw into their shells.
2. Some individuals can be heavy. Watch out for the hindlegs, which may push against your hands and push the body out of your grip.
3. Terrapins are known to carry *Salmonella* infection and you should take precautions to protect yourself from this zoonosis. This is important if you have to remove the animal from water.
4. This will prevent the terrapin from biting your fingers. If the terrapin has been in water it will be slippery. Some terrapins also have long claws, which can scratch.
5. The towel will cover the head, preventing the animal from biting.

6. To prevent damage to the carapace and to prevent you being bitten.

7. In any species of chelonian, extend the head by placing your finger and thumb behind the occipital condyle and pulling slowly against the action of the retractor muscles of the neck.

8. Forcing the hindlegs into the inguinal region may bring the head and forelegs out.

7. Gentle but firm and constant pressure must be applied. The muscles will become tired and relax. Holding a tortoise with its forelegs against the shell and its body downwards may induce the head to come out far enough for you to grasp it.

8. The use of padded forceps may help extraction of the head, but be careful not to cause any damage.

PROCEDURE: TO ADMINISTER FLUIDS OR LIQUID MEDICATION

ACTION

1. Select an appropriate type of stomach tube and lubricate it.

2. Calculate the required dose of fluid or medication and fill a syringe of an appropriate size.

3. Holding the tortoise on its back for a short time, place the tube along the length of the plastron and mark the approximate position of the stomach on the tube using a ballpoint pen (Fig. 12.16).

4. Restrain the tortoise so that it is resting on its caudal scutes and extend the head and neck.

RATIONALE

1. Tubes designed for use in chelonians are available, but small dog catheters can be used.

2. It is good practice to have all equipment ready before you begin to handle the tortoise, as this reduces the stress caused by the procedure.

3. The stomach lies under the abdominal scute of the plastron. Lay the tube from the gular notch to the caudal border of the abdominal scute. (Fig. 12.16).

4. If the patient withdraws into its shell you may need to ask for assistance.

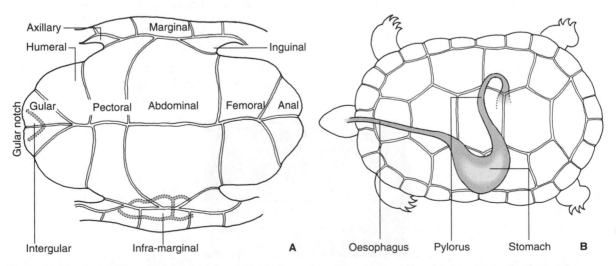

Figure 12.16 The position of the stomach in relation to the scutes of the plastron (A) and the carapace (B) of a tortoise.

5. Pull the mandible down with one finger and insert your index finger into the commissure of the lips.

6. Slide the lubricated tube towards the back of the mouth, down the oesophagus and into the stomach.

7. Introduce the fluid in the syringe slowly.

8. Gently withdraw the catheter and observe the patient.

Note. This method is suitable for all types of chelonian.

5. Your index finger acts as a gag. Tortoises have a beak but no teeth and placing your finger at the angle of the lips is unlikely to be painful.

6. The glottis is easy to see and to avoid. You will feel the tube pass through the cardiac sphincter into the stomach. The ballpoint pen mark will lie at the mouth.

7. If you introduce the fluid too quickly the pressure applied may cause the fluid to spurt out of the junction with the syringe.

8. To check that there are no adverse effects.

PROCEDURE: INTRAVENOUS INJECTION OR BLOOD SAMPLING

ACTION

1. Restrain the tortoise appropriately. You may need an assistant to hold the body.

2. To use the jugular vein, extend the head and neck fully by placing your finger and thumb behind the occipital condyle and pulling slowly against the action of the retractor muscles of the neck (Fig. 12.17).

3. Ask your assistant to raise the vein by applying pressure at the base of the neck.

4. Insert a small needle parallel to the neck, pointing towards the body (Fig. 12.17) and draw back on the syringe.

5. To use the dorsal venous sinus, extend the tail fully.

RATIONALE

1. The sites most commonly used in chelonians are the jugular and the dorsal venous sinus. If an assistant is not available, you can hold the shell between your knees.

2. The jugular vein runs from the level of the eardrum to the base of the neck and may be visible (Fig. 12.17).

3. The jugular vein carries blood from the head and neck towards the heart.

4. If blood appears in the hub of the needle, the needle is correctly placed.

5. The vein is located in the dorsal midline of the tail. This is the site of choice in the Mediterranean tortoise.

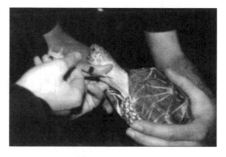

Figure 12.17 Intravenous injection in a tortoise using the jugular vein.

6. Insert a small needle in the exact midline at an angle of 45° and advance the needle until it touches the bone. Aspirate the syringe and withdraw the needle slightly until blood appears in the hub of the needle.

7. At both sites inject the drug slowly.

8. If blood is to be collected, withdraw the required amount of blood and place in a lithium heparin tube.

9. After the procedure is complete, withdraw the needle and apply gentle pressure over the site.

Note. The total volume of blood is approximately 5–8% of bodyweight. This is about 70 ml/kg and, of this, 10% can be collected in one withdrawal.

Sites for the administration of parenteral drugs. These are:

- subcutaneous—use the loose skin around the neck
- intramuscular—triceps muscle in the forelimb; pectoral muscles at the angle of the forelimb and neck; muscles of the hindlimb.

6. At first the needle goes through the sinus but, as you withdraw the needle, it re-enters the sinus and blood is aspirated.

7. If you apply too much pressure, the drug may spurt out of the junction between the needle and syringe.

8. EDTA lyses the blood cells.

9. To prevent the formation of a haematoma.

Injections may be given into the hindlimb, but chelonians have a renal portal venous system in which blood flows from the hindlimbs to the kidneys before returning to the heart. Any drug injected into the hindlimbs and tail may be eliminated by the kidneys without being absorbed. Nephrotoxic drugs must not be injected into the hindlimb.

Lizards

PROCEDURE: TO RESTRAIN A LIZARD

ACTION

1. Identify the species of lizard and ask the owner whether it is used to being handled.

2. Place your hand around the shoulders and lift the animal clear of the cage.

RATIONALE

1. There are many species of lizard commonly kept as pets. They vary in size and in nature. Most are amenable to handling but some, notably the Tokay gecko, are aggressive. There are only two venomous lizards—*Heloderma suspectum* (the gila monster) and *Heloderma horridum* (the beaded lizard)—but neither are particularly aggressive.

2. Never lift a lizard by the tail. Many species are able to shed their tails as a means of defence—a process known as autotomy. The tail will regrow but it never looks the same again.

3. Restrain the lizard by placing one hand around the pectoral girdle and the other around the pelvic girdle and hindlegs. Hold the hindlegs against the tail.
4. You may need to wear gloves when handling larger lizards.
5. More aggressive specimens can be induced to lie still by placing a towel over the head.

3. In this position the lizard is unable to struggle or to thrash its tail around.

4. Some species may bite or scratch, lash out with their tails or graze you with their scales.
5. If the head is in the dark, the lizard will remain motionless, so the body can be examined.

PROCEDURE: TO ADMINISTER FLUIDS OR LIQUID MEDICATION

ACTION

1. Select a 5–8F catheter and lubricate it.

2. Lay the catheter along the outside of the lizard. Mark the approximate position of the stomach on the catheter using a ballpoint pen.
3. Select an appropriate size of syringe and fill with fluid.

4. With the lizard on a table, restrain the body and open the mouth using a blunt metal spatula.
5. Use a mouth gag if necessary.

6. Slowly insert the catheter into the back of the mouth and down the oesophagus.

7. Insert the catheter to the level of the stomach.
8. Introduce the fluid in the syringe slowly.

9. Gently withdraw the catheter and observe the lizard.

RATIONALE

1. The type used for dogs and cats is appropriate. Lubrication aids the introduction of the catheter.
2. The stomach lies at a point just caudal to the caudal border of the ribs.

3. It is good practice to have all equipment ready before you begin to handle the lizard as this reduces the stress caused by the procedure.
4. Take steps to avoid being bitten.

5. Most lizards will open their mouths quite easily when gentle pressure is applied. Make a gag by folding a small piece of radiographic film and cutting a hole in the centre. The catheter is passed through the hole.
6. The glottis, leading to the trachea and lungs, sits forward in the oral cavity. It is easy to see and there is little risk of the catheter entering it.
7. The ballpoint pen mark will lie at the level of the mouth.
8. If you introduce the fluid too quickly the pressure applied may cause the fluid to spurt out of the junction with the syringe.
9. To check that there are no adverse effects.

PROCEDURE: INTRAVENOUS INJECTION OR BLOOD SAMPLING

ACTION	RATIONALE
1. Restrain the lizard appropriately.	1. The site most commonly used in large lizards is the ventral venous sinus lying in the midline of the ventral surface of the tail. In smaller species a toenail can be clipped to provide enough blood to fill a capillary tube.
2. Prepare the site aseptically using povidone-iodine or 70% ethanol.	2. To prevent the introduction of infection.
3. Select a small needle and syringe.	3. The needle must be small enough to enter the vein.
4. Introduce the needle in the exact midline of the ventral surface of the tail distal to the vent, at an angle of 45°. Advance the needle until you touch bone.	4. The needle will go through the sinus and touch the underlying vertebra.
5. Slowly withdraw the needle and aspirate the syringe at the same time until blood appears in the hub of the needle.	5. As you pull the needle back, it will re-enter the sinus and blood will be aspirated into the syringe.
6. Collect the sample into a lithium heparin tube.	6. EDTA lyses the cells.
7. A drop of blood can be used to make a blood smear.	7. This is useful for haematology.
8. If giving medication, slowly introduce the drug into the vein.	
9. Withdraw the needle.	

Note. The total volume of blood is approximately 5–8% of bodyweight. This is about 70 ml/kg and, of this, 10% can be collected in one withdrawal.

Sites for the administration of parenteral drugs. These are:

- Subcutaneous—under the loose skin of the ribs
- Intramuscular—into the caudal muscles of the forelimb; into the tail, but care must be taken in those species that show autotomy as they may slough their tails.

Injections may be given into the hindlimb, but lizards have a renal portal venous system in which blood flows from the hindlimbs and tail to the kidneys before returning to the heart. Any drug injected into the hindlimbs may be eliminated by the kidneys without being absorbed. Nephrotoxic drugs must not be injected into the hindlimb.

General anaesthesia

General points to be considered for all species of reptile

PROCEDURE: INDUCTION OF ANAESTHESIA

ACTION	RATIONALE
1. Have all anaesthetic equipment ready, organise assistance if required and be familiar with all the procedures involved before you get the patient from the cage.	1. This will minimise the stress caused to the patient. Reptiles are not as used to being handled as dogs and cats and this increase in stress will increase the risks of anaesthesia.
2. Small species of reptile do not need to be starved before an anaesthetic. Starve larger lizards and chelonians for 18 hours, and large snakes for 72–96 hours. Avoid feeding live insects just before an anaesthetic.	2. The presence of live insects in the stomach may cause a problem. Vomiting does not occur in reptiles.
3. Weigh the animal accurately.	3. This enables you to calculate an accurate dose of anaesthetic and the replacement fluid requirement.
4. Sedatives may be used as premedication but the use of atropine to reduce the production of saliva is unnecessary.	4. The use of sedatives will facilitate handling and reduce the stress caused to the patient. Salivary secretions do not cause a problem in reptiles.
5. Induce anaesthesia using injectable agents administered by the appropriate method.	5. For drugs and dose rates see Table 12.8.
6. Induce anaesthesia by inhalational agents, using a mask for large lizards and for snakes but not for chelonians.	6. The use of a mask may be difficult in chelonians. For drugs and dose rates see Table 12.8.
7. Induction chambers can be used to deliver inhalational agents for most reptiles except terrapins.	7. Terrapins are aquatic chelonians and are able to hold their breath and revert to anaerobic metabolism for up to 27 hours. This delays the uptake and activity of the anaesthetic agent.

Table 12.8 Anaesthetic agents for use in reptiles

Anaesthetic agent	Dose rate and site of administration	Comment
Alphaxalone/alphadolone (Saffan)	6–9 mg/kg i.v. or 9–15 mg/kg i.m.	Used for most species. Results are variable. May be a violent recovery
Alphaxalone/alphadolone (Saffan)	9 mg/kg i.v. or intracardiac	Recommended for snakes. Induction in minutes. Good muscle relaxation. Minimal result if given i.m.
Alphaxalone/alphadolone (Saffan)	15 mg/kg i.m.	Used for lizards and induction of chelonians. Lasts for 15–35 minutes Variable results
Isoflurane	3–5% induction; 1.0–3.0% maintenance	Drug of choice for all species. Induction takes 6–20 minutes, recovery takes 30–60 minutes. Smooth recovery
Ketamine	22–44 mg/kg s.c. i.m.	Provides sedation in most species
Propofol (Rapinovet)	5–10 mg/kg i.v. or intracardiac	Snakes
Propofol (Rapinovet)	3–5 mg/kg i.v., i.o.	Lizards—used for intubation and minor diagnostic procedures

8. Reptiles can be intubated relatively easily using an uncuffed tube. The glottis is easily visualised in snakes but the large fleshy tongue of some lizards and chelonians may obscure the view.
9. Dehydration may increase the risk of anaesthesia.
10. Reptiles should be kept at their preferred body temperature throughout the anaesthetic and during the recovery period.

8. Reptiles have complete tracheal rings, which may be ruptured by inflation of a cuff. Use a gag to keep the mouth open. Dog and cat intravenous catheters can be used to intubate small reptiles.
9. Correct fluid inbalance before anaesthesia.
10. All reptiles have their own preferred body temperature (PBT) at which the metabolic rate is at its most efficient. If the PBT is too low, the rate of recovery and healing will be reduced.

PROCEDURE: MAINTENANCE AND MONITORING OF ANAESTHESIA

ACTION

1. Closed anaesthetic circuits are commonly used in reptile anaesthesia.

2. IPPV may be used as a continuous means of ventilation during the anaesthetic.

3. Monitor the respiratory rate by observation.

4. The corneal and palpebral reflexes may be used to monitor the depth of anaesthesia, except in the snake.

5. The tongue withdrawal reflex is a useful means of monitoring the depth of anaesthesia in snakes and in some lizards.
6. Monitor jaw tone, pedal and tail reflexes.

7. Monitor the heart rate by oesophageal stethoscope, Doppler ultrasound or electrocardiography.

RATIONALE

1. The respiratory rate required to maintain an adequate level of anaesthesia is often greater than the rate shown by a conscious animal. A closed circuit will keep gas concentration higher than a semi-closed circuit.

2. Reptiles have a low respiratory rate and apnoea is common. Administer at the rate of 2 breaths/min.

3. Observation of the respiratory rate may be difficult, as the rate is often slow.

4. Snakes have no eyelids and the cornea is covered in a transparent skin scale known as a spectacle. The palpebral reflex is lost when the surgical plane of anaesthesia is reached.

5. Pull out the tongue gently and note whether it flicks or is withdrawn. This is lost when the surgical plane of anaesthesia is reached.

6. The pedal and tail reflexes are lost when the surgical plane of anaesthesia is reached.

7. During deep anaesthesia the heart rate slows and the pupils become fixed and dilated.

PROCEDURE: POST-OPERATIVE CARE

ACTION

1. If a reptile has been induced with an injectable anaesthetic agent it may take hours to regain complete consciousness.
2. Continue to give oxygen by IPPV until the reptile has begun to breathe spontaneously.
3. Keep the patient warm at all times. Once the surgical procedure is complete, transfer it to its vivarium maintained at its PBT. Monitor the environmental temperature to avoid overheating.
4. Monitor the respiratory rate until the patient is fully conscious and moving around.
5. Give replacement fluid therapy orally, intravenously or intraperitoneally—up to 4% of bodyweight.
6. Monitor the patient until it is fully conscious.

RATIONALE

1. Reptiles have a slow metabolic rate so anaesthetic drugs are broken down slowly and recovery will be slow.
2. To maintain adequate levels of oxygen to the tissues.
3. Reptiles are cold-blooded and the environmental temperature influences their metabolic rate. If the reptile is kept at its PBT, the recovery will occur more quickly than if the reptile is cold.
4. Respiratory stimulants, e.g. Doxapram can be used.
5. Dehydration can lead to visceral gout—the build-up of urates in the visceral organs.
6. Problems may occur during the post-operative period. Appetite is often difficult to measure, as many reptiles eat infrequently.

FURTHER READING

Anderson RS, Edney ATB (eds) 1991 Practical Animal Handling. Pergamon, Oxford

Beynon PH (ed.) 1991 Manual of Exotic Pets. BSAVA, Gloucester

Beynon PH (ed.) 1994 Manual of Reptiles. BSAVA, Gloucester

Beynon PH (ed.) 1996 Manual of Psittacine Birds. BSAVA, Gloucester

Hillyer EV, Quesenberry KE 1997 Ferrets, Rabbits and Rodents: Clinical Medicine and Surgery. WB Saunders, Philadelphia

Hotson Moore A (ed.) 1999 Manual of Advanced Veterinary Nursing. BSAVA, Gloucester

Laber-Laird K, Swindle M, Flecknell P 1991 Handbook of Rodent and Rabbit Medicine. Pergamon, Oxford

Index